Current Topics in Microbiology and Immunology

Volume 379

For further volumes:
http://www.springer.com/series/82

Current Topics in Microbiology and Immunology

Bernard Malissen
Centre d'Immunologie de Marseille-Luminy, Parc Scientifique de Luminy, Case 906, 13288 Marseille Cedex 9, France

Michael B. A. Oldstone
Department of Immunology and Microbial Science, The Scripps Research Institute, 10550 North Torrey Pines Road, La Jolla, CA 92037, USA

Rino Rappuoli
Novartis Vaccines, Via Fiorentina 1, Siena 53100, Italy

Peter K. Vogt
Department of Molecular and Experimental Medicine, The Scripps Research Institute, 10550 North Torrey Pines Road, BCC-239, La Jolla, CA 92037, USA

Honorary Editor: Hilary Koprowski (deceased)
Formerly at Biotechnology Foundation, Inc., Ardmore, PA, USA

For further volumes:
http://www.springer.com/series/82

G. Balakrish Nair · Yoshifumi Takeda
Editors

Cholera Outbreaks

Responsible Series Editor: Klaus Aktories

Springer

Editors
G. Balakrish Nair
Translational Health Science and Technology Institute
Gurgaon, Haryana
India

Yoshifumi Takeda
National Institute of Infectious Diseases
Tokyo
Japan

ISSN 0070-217X ISSN 2196-9965 (electronic)
ISBN 978-3-642-55403-2 ISBN 978-3-642-55404-9 (eBook)
DOI 10.1007/978-3-642-55404-9
Springer Heidelberg New York Dordrecht London

Library of Congress Control Number: 2014941200

Printed on acid-free paper

Springer is part of Springer Science+Business Media (www.springer.com)

Preface

As we place our thoughts together to write the Preface of this book on "Cholera Outbreaks," we are constantly reminded through all forms of media of the impending outbreak of cholera in Sudan. The country is in the midst of armed conflict resulting in the formation of temporary camps of thousands of displaced people living in poor sanitary conditions and overcrowding; the perfect recipe to initiate an outbreak of cholera. The World Health Organization has dipped into the newly launched stockpile of cholera vaccine and is creating history of sorts in attempting to preempt the outbreak by vaccinating people in these camps using the WHO prequalified bivalent oral cholera vaccine. In many ways this is not "new" news, instead this is news that is retold with remarkable regularity with the only difference being that the name of the country differs each time. Cholera has been exceptionally pervasive during the past three decades, particularly since the beginning of this millennium. The Sudan outbreak was preceded by the Haiti outbreak, which stupefied the world just by its scale, its enormity, and the disputes that arose in its wake. Cholera has this penchant of being in the forefront of news.

What remains a continuing enigma, however, is that we allow it to happen time and again despite the enormous body of knowledge on the pathogen *Vibrio cholerae* and on the disease cholera. Yet we are unable to accurately predict and preempt outbreaks of cholera. The complete genome sequence of more than 150 strains of *Vibrio cholerae* are available in international databases, which have been thoroughly analyzed, explored, teased, and interpreted, we know the epidemiology of the disease through decades of painstaking work; the ecology of the pathogen and the impact of climate change has been thoroughly investigated. We are also aware of simple ways to treat the disease. However, we have not been able to decipher the reason for the ferocious spread of the pathogen during outbreaks of cholera nor have we been able to predict accurately where an outbreak will occur. Ironically, what is most predictable about cholera is its unpredictability.

The genesis of this book is the reaction to a lecture on cholera at the 85th Annual Meeting of Japanese Society of Bacteriology held in Nagasaki from March 27 to 29, 2012. Professor Dr. Klaus Aktories of the Albert-Ludwigs-Universitat Freiburg was in the audience. The lecture evoked his interest and he requested us whether we would be interested to edit a volume on Cholera in the series Current Topics in Microbiology and Immunology. We accepted the offer and are grateful to Professor Aktories for having initiated our thoughts to edit this book. We chose the topic of cholera outbreaks as the theme because we felt that there is a hiatus in information in the area of cholera outbreaks. Besides, for those who have worked on cholera and were involved in cholera outbreaks in any capacity, it is a life-changing experience.

The book starts with a chapter on cholera outbreaks in the times when classical biotype of *Vibrio cholerae* O1, acknowledged as the more virulent biotype, prevailed. To bring about the contrast between biotypes in relation to cholera outbreaks, "Cholera Outbreaks in the El Tor Biotype Era and the Impact of the New El Tor Variants" focuses on the El Tor biotype and its recent variants including O139, the altered El Tor and the hybrid El Tor, all of which are a testimony to the subtle changes taking place in the rapidly evolving genome of El Tor *Vibrio cholerae*. We have then focused on an overview of outbreaks of cholera in India, Southeast Asia, Africa, and America to give a continent-wise flavor. There is increasing evidence that the incidence of cholera and the factors that cause cholera outbreaks vary between Asia and Africa. An analysis of a huge outbreak of cholera in Haiti in "The Cholera Outbreak in Haiti: Where and How did it Begin?" provides an insight into how an outbreak of cholera can overwhelm a country and the controversies that it can generate. The role lytic phages play in modulating cholera epidemics and enhance *Vibrio cholerae* evolution through a bactericidal selection process is highlighted in "Role of Phages in the Epidemiology of Cholera". The fate of circulating clones of *Vibrio cholerae* during cholera outbreaks including genetic changes as a result of mutations or acquisition of new genetic sequences is discussed in detail in "Circulation and Transmission of Clones of *Vibrio cholerae* During Cholera Outbreaks". Of late, there has been concerted efforts to use mathematical models to synthesize knowledge on cholera into a quantitative framework with an effort to predict and manage cholera, which is discussed in "Modelling Cholera Outbreaks." The past two decades have seen a quantum leap in Genomic sciences and "Genomic Science in Understanding Cholera Outbreaks and Evolution of *Vibrio cholerae* as a Human Pathogen" collates this information and extols how this information could be useful from a cholera control viewpoint or from the way clones of the pathogen spread across the globe. The precision of SNP analysis across the whole genome in tracking the spread of the clones of the pathogen is highlighted in great detail. The last chapter analyzes circumstances of when the available cholera vaccines can be used to interrupt cholera outbreaks.

We hope the information provided by domain experts will give you a comprehensive overview on cholera outbreaks and their consequences. It is also in a way to remind the readership that cholera is not an antiquated disease; it is still very much there and will be there in places where hygiene and sanitation is compromised. Putting this book together has been a delightful assignment. We are indebted to all the authors and coauthors of the 11 chapters for their cooperation and for all the effort to prepare the chapter. Without their contribution, this book would not exist. We applaud their expertise and acknowledge their efforts.

Finally, the book is a celebration of collaboration between the two Editors for more than three decades—a collaboration bonded by research on cholera. The 30-

plus years have been humbling and a learning experience. Cholera continues to persist and devastate especially among the marginalized section of the world. It is like a fire that cannot be put off.

G. Balakrish Nair
Yoshifumi Takeda

Contents

Cholera Outbreaks in the Classical Biotype Era

A. K. Siddique and Richard Cash

Abstract In the Indian subcontinent description of a disease resembling cholera has been mentioned in Sushruta Samita, estimated to have been written between ~400 and 500 BC. It is however not clear whether the disease known today as cholera caused by *Vibrio cholerae* O1 is the evolutionary progression of the ancient disease. The modern history of cholera began in 1817 when an explosive epidemic broke out in the Ganges River Delta region of Bengal. This was the first of the seven recorded cholera pandemics that affected nearly the entire world and caused hundreds of thousands of deaths. The bacterium responsible for this human disease was first recognised during the fifth pandemic and was named *V. cholerae* which was grouped as O1, and was further differentiated into Classical and El Tor biotypes. It is now known that the fifth and the sixth pandemics were caused by the *V. cholerae* O1 of the Classical biotype and the seventh by the El Tor biotype. The El Tor biotype of *V. cholerae,* which originated in Indonesia and shortly thereafter began to spread in the early 1960s. Within the span of 50 years the El Tor biotype had invaded nearly the entire world, completely displacing the Classical biotype from all the countries except Bangladesh. What prompted the earlier pandemics to begin is not clearly understood, nor do we know how and why they ended. The success of the seventh pandemic clone over the pre-existing sixth pandemic strain remains largely an unsolved mystery. Why classical biotype eventually disappeared from the world remains to be explained. For nearly three decades (1963–1991) during the seventh pandemic, cholera in Bangladesh has recorded a

A. K. Siddique (✉)
ICDDR,B, 68. Shahed Tajuddin Ahamed Sarani, Mohakhali, Dhaka 1212, Bangladesh
e-mail: siddique@icddrb.org

R. Cash
Department of Global Health and Population, Harvard School of Public Health, 665 Huntington Avenue, Boston, MA 02138, USA
e-mail: racash@hsph.harvard.edu; richard.cash@phfi.org

Public Health Foundation of India, PHD Chambers, August Kranti Marg, New Delhi 110016, India

Current Topics in Microbiology and Immunology (2014) 379: 1–16
DOI: 10.1007/82_2013_361

Published Online: 25 December 2013

unique history of co-existence of Classical and El Tor biotypes of *V. cholerae* O1 as epidemic and endemic strain. This long co-existence has provided us with great opportunity to improve our understanding of the disease itself and answer some important questions.

Contents

1 Introduction

A description of cholera would be incomplete in the absence of a historical account of the disease including its origin, emergence as an epidemic disease and its devastating spread throughout the world that killed millions. There is little disagreement among cholera historians about the existence of cholera-like diseases during ancient times in Asia, China and Europe. It is not clear, however, whether the disease known today as cholera caused by *Vibrio cholerae* O1 is the evolutionary progression of the ancient disease.

In the Indian subcontinent, *Visuchica* a Sanskrit word describing a disease that closely resembles a case of cholera has been mentioned in *Sushruta Samita* which is estimated to have been written between ~400 and 500 BC (Bhishagrant 1963). Proof of its presence in historical times has been furnished by the early Europeans who arrived in India in the fourteenth century. When the Portuguese landed in the south western or Malabar coast of India in 1498, cholera existed in the region. In 1503, about 20,000 men of Calicut died of an epidemic of the disease having symptoms resembling cholera as described by Gasper Correa, an officer of Vasco da Gama (Peters 1885). This was one of the earliest published descriptions of the Asiatic cholera written by an European. The modern history of cholera began in 1817 when a violent epidemic of the disease broke out in the Ganges River Delta region of Bengal (Pollitzer 1959). This was the first of the recorded cholera pandemics (Barua 1992).

It originated in the lower Ganges River Delta and spread beyond India in three directions, continuing for 7 years (1817–1823). Its spread to the western direction affected Oman, Bahrain, and the Persian Gulf region, part of Iran, Iraq, Syria, Turkey and Egypt; spread to the eastern direction involving Burma, Thailand, Malacca, Penang, Singapore, and Indonesian archipelago, Philippines, China and Japan; and the southern movement affected the Indian Ocean islands of Ceylon, Mauritius, Re'union and Zanzibar (Pollitzer 1959).

The origin of the second pandemic (1829–1851) can also be traced back to Bengal when in 1826 there were signs of epidemic activities of the disease and a steady westward spread. By 1829, the epidemic invaded Afghanistan and Persia, spreading northward to Russia, northern and central Europe. Cholera appeared in England in 1831, and did not spare France, Italy, Spain, Portugal and North African countries (Pollitzer 1959). The disease also crossed the Atlantic to North America by ships carrying Irish immigrants and reached Canada (Chambers 1938). At about the same time, cholera appeared in New York, Philadelphia and extended across the southern US (Duffy 1971). The third pandemic (1852–1859) is thought to have started as a consequence of an upsurge of cholera in India. Beginning in 1853, epidemics of the disease were rampant in Persia and Mesopotamia, northern Europe, including England, Canada, the US, Mexico, Colombia and West Indies. In the east, China, Japan, Korea and the Philippines were also affected.

In 1863, during the fourth pandemic (1863–1879), a major epidemic occurred among the pilgrims in Mecca which resulted in nearly 30,000 deaths. The aftermath of this epidemic had a disastrous effect involving nearly the whole of Europe and Russia in 1866 (McNamara 1876) and over 417,000 people lost their lives. In addition to resurgence of epidemics in some of the previously infected countries, the fifth pandemic (1881–1896) largely affected the South American countries. The sixth pandemic (1899–1923) is believed to be connected to the resurgence of cholera in India (Pollitzer 1959) and struck central and southern Europe and Southeast Asia.

The bacterium responsible for this human disease was first recognised in 1884 (Koch 1884) during the fifth pandemic and was named as *V. cholerae* (Pollitzer 1959) which was grouped as O1 on the basis of their serological response to antiserum (Sakazaki 1992). *V. cholerae* O1 was further differentiated into Classical and El Tor biotypes on the basis of certain biological tests (Farmer 1985). Each biotype can be further classified into the serotypes Ogawa and Inaba. We know that the fifth and the sixth pandemics were caused by the *V. cholerae* O1 of the Classical biotype. However, the division between the six pandemics is not distinct and the cholera-free intervals between the individual pandemics were not always clear. It may be reasonable to consider that the first six pandemics were single continued pandemics. For nearly 80 years during the fifth and sixth pandemics of cholera, the Classical biotype of *V. cholerae* dominated the spectrum of cholera. What prompted the earlier pandemics and its spread is not well understood, nor do we know how and why they ended. Cholera did not persist in many of the countries invaded during the pandemics, though on other areas it continued as an endemic disease.

In 1906, Gotschlich isolated a new strain of *V. cholerae* at the El Tor Quarantine Station in the Sinai desert from Indonesian pilgrims who had died of a cholera-like illness. These organisms had all the characteristics of *V. cholerae* except they were haemolytic (Mosley 1969). They caused small outbreaks in Indonesia for nearly 30 years affecting Java, Sarawak, and Borneo. This strain designated El Tor, did not gain international notoriety, despite causing a large outbreak in Celebes, Indonesia in 1936 (De Moor 1938), until the early 1960s when for unknown reasons epidemic cholera caused by El Tor began to rapidly spread outward from Indonesia. This became the seventh cholera pandemic (Barua 1992). By the end of 1962, epidemics affected the entire South Asian archipelago and reached the Indian subcontinent, first affecting East Pakistan (now Bangladesh) in 1963 and Calcutta, India, in 1964. The epidemic then spread to Pakistan, Afghanistan, Iran, Iraq and Uzbekistan in 1965. In 1970, the epidemic affected Southern Europe and reached Africa, mainly sub-Saharan West Africa, where it caused epidemics resulting in 40,000 deaths (Goodgame 1975). One of the striking features of the seventh pandemic was its extension in 1991 to South and Central America, areas that had not seen cholera for nearly a hundred years. The epidemic was first reported in Peru in January 1991 (Levin 1991) and by November 1991 it had affected seven South American and nine Central American countries (PAHO 1991). Between 1991 and 1993, the seventh pandemic was responsible for over 951,000 reported cases of cholera and 8,700 deaths from 20 Latin American countries (Guthmann 1995).

Since the El Tor biotype first appeared, many clinical and epidemiological observations suggested that *V. cholerae* of the El Tor biotype, although better adapted to the environment, may be less virulent clinically. It was also suggested that El Tor strain had certain competitive advantages in comparison to the classical strain. One of these advantages was the greater prevalence of inapparent infections (35–100:1 vs. 4:1), indicating that many patients infected with El Tor strain have milder or asymptomatic infections than the classical strain (Bart 1970). However, infection with either biotype can be acute, severe and life-threatening, but in general fewer patients infected with El Tor strains presented with severe dehydration (Chandu 1971). The severity of the infection depends on many factors such as local intestinal immunity (from previous natural exposure), the size of inoculum, the adequacy of gastric-acid and the patient's blood group (Sack 2004). For unknown reasons, people of blood group O are at higher risk of severe cholera from El Tor vibrios than those of other blood groups (Glass 1985; Clemens 1989).

The seventh pandemic was strikingly different from the earlier pandemics in its rapidity of geographic spread and duration. Within the span of approximately 50 years the pandemic caused by *V. cholerae* O1, El Tor biotype invaded nearly the entire world. The El Tor biotype of *V. cholerae* O1 completely displaced the Classical biotype as the predominant epidemic strain from the countries where it existed within a year of its first appearance.

2 Cholera in the Ganges River delta

Historically, Asiatic cholera has always flourished in the Ganges river delta region though it is not known just how long it has been ravaging the population of the region (McNamara 1876). Few regions have a history of cholera that is more complex than the Ganges River delta region of Bengal. The land mass which lies between the two great rivers of the Indian subcontinent the Ganges and the Brahmaputra is known as the lower Ganges River delta region, the greater part of which is now Bangladesh. In the past, changes in the epidemiology of cholera in this region have greatly influenced its global spread. The great epidemic of 1817 which was the beginning of the first pandemic started in Jessore (now in Bangladesh), spread throughout the province of Bengal (British India) within 3 months involving an area of $\sim$507,500 km^2. Within 3 years the disease affected nearly every province of India (McNamara 1876). The region was implicated as the source of origin of all the cholera pandemics except the current seventh pandemic (Pollitzer 1959).

Available records of classical cholera deaths during the pandemic in the Indian subcontinent, was limited to the last 13 years of the sixth pandemic (1910–1923). However, records of classical cholera deaths beyond the sixth pandemic were available up to 1954 (Politzer 1959). Between 1910 and 1954, it is estimated that over 10 million cholera deaths occurred in pre-independence (British India) and post-independence India. Bengal accounted for the highest proportion (29 %), followed by Bihar and Orissa (25 %), United Provinces (17 %) and the Madras Presidency (14 %); that is these four provinces accounted for 85 % of the total reported cholera deaths during the 45-year period (Politzer 1959). Among a total of 171,000 deaths attributed to cholera between 1947 and 1954 in Pakistan, 96 % occurred in East Pakistan (present Bangladesh) (Pollitzer 1959).

One of the landmark events in the history of cholera in the lower Ganges delta region was the establishment of the Pakistan SEATO (South-east Asia Treaty Organization) Cholera Research Laboratory in Dacca in 1960. It was felt that in addition to the clinical, pathological and microbiological research on cholera, a field site for cholera studies including field-testing of existing and new cholera vaccine was needed. The search for such a field site led to the finding of Matlab, a cholera prone rural area, located at a distance of 57 km from Dhaka and accessible only by waterways. Thus in the fall of 1963, the Pakistan-SEATO Cholera Research Laboratory (PSCRL) established an epidemiological field study area in the home of Asiatic cholera. In 1964, the Government of East Pakistan made available an old barge (which previously served as a floating judge's quarters and a temporary jail for river pirates) for treatment of cholera patients in Matlab. The barge was soon abandoned as a treatment centre as a few rooms of the government PHC were given over to the PSCRL for that purpose. Over the last five decades, the PSCRL evolved to what is known to the world today as the "International Centre for Diarrhoeal Diseases Research, Bangladesh (ICDDR, B)". The ICDDR,B now runs a well-equipped hospital in Matlab that especially caters to diarrhoea and MCH activities and is the hub for the many studies now based in Matlab.

In the last several decades cholera has been the subject of numerous studies of ICDDR,B, both in Dhaka and Matlab, which have increased our understanding of all aspects of the cholera. A partial list of the hundreds of pre-1990 citations might include the following: epidemiology (Lindenbaum 1966; Khan 1967, 1980; McCormack et al. 1969a, b; Martin 1969; Glass 1981); pathogenesis (Greenough 1979; Cash 1969); microbiology, immunology (Mosley 1968; Bart 1970; Glass 1985; Khan 1987), and clinical management (Nalin 1968; Cash 1969, 1970; Greenough 1964, 1984; Rabbani 1986). In addition there have been numerous field trials of both parental and oral cholera vaccines. The results of these studies have greatly changed our understanding of cholera, both in terms of all these areas of study. The ICDDR,B has become the premier research institution in the world for the study of enteric diseases and many other health problems that affect low and middle income countries.

2.1 Disappearance of Classical Cholera from India

Since 1964, when *V. cholerae* O1 biotype El Tor first entered India, cholera cases due to Classical biotype were progressively displaced. By the end of 1964, the ratio between the Classical and El Tor cholera cases was 1:10 in Calcutta. In the state of Bihar the classical was completely displaced by the middle of 1964. At about the same period, the classical biotype accounted for 50 % cholera cases in the western coast of India during outbreaks in Surat, and Baroda of Gujrat State; the remainder were due to El Tor biotype. In the first 3 months of 1965, classical biotype of *V. cholerae* O1 completely disappeared from Baroda area. In the city of Bombay, in the latter half of 1964, during epidemic outbreaks both Classical and El Tor were equally distributed. In the Kottayam area of Kerala during an outbreak in 1965, no Classical strain was identified. By the end of 1966, epidemic strains of Classical cholera seem to have largely disappeared from India (Mukerjee 1965). However, a few Classical strains were occasionally identified between 1967 and 1969 mostly from West Bengal (Calcutta), Orissa (Puri, Cuttack, Balasore), Assam (Shillong, Gauhati, and Tripura (Agartala) (Sanyal 1972). The presence of classical biotype in India has not been reported after 1969 signifying the end of the sixth pandemic of cholera within the present boundary of India. From then on the El Tor biotype was the only strain detected during the epidemic outbreaks both in the eastern and western states indicating that the Classical biotype had disappeared from India (Mukerjee 1965). During this period, the reasons for disappearance of the classical strain from India were not fully explained.

2.2 *Classical Cholera in Bangladesh During the Seventh Pandemic*

The Ganges and the Brahmaputra Rivers which flow through Bangladesh before draining into the Bay of Bengal have resulted in geo-ecological differences within Bangladesh. The northern and the middle belt regions constitute the flood plains of these rivers, whereas the southern region constitutes the tidal plain of the Bay of Bengal. The ecological difference between different regions of the country was found to have implications on the epidemiology of cholera in Bangladesh in the past and the present. Understanding the epidemiology of cholera in the lower Ganges river delta of Bangladesh has always been an epidemiological challenge.

The El Tor biotype was first detected in Bangladesh (formerly East Pakistan) in 1963 at Chittagong and in Dhaka in 1964, but the first significant outbreak was not reported until 1968 (Bart 1970). Since then, for nearly three decades (1963–1991) cholera in Bangladesh has recorded a unique history of coexistence of Classical and El Tor biotypes of *V. cholerae* O1 as epidemic and endemic disease. Epidemics produced contrasting pictures of appearance and disappearance of Classical and El Tor biotypes and serotypes of *V. cholerae* O1 in different regions of the country, between different time periods and in comparison to other countries.

2.3 *What Prompted Disappearance and Reappearance and Persistence of Classical Cholera in Lower Ganges Delta of Bangladesh?*

The Classical biotype which was responsible for the fifth and sixth pandemics of cholera dominated the spectrum of cholera epidemics in Bangladesh up to 1972 (Glass 1982). For nearly 6 years between 1973 and 1978, the Classical biotype disappeared from Bangladesh (Glass 1982; Samadi 1983), this was thought to be a part of a global phenomenon occurring at that time (Barua 1992). In contrast to the findings of complete disappearance of Classical strain from the rest of the world; the Classical biotype of *V. cholerae* O1 re-emerged in Bangladesh in September 1982 and by the end of December the biotype accounted for 90 % of the cholera patients in Dhaka. In the Matlab treatment centre of ICDDR, B, Classical biotype accounted for 63.4 % of the cholera patients and the El Tor biotype the remaining 36.6 %. A total of 66 Classical biotypes were also isolated from four rural districts. All but one of the isolates was from the southern region of the country (Khan 1980; Samadi 1983; Shahid 1984). The classical biotype became the epidemic strain in Matlab between 1982 and 1984. The overall isolation rate of Classical biotype during this period was 74 % compared to 26 % for El Tor. Since then the Classical biotype has been progressively displaced by El Tor as the epidemic strain in Matlab. In the Dhaka Hospital of the ICDDR,B between 1986 and 1988, the Classical biotype accounted for 39.2 % of cholera cases in contrast to El Tor

(60.8 %). By 1991, Classical biotype was rarely isolated from either Matlab or Dhaka treatment centres.

Beginning in the latter part of 1984, as cholera epidemics spread throughout the country, ICDDR,B set up an 'Epidemic Control Preparedness Programme' (ECPP) to assist the Government of Bangladesh to control the spread of epidemics and prevent deaths by providing prompt treatment. Between 1985 and 1999, ECPP physicians conducted investigations and interventions of diarrhoea epidemics in over 400 rural subdistricts. The ECPP team examined nearly 60,000 diarrhoea patients in field conditions and at rural health facilities, collecting 9,100 rectal swabs for culture at the ICDDR, B laboratories in Dhaka (Siddique 1991, 1992). These investigations provided valuable insight relating to the magnitude of cholera epidemics and distribution of the disease in different regions of Bangladesh. The investigations also contributed to our understanding of the interplay between the classical and El Tor biotypes during the 30 years of their coexistence.

A simultaneous outbreak of cholera by both Classical and El Tor biotypes with contrasting drug resistance and sensitivity patterns was detected during 1989 in six southern districts and in one north-eastern district. Nearly all the Classical isolates were resistant to tetracycline but sensitive to ampicillin. In contrast, the El Tor isolates were sensitive to tetracycline and resistant to Ampicillin. This was a rare event during the period when the sixth pandemic of cholera was being replaced by the seventh (Siddique 1989). Investigations of outbreaks involving 24 rural districts between September, 1988 and October 1998 demonstrated geographic clustering of *V. cholerae* O1 biotypes. In seven southern districts, 79 % of the isolates were Classical biotypes, and only 21 % were El Tor biotype. By contrast in the 17 northern and middle belt districts nearly all (99 %) isolates were of the El Tor biotype (Siddique 1991).

Analysis of ECPP epidemic data collected between 1984 and 1989 showed a selective distribution of *V. cholerae* O1 biotypes (Fig. 1). During epidemics in the southern coastal regions more Classical biotype were isolated than El Tor biotype whereas in the north-eastern, north-western and middle belt regions the reverse was true (Siddique 1991, 1992). The presence of the classical biotype of *V. cholerae* O1 as the predominant epidemic strain in the southern coastal region raised the suspicion that it may have never disappeared from Bangladesh (Siddique 1991) as previously suggested (Glass 1982). This suspicion was confirmed when it was revealed that a group of Classical biotype isolated from patients in southern Bangladesh were clones of the Classical biotype of the sixth pandemic of cholera (Faruque et al. 1993).

Evidence accumulated by the ecological studies over the past decades show that *V. cholerae*, is an autochthonous inhabitant of riverine, brackish water and estuarine ecosystems (Colwell 1981). In coastal and estuarine environments vibrios are found either as individual cells in the water column or as biofilm-associated cells attached to surface (Colwel and Huq 1994; Faruque 1998). The biofilm forming ability of *V. cholerae* appears to increase their survival in natural habitats. The ability of *V. cholerae* to grow in aquatic habitats is often diminished by the low availability of carbon sources. The photosynthetic microorganisms (i.e. phytoplankton) excrete a variety of organic compounds, attachment of *V. cholerae* to these microorganisms provide access to those compounds facilitates its growth and survival. Similarly, attachment to zooplankton, rich in *N*-acetyl glucosamine provides close access to a compound that can serve as both a carbon and nitrogen source (Huq 1984). *V. cholerae* has also developed a remarkable ability to adapt to the constantly changing range of salinity and temperature in tidal estuaries. Growth pattern studies (Singleton 1982) have shown that *V. cholerae* has an absolute requirement for sodium (Na^+). Salinity in presence of certain concentrations of organic nutrient is a controlling factor for vibrio growth (Singleton 1982). *V. cholerae* can also grow in low salinity if the water temperature is relatively high and organic nutrients are present in high concentrations which can compensate to a degree to the lack of salt (Singleton 1982; Huq 1984). This may explain their survival and growth in non-coastal environments. Five major rivers of the Indian subcontinent which flow through thousands of acres of agricultural lands and numerous industrial plants, draining into the Bay of Bengal (Siddique 1994), provide nutrients sufficient to convert the coastal waters into the eutrophic conditions needed for survival and growth of *V. cholerae* (Colwell 1966).

The reason for existence of the classical strain for three decades during the seventh pandemic and the interplay between *V. cholerae* biotypes in Bangladesh is not clear. One possible reason lies in the ecological changes of various regions. For the past several decades, soil erosion and construction of barrages and dams in the river system have had their effects on the ecological balance of the area. In 1975, India built the barrier 'Farakka Barrage' across the Ganges River, before it enters Bangladesh, in Murshidabad district of West Bengal. This was done to control the water level for preservation and maintenance of the Calcutta port and for increasing navigational depth of the Bhagirathi-Hooghly waterway that leads to the Bay of Bengal especially, during the dry season (Abbas 1984). The north-western region of Bangladesh has been becoming more and more arid due to the reduction of the river flow. Increasingly severe flooding has prolonged the waterlogged period, mostly in the north-eastern and middle belt region. These ecological changes have coincided with the appearance of the El Tor biotype in Bangladesh. Since El Tor is hardier and more viable in water than the Classical biotype (Felsenfeld 1963), the flood-vulnerable middle and north-eastern areas of the country may have been a more suitable habitat for El Tor than Classical strains. Variations in the nutrient concentration or salinity may account for the selective distribution of *V. cholerae*. In the south, where flood drainage has been more efficient, the conditions were probably suitable for the Classical strain. The Farakka Barrage has been diverting more than half of the Ganges river flow through Bangladesh during the dry season (Bangladesh Ministry of Water Resources 1966). This drastic reduction of fresh water flow has changed the dry season hydrodynamics in southern Bangladesh and resulted in an increase in salinity and incursion of brackish water deeper inland. The Classical biotype in the south adapted to this changing environment and thus improved its survival ability.

An important finding related to the ecology of cholera was the observation that *V. cholerae* O1 and non-O1 had the ability to become into a viable but

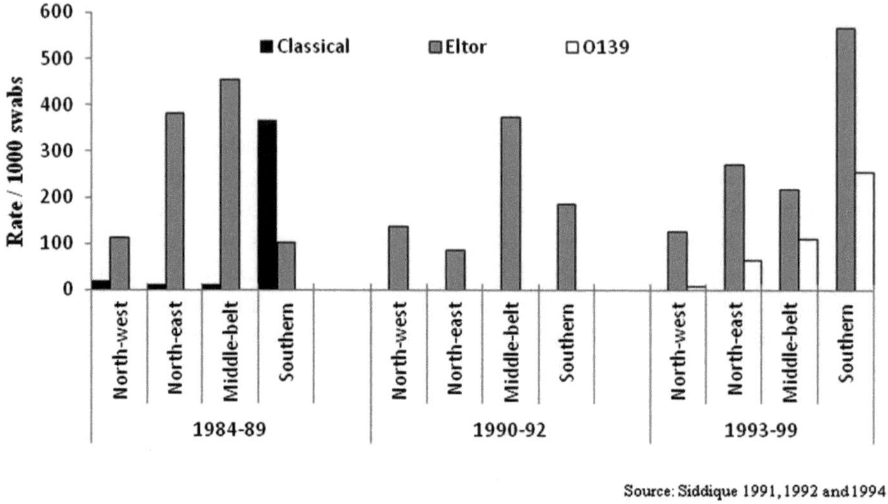

Fig. 1 Epidemic Strains of *V. cholerae* isolated in Bangladesh by region: 1984–1999

non-culturable state in response to nutrient deprivation and when environmental odds are against it (Cowell 1985; Xu 1982; Islam 1994). This has improved our understanding of epidemiology of *V. cholerae,* especially, in cholera endemic regions such as Bangladesh. It could explain the absence of the Classical strain from Bangladesh between 1973 and 1978. This assumption was further strengthened by the observation that the Classical strain which survived in the southern coastal region (Siddique 1991) was the clone of the classical biotype of the sixth pandemic of cholera (Faruque et al. 1993) suggesting that the Classical strain had never completely disappeared from Bangladesh. The apparent disappearance during that 6-year period could be interpreted as the Classical strain transformed into a viable but non-culturable state. It has been demonstrated that when environmental conditions are favourable, *V. cholerae* can revert to culturability from non-culturable state (Huq 1990). The re-emergence of classical strain in 1984 might then have occurred because environmental conditions became suitable for *V. cholerae* to revert to culturability from a non-culturable state.

Historically, the southern coastal region of Bangladesh has been one of the highest endemic and epidemic cholera regions in the lower Ganges delta (Pollitzer 1959). The average death rate from cholera in the five southern districts between 1901 and 1910 was 3.02/1,000 population (range: 2.63–3.47). In recent decades the coastal aquatic ecosystem of southern Bangladesh has been the hub for changes in the epidemiology of cholera. The epidemic strain of the Classical biotype continued to survive as the predominant epidemic strain and coexisted with El Tor biotype despite its disappearance from the rest of the country (Fig. 1). Within a span of 3 years a major change in the epidemiology of cholera has been noted in southern Bangladesh (Fig. 2). In 1991, the Classical strain completely disappeared from its last habitat in southern Bangladesh. In 1992 the El Tor biotype was found

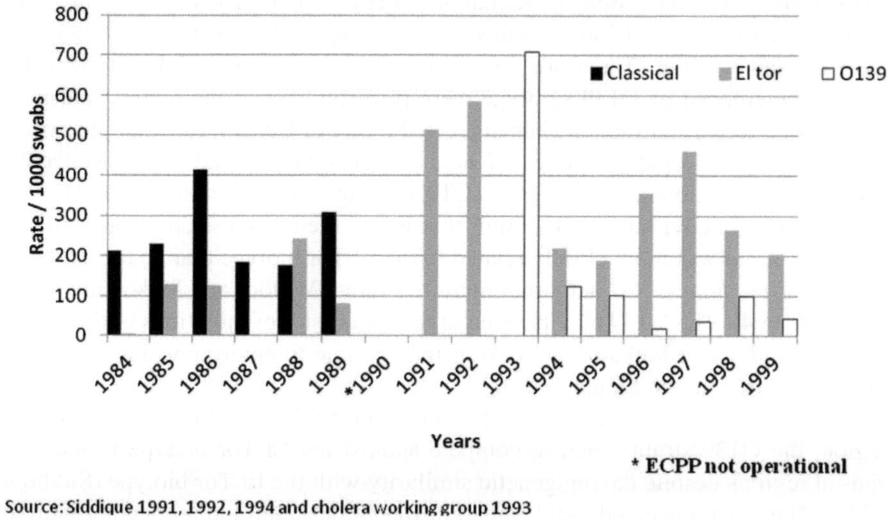

Fig. 2 Isolation rate of epidemic strain of *V. cholerae* in Southern Bangladesh: 1984–1999

to be the only epidemic strain in the region. For the first time in history, during the cholera epidemic in 1993, both biotypes (Classical and El Tor) of *V. cholerae* O1 had been completely replaced by a new strain of *V. cholerae* non-O1 (Siddique 1994) designated O139 Bengal (Albert 1993; Cholera working group 1993). Although the reasons for these changes are not clearly understood, epidemiological findings suggest that environmental changes in the Bay of Bengal may have been responsible. Between 1985 and 1992, during epidemic investigations, a few *V. cholerae* non-O1 were consistently isolated from acute diarrhoea patients from the southern coastal region. As these isolates have not been further studied, it was not known whether they played any role in the emergence of the non-O1 epidemic strain *V. cholerae* O139 (Siddique 1994).

The Bay of Bengal is subject to frequent violent atmospheric turbulence in the form of cyclones. In April 1991 a disastrous cyclone occurred when a great tidal surge flooded the entire coastal areas. This may have affected the estuarine water quality by mixing the sediments dislodged by the force of the tidal surge (Cowell R.R, vs Siddique A.K: personal communication) and altered the aquatic ecosystem. We assume that this may have led to disappearance of the both biotypes *V. cholerae* O1 from the cyclone affected areas. The disappearance of the Classical strain, however, was a permanent phenomenon since this area had been its last known habitat. The vacuum left by the Classical strain was filled by the El Tor strain, emigrating from the non-coastal regions where it had existed in endemic and epidemic form. Thus the El Tor biotype became the only epidemic strain in southern Bangladesh in 1992. The reason for the emergence of a new strain (O139) that caused a large epidemic in southern Bangladesh in late 1992 and 1993 was not clear. *V. cholerae* O139 was also the dominant organism in epidemics on the west coast of India and West Bengal (Ramamurthy et al. 1993). The organism involved in both Bangladesh and India seemed to be a single clone (Shamida 1993) and have the same origin. Therefore, the observed disappearance of *V. cholerae* O1 and the emergence of O139 serotype were probably due to the factors that were common to both. Environmental changes in the Bay of Bengal, for example, would be shared by the epidemic affected areas of Bangladesh and India. Molecular studies linking cholera toxin genes (CTX), chromosomal organization of virulence, gene and environmental stimuli that led to their expression, suggested that the O139 strain was more closely related to the El Tor biotype than to the Classical biotype of *V. cholerae* O1 and other non-O1 strains (Waldor and Mekalonos 1994; Faruque 1994). The O139 may have emerged as a result of mutations of the El Tor vibrio (Waldor and Mekalonos 1994) or may be due to environmental changes in the Bay of Bengal (Siddique 1994).

Despite its initial success as the predominant epidemic strain in the southern region, the O139 strain failed to compete against the El Tor biotype in the non-coastal regions despite having genetic similarity with the El Tor biotype (Siddique 1996). The emergence and rapid spread in Bangladesh and India, together with its detection in several countries have raised the question whether this constituted the threat of an eighth pandemic of cholera. However, such a threat did not materialise. Although it continues to be recovered sporadically in Bangladesh and in other regions of South Asia, O139 has remained as a relatively minor contributor to the overall cholera burden (Siddique 2010).

3 Why Classical Biotype of *V. cholerae* O1 Disappeared as the Global Pandemic and Endemic Strains

During the seventh pandemic the classical biotype of *V. cholerae* O1 was completely displaced by the El Tor biotype. The reasons for disappearance of Classical biotype from all countries where they had been existing, remains to be explained. Although, *V. cholerae* has been recognised as part of the normal free-living bacterial flora in the riverine and estuarine ecosystem, non-pathogenic strains are more frequently found in these areas than pathogenic strains. There are more than 200 serogroups of *V. cholerae* of which only two (O1 and O139) are associated with endemic and epidemic cholera because they carry CTX and TCP, but many O1 strains, particularly those in the environment do not. Both Classical and El Tor biotypes of *V. cholerae* carry CTX and TCP, so the explanation for the evolutionary success of the seventh pandemic clone over the pre-existing sixth pandemic strains remains largely an unsolved mystery.

In recent decades striking progress has been made in genetics, ecology and molecular epidemiology of *V. cholerae* which has improved our understanding of how newly emerged strains replace the old strains, their survival strategy and competition in the environment, and the genetic determinants of epidemic and pandemic properties. Bacterial viruses infecting *Vibrio* species (vibriophage) play a critical role in the transmission of virulent genes. This has been shown by studies of pathogenicity islands and the discovery of CTXØ (a lysogenic filamentous bacteriophages), which has also increased our understanding of the molecular basis for emergence of pathogeneses and control of conservation of particular genetic traits (Waldor and Mekalanos 1996; Faruque 1998). The role of vibriophages in the evolution of *V. cholerae* is not limited only to transfer of virulence genes. The revelation that phage predation may play a role in controlling cholera epidemics (Faruque 2005) also suggest that changes in the organism may be induced by factors outside human hosts. The emergence of certain strains are likely to be enhanced by phages through the bactericidal mechanism in which phage sensitive strains are killed while providing a selective advantage to phage resistant strains. This view was supported recently in a study which indicated that the elimination of the classical biotype of *V. cholerae* O1 during the seventh pandemic may have been induced by an environmental bacteriophage designated JSF9 to which the classical biotype of *V. cholerae* was sensitive (Zahid 2011). Because of its ability to resist the predation by JSF9 phage, the El Tor biotype emerged as the ultimate surviving epidemic strain during the seventh cholera pandemic.

In recent years unexplained genetic changes in *V. cholerae* have been observed in Bangladesh. In the mid-1990s, mutant strains of *V. cholerae* having characteristics of both El Tor and Classical types were isolated and termed as Matlab variant (Nair 2002). These appeared to be unusual strains for Bangladesh at that time (Nair 2006). During epidemics of cholera in 2006, at two rural health facilities (Bakerganj and Marhbaria) in southern Bangladesh, a much higher proportion of patients (79, 70 %) came for treatment with severe dehydration, which had not been seen before. *V. cholerae* isolated from these patients was found to be El Tor in its phenotype, but its cholera toxin (CT) was determined to be that of Classical biotype (Siddique 2010).

4 Conclusion

The constantly changing spectrum of cholera in the lower Ganges river delta of Bangladesh, known as the home of Asiatic cholera, reflects the unpredictable and poorly understood behaviour of this organism. Despite many years of study that have led to a far better understanding of the organism, we still do not know precisely how cholera spreads around the world and what determines its seasonality. Nor can we precisely predict the onset of an epidemic or pandemic. *V. cholerae,* one of the surviving primitive microorganisms, has remained as elusive as ever.

References

Abbas BM (1984) The Ganges water dispute. University Press Limited, Dhaka

Albert MJ, Siddique AK, Islam MS, Faruque ASG, Ansaruzzaman M, Faruque SM, Sack RB (1993) A large outbreak of clinical cholera due to *Vibrio cholerae* non-O1 in Bangladesh. Lancet 341:704

Bangladesh Ministry of Water Resources (1966) Adverse impact on Bangladesh due to withdrawal of dry season Ganges flow at Farakka and upstream. Bangladesh Ministry of Water Resources, Dhaka

Barua D (1992) History of cholera. In: Baru D, Greenough WB III (eds) Cholera. Plenum Medical Book Company, New York, pp 1–36

Bhishagranta K (1963) An english translation of the Sushruta Samhita, vol 3. The Chowkhamba Sanskrit Series Office, Varanasi, pp 352–356

Burt KJ, Huq I, Khan M, Mosley WH (1970) Seroepidemiologic Studies during a simultaneous epidemic of infection with El Tor Ogawa and Classical Inaba *Vibrio cholerae*. J Infect Dis 121:517–524

Cash RA (1969) Aspect of the current understanding of the pathphysiology of cholera. J Pak Med Assoc 1969(19):345–348

Cash RA, Nalin DR, Rochat R, Rellar B, Haque B, Rahman ASMM (1970) A clinical trial of oral therapy in a rural cholera treatment centre. Am J Trop Med Hyg 1970(19):653–656

Chambers JS (1938) The conquest of cholera. Macmillan, New York, pp 24–44

Chandu MG (1971) The seventh cholera pandemic. WHO Chronicle 25:155–160

Cholera working Group, International Centre for Diarrhoeal Disease Research, Bangladesh (1993) Large epidemic of cholera-like disease in Bangladesh caused by Vibrio cholerae O139 synonym Bengal. Lancet 342:30–431

Clemens JD, Sack DA, Harris JR et al (1989) ABO blood groups and cholera: new observations on specificity of risk and modification of vaccine efficacy. J Infect Dis 1989(159):770–773

Colwel RR, Huq A (1994) Environmental reservoir of V. cholerae. The causative agent of cholera. Ann N Y Acad Sci 740:44–45

Colwel RR, Siddler RJ, Kaper J, Joseph SW, Garges S, Lockman H, Maneval D, Bradford H, Roberts N, Remmers E, Huq I, Huq A (1981) Occurence of vibrio cholerae Serotype O in Maryland and Louisiana estuaries. Appl Environ Microbiol 41:555–558

Colwell RR (1966) Global climate and infectious disease: the cholera paradigm. Science 274(5295):2025–2031

Colwell RR, Bryton PR, Grimes DJ et al (1985) Viable but non-culturable *Vibrio cholerae* and related pathogens in the environment: implications for release of genetically engineered microorganisms. Bio Technology 3:817–820

De Moor CE (1938) Un vibrio du type El Tor responsible dans la sud de Celebes d'une epidemie presentant les apparences compl'etes due cholera. Bulletin Officiel International d'Hygiene Publique 30:1510–1519

Duffy J (1971) The history of Asiatic cholera in the United States. Bull N Y Acad Med 47:1152–1168

Farmer JJ, Hickman-Brenner FW, Kelly MT (1985) Vibrio. In: Lennette GH, Balows A, Hausler WJ, Shadony HJ (eds) Manual for clinical microbiology, 4th edn. American Society for Microbiology, Washington DC, pp 282–301

Faruque SM, Abdul Alim AR, Rahman MM, Siddique AK, Sack RB, Albert MJ (1993). Clonal relationships among classical *Vibrio cholerae* O1 strains isolated between 1961 and 1992 in Bangladesh. J Clin Microbiol 31(9):2513–2516

Faruque SM, Abdul Alim ARM, Roy SK, Khan F, Nair GB, Sack RB, Albert MJ (1994) Molecular analysis of rRNA and cholera toxin genes carried by the new epidemic strain of *Vibrio cholerae* O139 synonmy Bengal. J Clin Microbiol 32:2513–2516

Faruque SM, Albert MJ, Mekalanos JJ (1998) Epidemiology, genetics, and ecology of toxigenic *Vibrio cholerae*. Microbiol Mol Biol Rev 62:1301–1314

Faruque SM, Naser IB, Islam MJ, Faruque AS, Ghosh AN, Nair GB, Sack DA, Mekalonos JJ (2005) Seasonal epidemics of cholera inversely correlate with prevalence of environmental cholera phages. Proc Natl Acad Sci U S A 102:1702–1707

Felsenfeld O (1963) Some observation on the cholera (El Tor) epidemic in 1961–62. Bull WHO 28:289–296

Glass RI, Backer S, Huq MI, Stoll BJ, Khan MU, Merson MH, Lee JV, Black RE et al (1982) Endemic cholera in rural Bangladesh, 1966–1980. Am J Epidemiol 116(6):957–970

Glass RI, Holmgren J, Haley CE et al (1985a) Predisposition for cholera of individuals with O blood group: possible evolutionary significance. Am J Epidemiol 121:791–796

Glass RI, Svennerholm AM, Khan MR et al (1985b) Sero-epidemiological studies of El Tor cholera in Bangladesh: association of serum antibody with protection. J Infect Dis 151:236–242

Goodgame RW, Greenough WB III (1975) Cholera in Africa: a message for the West. Ann Int Med 82:101–106

Greenough WB III (1984) Oral rehydration therapy: scope and horizons. Al-Faisal Med J 10:4–6

Greenough WB III (1979) Vibrio cholerae. International Centre for Diarrhoeal Disease Research, Dhaka (Scientific report no. 22)

Greenough WB III, Gordon RS, Rosenberg IS, Davis BI, Benenson AS (1964) Tetracycline in the treatment of cholera. Lancet 1:340–342

Guthmann JP (1995) Epidemic cholera in Latin America: spread and routes of transmission. J Trop Med Hyg 98:419–427

Huq A, West PA, Small EB, Huq MI, Colwell RR (1984) Influence of water temperature, salinity, and pH on survival and growth of toxigenic *Vibrio cholerae* serovar O1 associated with live copepods in laboratory microcosms. Appl Environ Microbiol 48:420–424

Huq A, Colwell RR, Rahman R, Ali A, Choudhury MAR, Parveen S, Sack DA, Russek-Cohen E (1990) Detection of Vibrio cholerae O1 in the aquatic environment by fluorescent-monoclonal antibody and culture methods. Appl Environ Microbiol 56:2370–2373

Islam MS, Miah MA, Hassan MK, Sack RB et al (1994) Detection of non-culturable *Vibrio cholerae* with cyanobacterium from aquatic environment in Bangladesh. Trans R Soc Trop Med Hyg 88:298–299

Khan AQ (1967) Role of carriers in the intra-familial spread of cholera. Lancet 1:245–246

Khan M, Shahidullah M et al (1980) Cholera due to the El Tor biotype equals the classical biotype in severity and attack rates. J Trop Med Hyg 83(1):35–39

Khan MU, Barua DK, Begum T et al (1987) Vibriocidal titre in cholera cases and contacts: its value in assessing endemicity of cholera of or susceptibility to cholera. Trop Geogr Med 1987(39):271–275

Koch R (1884) An address on cholera and its bacillus. Br Med J 2:403–407

Levin MM (1991) South America: the return of cholera. Lancet 338:45–46

Lindenbaum J, Gordon RS, Hirschhorn N et al (1966) Cholera in children. Lancet 1:340–342

MacNamara C (1876) A history of Asiatic cholera. MacMillan and Co, London

Martin AR, Mosley WH, Sau BB et al (1969) Epidemiologic analysis of endemic cholera in urban East Pakistan. Am J Epidemiol 1969(89):572–582

McCormack WM, Islam MS, Fahimuddin M, Mosley WH (1969a) A community study of inapparent cholera infections. Am J Epidemiol 1969(89):658–664

McCormack WM, Mosley WH, Fahimuddin M, Benenson AS (1969b) Endemic cholera in rural East Pakistan. Am J Epidemiol 1969(89):393–404

Mosley WH (1969) Worldwide cholera surveillance and control. Pakistan Med Forum 2:87–85

Mosley WH, Benenson As, Barui R (1968) The distribution of antibody in the control population of a cholera-vaccine field-trial area and the relation of antibody titre to the pattern of endemic cholera. Bull WHO 38:327–34

Mukerjee S, Basu S, Bhattacharya P (1965) A new trend in cholera epidemiology. Brit Med J 2:837–839

Nair GB, Faruque Shah M, Bhuyan NA, Kamruzzaman M, Siddique AK, Sack DA (2002) New variant of *Vibrio cholerae* O1 Biotype El Tor with attributes of classical biotype from hospitalized patients with acute diarrhoea. J Clin Microbiol 40:3296–3299

Nair GB, Qadri F, Holmgren J, Svennerholm A-M, Safa A, Bhuiyan NA, Ahamed QS, Faruque SM, Faruque ASG, Takeda Y, Sack DA (2006) Cholera due to altered El Tor Strains of Vibrio cholerae O1 in Bangladesh. J Clin Microbiol 44:4211–4213

Nalin DR, Cash RA, Islam R et al (1968) Oral maintenance therapy for cholera in adults. Lancet 2:370–373

Pan American Health Organisation (1991) Cholera situation in the Americas. Epidemiol Bull 12:1–4

Peters JC (1885) Early history of Asiatic cholera as Known to Europeans A.D. 1500–1800. In: Wendt EC (ed) Asiatic Cholera. William Wood, New York

Pollitzer R (1959) Cholera. World Health Organization, Geneva

Rabbani GH (1986) Cholera. Clin Gastroentrology 15:507–528

Ramamurthy T, Grag S, Sharma S, Bhattacharya SK, Nair GB, Shimada T, Takeda T, KarasawaT, Kurazano H, Pal S, Takeda Y (1993) Emergence of a novel strain of Vibrio cholerae with epidemic potential in Southern and Eastern India. Lancet 341:703–704

Sack David A, Bradley Sack R, Balakrish Nair G, Siddique AK (2004) Cholera. Lancet 363:223–233

Sakazaki R (1992) Bacteriology of *Vibrio* and related organisms. In: Barua D, Greenough WB III (eds) Cholera. Plenum Medical Book Company, New York, pp 37–55

Samadi AR, Huq MI, Shahid NS, Khan MU, Eusof A, Rahman ASMM, Yunus M, Faruque ASG (1983) Classical *Vibrio cholerae* biotype displaces El Tor in Bangladesh. Lancet i:853–807

Sanyal SC, Dutta NK, Mukerjee S (1972) Present status of classical cholera in India. Indian J Med Res 60:1564–1567

Shahid NS, Samadi AR, Khan MU, Huq MI (1984) Classical vs El Tor cholera: a prospective family study of a concurrent outbreak. J Diarrhoeal Dis Res 2(2):73–78

Shimada T, Nair GB, Deb BC, Albert MJ, Sack RB (1993) Outbreak of *Vibrio cholerae* non-O1 in India and Bangladesh. Lancet 341:1346–1347

Siddique AK, Zaman K, Majumder Y, Islam Q, Bashir I, Mutsuddy P, Eusof A (1989) Simultaneous outbreak of contrasting drug resistant classic and El Tor *Vibrio cholerae* O1 in Bangladesh. Lancet 2(8659):396

Siddique AK, Baqui AH, Eusof A, Haider K, Hossain MA, Bashir I, Zaman K (1991) Survival of classic cholera in Bangladesh. Lancet 337(8750):1125–1127

Siddique AK, Zaman K, Baqui AH, Akram K, Mutsuddy P, Eusof A, Haider K, Islam S, Sack RB (1992) Cholera epidemics in Bangladesh: 1985–1991. J Diarrhoeal Dis Res 10(2):79–86

Siddique AK, Zaman K, Akram K, Mutsuddy P, Eusof A, Sack RB (1994) Emergence of a new epidemic strain of *Vibrio cholerae* in Bangladesh: an epidemiological study. Trop Geogr Med 46(3):147–150

Siddique AK, Akram K, Zaman K, Mutsuddy P, Eusof A, Sack RB (1996) *V. cholerae* O139: How great is the threat of a Pandemic? Trop Med Int Health 1(3):393–398

Siddique AK, Nair GB, Alam M, Sack DA, Huq A, Nizami A, Longini IM, Qadri F, Faruque SM, Colwell RR, Ahamed S, Bhuiyan NA, Sack RB (2010) El Tor cholera with severe disease: a new threat to Asia and beyond. Epidmiol Infect 138:347–352

Singleton FL, Attwell R, Jangi S, Colwell RR (1982) Effect of temperature and salinity on Vibrio cholerae growth. Appl Environ Microbiol 44(5):1047–1058

Waldor MK, Mekalanos JJ (1994) ToxR regulates virulence gene expression in non-O1 strains of vibrio cholerae that cause epidemic cholera. Infect Immun 62:72–78

Waldor MK, Mekalanos JJ (1996) Lysogenic conversion by a filamentous phage encoding cholera toxin. Science 272:1910–1914

Xu H-S, Roberts N, Singleton FL, Attwell RW et al (1982) Survival and viability of non-culturable *Escherichia coli* and *Vibrio cholerae* in the estuarine and marine environment. Microb Ecol 8:313–323

Zahid MSH, Wise Z, Kamruzzaman M, Ghosh AN, Nair GB, Khairul basher SAM, Mekalanos JJ, Faruque SM (2011) An experimental study of phage mediated bactericidal selection & emergence of the El Tor Vibrio cholerae. Indian J Med Res 133:118–124

Cholera Outbreaks in the El Tor Biotype Era and the Impact of the New El Tor Variants

Asish K. Mukhopadhyay, Yoshifumi Takeda and G. Balakrish Nair

Abstract *Vibrio cholerae* O1, the causative agent of the disease cholera, has two biotypes namely the classical and El Tor. Biotype is a subspecific taxonomic classification of *V. cholerae* O1. Differentiation of *V. cholerae* strains into biotype does not alter the clinical management of cholera but is of immense public health and epidemiological importance in identifying the source and spread of infection, particularly when *V. cholerae* is first isolated in a country or geographic area. From recorded history, till date, the world has experienced seven pandemics of cholera. Among these, the first six pandemics are believed to have been caused by the classical biotype whereas the ongoing seventh pandemic is caused by the El Tor biotype. In recent years, new pathogenic variants of *V. cholerae* have emerged and spread throughout many Asian and African countries with corresponding cryptic changes in the epidemiology of cholera. In this chapter, we describe the outbreaks during the seventh pandemic El Tor biotype era spanning more than five decades along with the recent advances in our understanding of the development, evolution, spread, and impact of the new variants of El Tor strains.

A. K. Mukhopadhyay (✉)
National Institute of Cholera and Enteric Diseases, P 33, CIT Road, Scheme XM, Beliaghata, Kolkata 700010, India
e-mail: asish_mukhopadhyay@yahoo.com

Y. Takeda
National Institute of Infectious Diseases, Tokyo, Japan

G. Balakrish Nair
Translational Health Science and Technology Institute, Faridabad, India

Current Topics in Microbiology and Immunology (2014) 379: 17–47
DOI: 10.1007/82_2014_363

Published Online: 13 February 2014

Contents

1 Introduction

Cholera, an intestinal infection spread by contaminated water and food, is a substantial health burden in countries where sanitation and availability of clean drinking water is limited. Recent years have witnessed a remarkable resurgence in the global incidence of cholera. The devastating and ongoing cholera outbreak in Haiti from 2010, for the first time in almost a century, placed this ancient scourge at the forefront of the global public health agenda. This dreadful diarrheal disease is caused by the Gram-negative toxigenic bacterium *Vibrio cholerae* O1 and O139. Based on certain phenotypic and genetic properties, *V. cholerae* O1 can be divided into two biotypes; classical and El Tor. From recorded history, till date, the world has experienced seven pandemics of cholera. Among these, the first six pandemics are believed to have been caused by the classical biotype whereas the ongoing seventh pandemic is caused by the El Tor biotype. In recent years, new pathogenic variants of *V. cholerae* have emerged and spread throughout many Asian and African countries with corresponding cryptic changes in the epidemiology of cholera. These strains include the Matlab variants from Bangladesh, the Mozambique variants, the altered El Tor type from various parts of the world, and very recently the Haitian variants of the El Tor biotype. These variants display a mix of phenotypic and genotypic traits from the two main biotypes, suggesting that they are genetic hybrids. Classical and El Tor biotypes have been the most epidemiologically successful cholera strains during the past century, and it is believed that the new variants are likely to develop successfully in a manner similar to these biotypes. Here, we describe the outbreaks during the seventh pandemic El Tor biotype era along with the recent advances in our understanding of the development, evolution, spread, and impact of the new variants of El Tor strains.

2 Biotypes of *Vibrio cholerae*

Biotype is a subspecific taxonomic classification of *V. cholerae* O1. Differentiation of *V. cholerae* strains into biotype does not alter the clinical management of cholera but is of immense public health and epidemiological importance in identifying the source and spread of infection, particularly when *V. cholerae* is first isolated in a country or geographic area. *V. cholerae* strains are classified into serogroups on the basis of epitopic variations in the cell surface lipopolysaccharide (Yamai et al. 1997), which identifies over 200 serogroups. However, the strains that have epidemic and pandemic potential belong to only two serogroups namely, O1 and O139. *Vibrio cholerae* O1 has two well-established biotypes, namely, classical and El Tor, that are differentiated primarily based on number of phenotypic traits like susceptibility to polymyxin B, chicken cell (erythrocytes) agglutination (CCA), hemolysis of sheep erythrocytes, Voges–Proskauer (VP) test, which measures the production of acetylmethylcarbinol, and phage susceptibilities (Faruque et al. 1998; Kaper et al. 1995). Conventionally, at least two or more of the phenotypic tests mentioned above should be included to determine the biotype, since results can vary between individual isolates. While El Tor strains are resistant to polymyxin B (50U), classical strains are susceptible to this antibiotic. El Tor strains yield a positive reaction in VP test indicating that the strains produce 2, 3-butanediol instead of producing organic acids as their fermentation end product and thus grow to much higher densities in media containing carbohydrates (Yoon and Mekalanos 2006); classical strains give negative VP reaction.

Another distinction among El Tor strains is the ability to agglutinate erythrocytes from several animal species like chicken, goat, or sheep, though classical strains are devoid of this capability. It has also been reported that the chicken blood cell-positive biotype of *V. cholerae* strains are observed to attach to the scattered erythrocytes and to propel them with a characteristic flipping motion when observed under a dark-field microscope (Mackowiak and Huq 1974). Based on phage-typing, El Tor strains are susceptible to El Tor-specific bacteriophage V, but are resistant to classical bacteriophage IV whereas classical strains show the reverse traits (Mukerjee 1963). El Tor strains were identified historically by its ability to hemolyze sheep erythrocytes, while classical strains were nonhemolytic. But by 1972, nearly all El Tor isolates become nonhemolytic worldwide (Barrett and Blake 1981). Exceptions are found in isolates from the U.S. Gulf Coast and from Australia (Barrett and Blake 1981). Thus, hemolysis of erythrocytes continues to be a useful phenotypic characteristic for differentiating the Gulf Coast clones of *V. cholerae* O1 El Tor from those isolated in the rest of the world, including Latin America.

Comparative genetic analyses have recently revealed a high degree of conservation among diverse strains of *V. cholerae* but have also shown genes that differentiate classical biotype from El Tor biotype (Dziejman et al. 2002). Molecular biotyping of *V. cholerae* O1 using multiplex PCR (*ctxA–tcpA*) exploits the nucleotide sequence differences of the major subunit protein of the toxin coregulated pilus (TCP) gene (*tcpA*) to differentiate between classical and El Tor biotypes (Keasler and Hall 1993). Only in toxigenic *V. cholerae* O1 El Tor and O139 strains, cholera toxin prophage region (CTXΦ) is often flanked by an element termed RS1 containing *rstC* gene (Waldor et al. 1997). The only difference between RS1 and RS2 is the presence of *rstC* gene in RS1 alone (Waldor et al. 1997; Davis et al. 2000). Another virulence-associated protein known as repeat in toxin (RTX) encoded by a cluster of genes of 10 kb size, comprising four ORFs, *rtxABCD*, of which the *rtxC* gene has been observed only in El Tor biotype (Lin et al. 1999). Nucleotide sequence comparison of hemolysin encoding *hlyA* gene from classical and El Tor strains reveal the presence of an 11-base-pair deletion in classical strains that results in a truncated protein product of 27 kDa in classical strains rendering it nonhemolytic, whereas in El Tor strains the HlyA is intact 82 kDa and biologically active (Rader and Murphy 1988). On the basis of differences in the sequences of *hlyA* genes, a 19-base-pair oligodeoxynucleotide probe has been developed to distinguish between the two biotypes of *V. cholerae* serogroup O1 (Alm and Manning 1990). This gene marker was found to be very useful to differentiate the biotypes than the other commonly used methods, which are less reliable and often difficult to interpret (Alm and Manning 1990). Recently, comparative genomic studies using a *V. cholerae* DNA microarray on 11 epidemic isolates identified two regions, *Vibrio* seventh pandemic island I (VSP-I), encompassing VC0175–VC0185 and VSP-II, encompassing VC0490–VC0497, that were found exclusively among El Tor biotype isolates (Dziejman et al. 2002). Subsequently, it was shown that the VSP-II region actually encompassed a 26.9 kb region (VC0490–VC0516) in *V. cholerae* biotype El Tor and O139 serogroup isolates (O'Shea et al. 2004). Besides these phenotypic and genotypic differences, there are also dissimilarities in the infection pattern of disease caused by the two biotypes (Nair et al. 2008). Epidemiological studies proved occurrence of more asymptomatic carriers among El Tor cholera cases that outnumber active cases by a ratio of up to 50:1 (Sack et al. 2004), better survival of El Tor strains in the environment and in the human host, and more efficient host-to-host transmission of El Tor strains than of classical strains (Finkelstein 1996).

Cholera toxin (CT), the primary toxin produced by *V. cholerae* O1 and O139, is responsible for most of the manifestations of the disease cholera. Based on the B subunit of CT, two immunologically related but not identical epitypes have been designated: CT1 is the prototype elaborated by classical biotype strains and by U.S. Gulf Coast strains, while CT2 is produced by the El Tor biotype and O139 strains (Finkelstein et al. 1987). Another classification identifies three types of *ctxB* genes based on three non-random base changes resulting in changes in the deduced amino acid sequence. Genotype 1 is found in strains of the classical biotype worldwide and in US Gulf Coast, genotype 2 is found in El Tor biotype strains from Australia, and genotype 3 is found in El Tor biotype from the seventh pandemic and the Latin American epidemic strains (Olsvik et al. 1993). Thus, the *V. cholerae* O1 El Tor biotype of the ongoing seventh pandemic produces CT of the CT2 epitype and genotype 3, while the classical biotype CT belongs to the CT1 epitype and genotype 1.

However, over time, especially after the emergence of El Tor variant strains, many of the phenotypic and genotypic tests have proven to be inadequate for classifying strains of *V. cholerae* O1 strains into their biotype. Thus, revision of the conventional tests used for the identification of biotypes of *V. cholerae* O1 strains are necessary and an amendment of the existing biotyping scheme has been proposed (Raychoudhuri et al. 2008).

3 Origin of El Tor Biotype and Seventh Pandemics of Cholera

Although the Ganges delta has been considered as the cradle of cholera for many centuries, the seventh pandemic began in Sulawesi island of Indonesia (Barua 1972). This pandemic now has involved almost the whole world, and the causative agent was a biotype of *V. cholerae* serogroup O1 called El Tor. It was first isolated in 1905 from Indonesian pilgrims traveling to Mecca at a quarantine station in the village of El Tor, Egypt by a German physician, E. Gotschlich (Pollitzer 1959) and found again in an outbreak in 1937 in Sulawesi, Indonesia (Tanamal 1959). It caused four outbreaks in Sulawesi during 1937–1958, where it was endemic. During mid-1961, a few cases of cholera caused by the El Tor *V. cholerae* was reported in Java, and Samarang in Indonesia and then the infection spread out like a wild fire to neighboring countries, and went on a pandemic rampage (Barua 1992). The extent of the pandemic was due to the relative mildness (lower expression level) of El Tor and the disease has many more asymptomatic carriers (Sack et al. 2004).

4 Cholera Outbreaks in the 1960s

The factors that provoked the El Tor biotype of *V. cholerae* O1 to spread from its endemic focus in Sulawesi (Celebes), where it began to be more active than usual in January, 1961, will probably be never known. The increase in population movement due to political unrest and the availability of the faster transport systems may have contributed for the dissemination of the infection. The seventh pandemic El Tor cholera spread during 1961–1962 from Sulawesi to involve the other islands of Indonesia, including Java, Sarawak, and Borneo (Kamal 1974). El Tor cholera then spread to the Philippines, Sabah, Taiwan, and Irian Barat, thereby affecting virtually the entire Southeast Asian archipelago. In 1963, the pandemic strain reached Chittagong, Bangladesh, Cambodia, Thailand, Singapore, west Malaysia (Kaper et al. 1995). India was invaded in 1964 through the port of Madras, and within 1 year El Tor cholera had disseminated throughout the country. In 1965, the pandemic spread further westward and invaded West

Pakistan, Nepal, Brunei, Afghanistan, Iran and a limited area of Uzbekistan (USSR). Local outbreaks and sporadic cases of cholera followed subsequently in Uzbekistan (1968), Turkmenistan (1969) and some parts of Russia (1969). During this time a number of cholera strains were isolated, mainly from surface water in these areas as well as in Azerbaijan and in the Krasnodar region (Narkevich et al. 1993). From the time that El Tor cholera reached Pakistan, its spread became even more accelerated. In the space of a few months, Afghanistan, Iran, and nearby republics within the Soviet Union experienced outbreaks. Iraq reported El Tor cholera during the following year in 1966 (Kaper et al. 1995). A large outbreak of classical cholera was recorded in West Pakistan in 1968, and then spread with more vigor to the other countries. Laos reported cholera for the first time during this era. Hong Kong, Macao, and the Republic of Korea got affected again after remaining practically free from the disease since 1965. At the same time, Nepal, Malaysia, and Myanmar reported higher incidence of cholera than the previous years.

5 Cholera Outbreaks in the 1970s

The seventh El Tor pandemic gained its entry and caused explosive outbreaks of cholera in the Middle East and West Africa in 1970. El Tor cholera had touched the Arabian Peninsula, Syria, and Jordan by 1970 and a limited outbreak was recorded in Israel (Cohen et al. 1971). At this time, resurgence of El Tor Inaba serotype was documented in Iran and the southern Soviet Union. It is of interest that in Lebanon and Syria the epidemic strain was El Tor Ogawa, whereas in nearby Israel and Jordan and in Dubai and Saudi Arabia the epidemic organism was El Tor Inaba. The invasion of El Tor Ogawa cholera into the sub-Saharan West Africa was a momentous epidemiologic event (Goodgame and Greenough 1975). Following its introduction in Guinea in August 1970, probably by means of a returning asymptomatic traveler from the Asian continent, cholera subsequently spread along waterways along the coast and into the interior along rivers ((Swerdlow and Isaäcson 1994; Isaäcson et al. 1974). Subsequent dissemination into the interior of the Sahelian states occurred by land travel fostered by the movement of nomadic tribes (Kaper et al. 1995). It is estimated that the outbreak during 1970–1971 in West Africa sickened more than 400,000 persons. Within a year, 25 African countries were affected by cholera with a high case fatality rate (CFR) of 16 % (WHO 1991). In the following years (1972–1991), cholera swept in most of the African countries with case fatality ranging from 4 to 12 % (WHO 1991). Due to the lack of background immunity in the population, insufficient transport to move severe cases to treatment facilities, and inadequacies in the health care infrastructure, case fatality in West Africa was high (Kaper et al. 1995). According to WHO records, of the 36 countries that reported cholera in 1970, 28 were newly affected countries and 16 were in Africa. As epidemic cholera stormed in West Africa in 1970, epidemiologists and public health officials in South

America and elsewhere in Latin America restrained themselves and their communities for what was deemed to be the inevitable passage of cholera westward across the South Atlantic. The scenario of introduction of cholera into the Americas was considered particularly likely to occur once cholera hit Angola, since an estimated 40,000 Cuban troops were in that country. Yet, inexplicably, cholera did not cross the South Atlantic during the next 20 years.

In West Africa, cholera epidemic occurred in Togo during 1970–1973, affecting more than 1,000 people with CFR of 4–10 % (Bockemühl and Schröter 1975). Cameroon first reported cholera cases in 1971 when the current pandemic hit the African continent. More than 2,000 cases were reported in 1971 with a high case fatality rate (CFR) of 15 % (WHO 2012). Since the first outbreak in 1970 in Guinea, cholera recurred every 8 years till 1994 (Boiro et al. 1999). Based on the reported cases, cholera first appeared in Burundi, Zaire, and Congo during 1978–1979 (Yala et al. 1982) and in South Africa in 1980 (Küstner et al. 1981). *Vibrio cholerae* O1 Inaba was associated with African cholera for many years (Mugoya et al. 2008). Early cholera outbreaks (1971–1975) in Algeria were caused by the serotype Ogawa (Guechi and Mered 1978). In Zaria, Nigeria, Hikojima serotype that reacts with both Ogawa and Inaba antisera was prevalent from 1976 to 1978, but Ogawa became dominant from 1984 to 1986 (Onyemelukwe and Lawande 1991).

In USSR, cholera spread intensively between 1970 and 1977 and more than 80 regions of the country reported outbreaks. The peak occurred in 1970 when 3,989 cases and carriers were reported; this coincided with intensification of the global pandemic. The infection was introduced to Odessa, Kerch, Astrakhan (Pavlov 1976; Sergiev et al. 1981) and Batumi in 1970, followed by its spread from these foci to 38 cities in the same year, despite cholera control measures. Cholera was also imported to Azerbaijan from India, Jordan, and Iran (1970–1972), and to the Kemerovo region from Egypt (1975). Large-scale outbreaks occurred in 1970–1971 along the river Volga (5,584 cholera cases and carriers) and also in the Ukraine, Georgia, Azerbaijan, and Tajikistan. Subsequently, cholera spread into new territories, causing outbreaks in the north Caucasus, in the region of the rivers Volga and Viatka, and in western Siberia. The annual incidence of cholera in the USSR varied from 0.001 per 100,000 in 1977 to 0.8 per 100,000 in 1979. In India, the classical biotype was replaced by the El Tor from 1965 (Datta and Singh 1990). In some areas in India such as Raipur, the classical cholera prevailed till 1970 and the subsequent cholera outbreaks in 1975, 1977, and 1979–1981 were caused by El Tor vibrios (Darbari et al. 1982).

In Asia, Sri Lanka reported cholera for the first time since 1953; the Philippines reported 5,600 cases in 1972 and 2,075 in 1973, and Indonesia reported 44,300 cases in 1972; 52,000 cases in 1973; 41,000 cases in 1976, and 17,000 cases in 1977 (Barua and Burrows 1974).

In developed areas as Japan, Northern Europe, and North America, cholera has been introduced repeatedly in recent years, but had not caused devastating outbreaks. However, Japan also reported a limited outbreak in Wakayama Prefecture in 1977 and, in 1978, the United States experienced an outbreak of about 12 cases in Louisiana. In that outbreak, sewage was infected, and infected shellfish apparently were involved. Interestingly, the hemolytic vibrio strain implicated was identical to one that caused an unexplained isolated case in Texas in 1973 (Finkelstein 1996). In 1973, Italy suffered serious losses in its tourist trade when cholera broke out in August around Naples and Bari with some sporadic cases in other parts of the country (Baine et al. 1974). Cholera was reported again in 1979 in Italy and in eight districts of Spain.

6 Cholera Outbreaks in the 1980s

Intermittent appearance of classical cholera was recorded during 1979–1981 (Samadi et al. 1983a, b). Classical cholera appeared in the form of large epidemic starting from Matlab, Comilla, and Dhaka during late 1982 and spread to other districts replacing the El Tor biotype (Khan et al. 1984; Samadi et al. 1983a, b). Phenotypically, the new classical strains were identical to the one that prevailed a decade earlier and the virulence features and seasonality resembled that of El Tor strains prevailing at that time. It was hypothesized that the classical strains of *V. cholerae* O1 were indigenous to Bangladesh (Huq et al. 1983). Cholera due to classical biotype was predominant (79 %) in southern regions of Bangladesh during 1988–1989 (Siddique et al. 1991).

A 33-year (1966–1998) data analysis provided much information from Bangladesh (Longini et al. 2002). Between 1966 and 1988, both classical and El Tor biotypes had alternated and persisted and by 1988, the classical biotype disappeared. Both the Ogawa and Inaba serotypes circulated the entire time. The serotype prevalence during 1988–1989 was interesting as El Tor belonged to Inaba, whereas the classical strains to Ogawa type (Longini et al. 2002). Studies conducted from 1985 to 1991 in Bangladesh indicated that the incidence of cholera was among children below 5 years (24 %) and children below 2 years of age accounted for 10 % of the cases (Siddique et al. 1992). The overall case fatality during epidemics was 4.0 %. China also reported cholera in 1980. Large number of cases was reported by Indonesia, Iran, Jordan, and Yemen during in the early 1980s.

In Africa, large epidemics raged during 1984–1986 in the drought-affected countries of Burkina Faso, Niger, Mali, Mauritania, Senegal, Ghana, and the United Republic of Tanzania. Cameroon was also affected by the epidemic in 1985. A cholera epidemic in South Africa occurred in the 1980s, with over 20,000 culture-confirmed cases being documented. KwaZulu-Natal was the worst-affected province, although cases were described in Limpopo and Mpumalanga. This epidemic was primarily due to *V. cholerae* O1 Inaba (Küstner and Du Plessis 1991). This followed an outbreak of cholera in Maputo in Mozambique between 1980 and 1981 (Swerdlow and Isaäcson 1994).

Vibrio cholerae O1 was introduced in northern Somalia from Ethiopia during the early 1980s (Coppo et al. 1995). Recurrent cholera epidemics were reported during rainy hot seasons since 1987 in Angola (Colombo et al. 1993). In Malawi, cholera cases were reported with high attack rate (2.6 %) with CFR of 3.3 % during 1988 (Moren et al. 1991). This outbreak was related to consumption of contaminated shallow waters.

Seventh pandemic of cholera extended to Swaziland in 1981, the Trust Territory of the Pacific islands in 1982, and Equatorial Guinea in 1984 bringing the total number of countries affected by the seventh pandemic to 93 (Barua and Burrows 1974). Somalia reported a large number of cases in refugee camps in 1985 and 1986. Guinea-Bissau was affected in 1986 and Yugoslavia in Europe in 1989. During 1982–1987, the number of countries reporting cholera to WHO has varied between 30 and 37 each year as compared to 40 and 42 in 1980 and 1981.

In 1981, for the first time the health authorities in the Mecca pilgrimage waived the requirement of a cholera vaccination certificate. In 1986, for the first time, India also did not enforce the use of cholera vaccine during the country's largest religious congregation at Kumbh Mela, instead relied heavily on the success of surveillance and sanitation measures taken by the authority.

7 Cholera Outbreaks in 1990s

The 1990s was a significant decade in the history of cholera, as there was a remarkable upsurge in the global incidence of the disease. The number of cases and number of countries reporting cholera to the WHO showed a precipitous increase. In the July 1998 issue of the WHO Weekly Epidemiological Record, it was reported that "almost every developing country is now facing either a cholera outbreak or the threat of an epidemic" (WHO 1996). The striking events of the 1990s included the dramatic reappearance of epidemic cholera caused by *V. cholerae* O1 El Tor in Latin America in 1991 after its absence for 100 years in that continent (Tauxe and Blake 1992); the genesis in late 1992 in the Indian subcontinent of a new epidemic strain of *V. cholerae* non-O1 (Ramamurthy et al. 1993; Albert et al. 1993), presently classified as O139 Bengal (Shimada et al. 1993); the death in Africa in 1994 of as many as 14,000 Rwandan refugees due to cholera related to the poor quality of the water supply, sanitation, and treatment facilities (Siddique et al. 1995) and the dramatic cholera epidemic affecting the countries in the Horn of Africa in 1997 (WHO 1996). Clearly, there was a fresh resurgence of this ancient disease.

7.1 Latin America Epidemics of Cholera

The seventh cholera pandemic reached Latin America in January 1991 for the first time in more than a century. Nearly a million cases were reported from the epidemic of cholera in Latin America, and almost 9,000 people died between

January 1991 and December 1993 (Tauxe and Blake 1992; Tauxe et al. 1994). Latin America's cholera epidemic struck first on January 29 at the harbor city of Chimbote, Peru and caused a major outbreak along the Peruvian coast and it also spread inland through the Andes, as well as through the Peruvian Amazon, and by April, 1991 it had reached most of Peru (Tauxe et al. 1994).

The epidemic disseminated rapidly from country to country, and cholera first spread to neighboring Ecuador to the north, and then in Colombia. Later on, Guatemala, Brazil, Mexico, Bolivia, Chile, El Salvador, Venezuela, and Honduras were also affected. Notifications of cholera markedly diminished during the cool season in South America, but with the return of warm weather in December 1991, the incidence of cholera once again rose. By the end of 1993, all countries of Latin America except Uruguay and the Caribbean reported cholera cases. The greatest proportion of cholera cases and the highest incidence rate were in Peru (63.7 % and 26.9/1000, respectively) (Guthmann 1995). Most cholera cases were reported in 1991 and were concentrated in Peru (82.3 %). 45.5 % of all cholera deaths occurred in 1991 (Guthmann 1995). Central America had the highest case fatality rates. Actually, Peru accounted almost half of the cholera cases registered in Latin America (Kaper et al. 1995). The overall case fatality rate was only 0.92 %, mainly due to good oral rehydration treatment provided by local health services and the Pan American Health Organization. In each of these countries, cholera struck underprivileged low socioeconomic populations lacking unpolluted drinking water and proper sanitation (Pan American Health Organization. 1991).

The causative organism was *V. cholerae*, serogroup O1, serotype Inaba (and Ogawa) of the El Tor biotype. The cholera epidemic in Latin America was originally suspected to have come from Asia and to have been facilitated by the discharge of contaminated ballast water into Peruvian ports by international trade ships (Seas et al. 2000). Another view was that as the seventh pandemic spread through Africa during the 1970s, travel from Africa to South America and inadequate sanitation in parts of South America were thought to place the Latin American continent at particular risk (Wachsmuth et al. 1993).

Latin American isolates from Peru, Bolivia, Chile, Colombia, Guatemala, Ecuador, El Salvador, and Mexico were identical when isolates were compared by restriction enzyme *Hind*lll digestion and hybridization with probe *ctxA* or by *Bgl*l digestion and a 16S + 23S rRNA probe. When those isolates were compared with isolates from other parts of the world, they were clearly different from the Gulf Coast clone (Wachsmuth et al. 1993). From the result of their study, Wachsmuth et al. (1993) concluded that Latin American isolates are clonal, probably a variant of the seventh pandemic clone. Another study also showed that all *V. cholerae* O1 isolates tested from the Latin American epidemic were indistinguishable by their MEE, ribotype, or PFGE patterns (Cameron et al. 1994). Genetic characterization showed this strain to be unique, and the designation is reserved for the Latin American strain, distinguishing it from the other El Tor isolates from the seventh pandemic.

Recently, Lam et al. 2010 performed genome-wide single-nucleotide polymorphisms (SNPs) to track the evolution and spread of the seventh cholera pandemic and showed that the isolates from Latin American epidemic were closely related to isolates found in Africa in the 1970s and 1990s. This finding suggested that the strain that caused the epidemic in Latin America came from Africa rather than Asia. The outbreak in Peru occurred in parallel with the upsurge of cholera generally in Africa (Reeves and Lan 1998) and could have been imported at that time. However, the epidemic strain may have reached Latin America well before it caused the epidemic in 1990s, given the ability of the organism to persist in the marine environment for long periods (Seas et al. 2000). Phylogenomic analysis of 136 El Tor isolates clustered the Latin American epidemic strains with an Angolan strain isolated in 1989 (Mutreja et al. 2011). In this period, an increased circulation of people between Africa and Latin America was reported, due to the Cuban Angolan intervention (1975–1991).

At the late epidemic period (1994), in the state of Amapá, Brazil, outbreak was caused by the sucrose non-fermenting *V. cholerae* strain (Ramos et al. 1997; Garza et al. 2012) and Multi Locus Enzyme Electrophoresis (MLEE) later showed that this strain belonged to the same zymovar as the Latin American epidemic lineage, suggesting that this variation was the consequence of a mutation in the sucrose operon (Freitas et al. 2002).

Since the beginning of the 1990s, Kivu provinces have been identified as one of the most active foci of cholera in the world (Bompangue et al. 2009). In July 1994, 500,000–800,000 Rwandans crossed the border into the North Kivu region of Zaire (now called the Democratic Republic of the Congo, DRC). During the first month after the influx, almost 50,000 refugees died; an average crude mortality rate of 20–35 per 10,000 per day; and cholera was a major contributor (Goma Epidemiology Group 1995; Bhattacharya et al. 2009). The refugee camps located around Goma and Bukavu experienced the deadliest cholera epidemics recorded during the last hundred years. This explosive outbreak of cholera, which affected Rwandan refugees, resulted in about 70,000 cases and 12,000 deaths (Siddique et al. 1995).

7.2 *Genesis of* **Vibrio cholerae** *O139: A Bewildering Event in the History of Cholera*

The emergence of *V. cholerae* O139 Bengal as the second etiologic agent of epidemic cholera in 1992 in the south Indian coastal city of Madras has changed the long-held dogma that only *V. cholerae* belonging to serogroup O1 are capable of causing epidemic (and pandemic) cholera. The first report of an epidemic of "cholera-like" diarrhea was from a suburban area of north Madras, India, in September 1992 (Ramamurthy et al. 1993). In December 1992, there was an outbreak of "cholera-like" diarrhea in southern Bangladesh, which over the subsequent several months, spread to the entire country (Nair et al. 1994). Retrospective examination of all the *V. cholerae* isolates collected from 1992 at the Communicable Diseases Hospital in Madras showed that these strains belonged to *V. cholerae* O139 serogroup (Dhamodaran et al. 1995). This serogroup made its first appearance in January 1992 (Sharma et al. 1997a, b) and took almost 10 months for this serogroup to cause an epidemic. More than a year earlier, from April to July 1991 and again in September 1992, there had been an increase in the number of *V. cholerae* non-O1 isolates from patients with cholera at the Christian Medical College Hospital at Vellore, India, indicating an outbreak (John 1996). However, *V. cholerae* non-O1 strains isolated during 1991 were not stored for identification.

These strains of *V. cholerae* which did not agglutinate with antisera from O1 to O138 were included as a new serogroup O139 (Shimada et al. 1994). This serogroup had spread quickly to Bangladesh and to other states of India within a span of about 10 months (Albert et al. 1993; Nair et al. 1994). Since *V. cholerae* O139 was first discovered in the areas surrounding the Bay of Bengal (Tamil Nadu, Andhra Pradesh, West Bengal and Bangladesh), this serogroup was given a synonym "Bengal."

In a span of 1 year, this serogroup has been reported in many Asian countries including Bangladesh, Pakistan, Nepal, and China. The O139 infection produced severe dehydrating diarrhea, which is indistinguishable from clinical cholera and does not appear to confer any cross-protection from the O1 serogroup (Mahalanabis et al. 1994). Based on the clinical symptoms and severity of diarrhea, the disease caused by *V. cholerae* O139 is now considered as cholera (Bhattacharya et al. 1993) and the infections caused by the rest of the non-O1 and non-O139 serogroups are known as "cholera-like diarrhea."

Before its total replacement, the O139 prevailed along with the O1 serogroup in many countries. The affected age group by the O139 infection depends on the period and place of its occurrence. In Delhi the incidence of O139 and O1 cholera was frequent in children below 5 years of age (Singh et al. 1997). In this study, the incidence of both the serogroups was detected among 1.4 % of the children with cholera. A similar epidemiological observation was made in Karachi, Pakistan (Sheikh et al. 1997). The incidence of O139 among children during 2003 in Pakistan was 21 % and the infected patients were more likely to be febrile ($P < 0.001$) (Siddiqui et al. 2006).

After its initial explosive epidemic during late 1992 and early 1993, occurrence of O139 serogroup declined in many cholera-endemic regions (Faruque et al. 1996; Mukhopadhyay et al. 1996). The emergence of *V. cholerae* O139 initially caused a complete displacement of the O1 El Tor biotype strains in India and Bangladesh. However, *V. cholerae* O139 was again displaced in 1994 by a new genetic variant of the O1 strain, and this variant strain dominated until 1996 in India (Fig. 1). In August, 1996, a new variant of the O139 strain emerged, and cholera caused by the new O139 genetic variant dominated for a year, until September, 1997 in Calcutta. Similarly in neighboring Bangladesh, during 1994 and till the middle of 1995, in most northern and central areas of the country, the O139 vibrios were replaced by a new clone of *V. cholerae* O1 of the El Tor biotype, whereas in the southern coastal regions, the O139 vibrios continued to exist (Faruque et al. 1997a, 1999). During late 1995 and through 1996, cases of cholera caused by both *V. cholerae* O1 and O139 were again detected in various

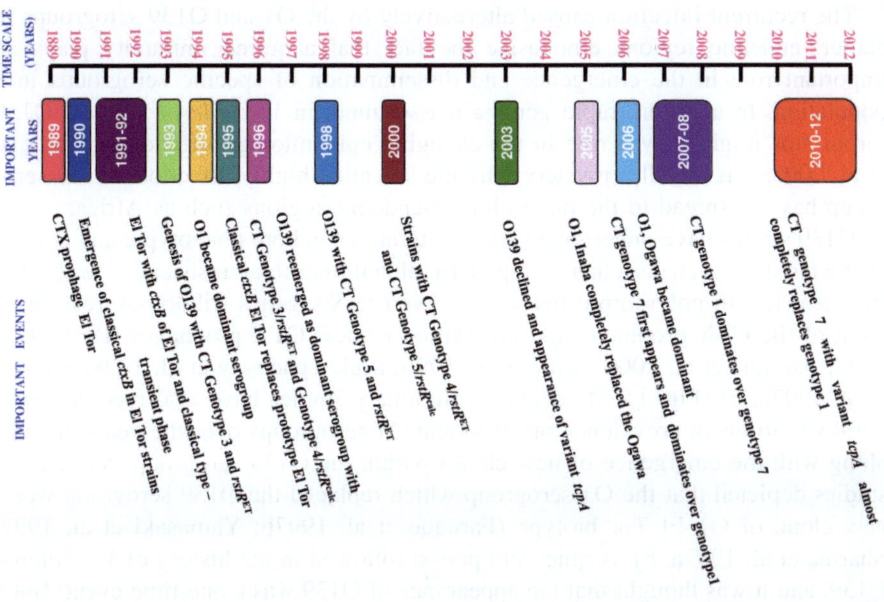

Fig. 1 Major events in the evolution of *Vibrio cholerae* O1 El Tor and O139 CTX prophases in Kolkata for the last two decades

regions of Bangladesh. However, since 1996, cholera in Bangladesh was caused mostly by *V. cholerae* O1 of the El Tor biotype, whereas only a few cases were caused by strains of the O139 serogroup. Between 1997 and 2000, incidence of cholera due to O139 serogroup decreased to 3.8 % in rural Bangladesh (Sack et al. 2003). This changing epidemiology of cholera shifted further, and a large outbreak of cholera caused predominantly by *V. cholerae* O139 occurred in the capital city of Dhaka and adjoining areas during the first half of 2002 (Faruque et al. 2003a). Resurgence of O139 cholera was also reported in other Asian countries including Pakistan (2000–2001), and India (1997, 2001), mostly affecting the older age groups (Jabeen and Hasan 2003; Mitra et al. 1996; Sundaram et al. 2002; Agarwal et al. 2003). From 1999 to 2000, most of the cholera outbreaks in India were caused by the O139 serogroup (Sinha et al. 2002). Investigations conducted in Indonesia revealed that the O139 serogroup had not invaded into this country till 1999 (Simanjuntak et al. 2001). The first incidence of O139 was recorded in Baghdad, Iraq, in 1999, though the numbers of cases were low (Al-Abbassi et al. 2005). In 1993, the first outbreak caused by serogroup O139 strains occurred in Xinjiang, China, where 200 cases were reported. In 1994, outbreaks of *V. cholerae* O139 were reported in six Chinese provinces. Imported cases of O139 cholera were reported soon after its emergence in Asia in California (CDC 1993) and other parts of the USA (Mahon et al. 1996), Japan (Kurazono et al. 1994), and Denmark (Dalsgaards et al. 1995).

The recurrent infection caused alternatively by the O1 and O139 serogroups in cholera-endemic regions emphasize the fact that acquired immunity plays an important role in the emergence and dissemination of specific serogroups in a population. In addition, rapid genetic reassortment in *V. cholerae* O1 and O139 serogroups might play a role in the changing epidemiology of cholera (Faruque et al. 2003a). It is still a mystery why the so-called highly infectious O139 serogroup has not spread to the other cholera-endemic regions such as Africa.

O139 strains have undergone various alterations in both phenotypic and genetic characteristics such as changing pattern of antimicrobial resistance, restriction fragment length polymorphisms in conserved rRNA genes (ribotype), rearrangement of the CTX prophage, and acquisition of new CTX prophages (Basu et al. 1998; Faruque et al. 2000; Mitra et al. 1996; Mukhopadhyay et al. 1998; Sharma et al. 1997a, b) (Fig. 1). Molecular evolutionary studies have also recorded temporal variations in prevalence of O139 and O1 serogroups over the years in India along with the emergence of new clones within the O139 serogroup. Subsequent studies depicted that the O1 serogroup which replaced the O139 serogroup was a new clone of O1 El Tor biotype (Faruque et al. 1997b; Yamasaki et al. 1997; Sharma et al. 1997a, b). A quiescent period followed in the history of *V. cholerae* O139, and it was thought that the appearance of O139 was a one-time event. But a resurgence of serogroup O139 occurred in 1996 in Kolkata (Mitra et al. 1996). Between December 1999 and December 2000, escalating events of O139 were recorded in several outbreaks occurring throughout India, including Kolkata (Sinha et al. 2002). After this period, *V. cholerae* O1 continued to be a dominant serogroup in Kolkata and the incidence of O139 gradually decreased over the years. The factor(s) contributing to the diminished isolation of O139 vibrios and the re-emergence of O1 EI Tor vibrios are not understood. The vibrios might have undergone changes that would have affected their ability to survive and compete in the environment. One study from Kolkata reported the appearance of new genotype of *ctxB* in 1996 with the re-emerged *V. cholerae* O139 strains that had CTX Calcutta phage and was designated as genotype 4 and in 1998, another new genotype designated as genotype 5 was detected that prevailed mostly in CTX phages with El Tor *rstR* (Raychoudhuri et al. 2010). During the course of appearance and disappearance over a decade, five types of O139 strains have been detected based on CT genotypes (Raychoudhuri et al. 2010). Frequent mutations thus acquired by *V. cholerae* O139 strains since its genesis may have an impact in their declining prevalence in cholera-endemic areas like Kolkata (Fig. 1).

8 Cholera Outbreaks in the Twenty-first Century

Among the 39 African countries that reported cases of cholera in any year from 2000 through 2005, 18 (46 %) countries reported cases in all 6 years: Benin, Burundi, Cameroon, Democratic Republic of the Congo, Ghana, Guinea, Liberia, Malawi, Mozambique, Niger, Nigeria, South Africa, Swaziland, Togo, Uganda,

United Republic of Tanzania, Zambia, and Zimbabwe. Countries with such high endemicity are found in East, Southern, Central, and West Africa (Gaffga et al. 2007). A total of 67,738 cases and 3,666 deaths (CFR 5.4 %) were reported between 2000 and 2005 in eastern provinces of DR Congo (Bompangue et al. 2008). During the period between 2000 and 2005, four countries in Africa had a cholera density greater than 200 cases per 1,000,000 people: Mozambique (793/million), Liberia (594/million), Somalia (441/million), and the Democratic Republic of the Congo (242/million) (Gaffga et al. 2007). In 2005, 31 (78 %) of the 40 countries that reported indigenous cases of cholera to WHO were in sub-Saharan Africa (Gaffga et al. 2007). The reported incidence of indigenous cholera in sub-Saharan Africa in 2005 (166 cases/million population) was 95 times higher than the reported incidence in Asia (1.74 cases/million population) and 16,600 times higher than the reported incidence in Latin America (0.01 cases/million population).

In 2004–2005, as part of a significant series of cholera outbreaks in West Africa, an epidemic took place in Senegal, resulting in 31,719 cases, i.e., 293 cases/100,000 habitants, with 458 deaths (case fatality rate (CFR) of 1.44 %) (de Magny et al. 2012; WHO 2008a). This epidemic was the largest recorded by the World Health Organization (WHO) for Africa during that time (WHO 2006). A large outbreak occurred in Cameroon during 2004, when 8,000 cases were reported in Littoral and West regions. The outbreak which started in Bepanda, an area located in the northwest of Douala, spread rapidly to other areas (New Bell and Nylon), and soon reached the entire town of Douala (WHO 2012). In 2005, Cameroon reported 2,847 cases including 110 deaths (CFR 3.86 %) with 70 % of the cases from the Littoral region (WHO 2012). In 2006, Cameroon reported 922 cases including 35 deaths (CFR 3.8 %). A first outbreak occurred from April to June in Bafoussam (Ouest province) and a second one occurred in the Far North region in November (WHO 2012). Over 25,000 cases of cholera have been reported in Sierra Leone and Guinea including 392 deaths since February 2012, when the epidemic was reported. It is the country's worst outbreak of cholera in 15 years.

A retrospective study on cholera outbreaks in Mali reported 12,176 recorded cholera cases, including 1,406 deaths, between 1995 and 2004 (Dao et al. 2009). South Africa experienced a cholera epidemic between the years 1997 and 2005 and the worst cholera epidemics in the country's recent history reached its peak in 2001 (Keddy et al. 2007). Initial reports of the cholera outbreak came from the largely rural and impoverished communities on the outskirts of the Ngwelezane Township, near the Empangeni town. The source of the epidemic was traced to the Mhlathuze River, also in the northern part of the KwaZulu-Natal Province. However by the end of the year 2000, the northern KwaZulu-Natal cholera outbreak had replicated itself in eight of South Africa's nine provinces and cases were identified in the Eastern Cape, Mpumalanga, Limpopo, and Gauteng. Over 100,000 cases were notified based on clinical diagnosis between 2000 and 2002 (Department of Health; http://www.doh.gov.za/facts/stat-notes-f.html). Initially, the causative organism was identified as *V. cholerae* O1, Ogawa. But in mid-2001,

O1, Inaba emerged in KwaZulu and subsequently, further isolates of *V. cholerae* O1 Inaba were identified from other provinces. It is noteworthy that during the 2001/2002 epidemic the death rate was less than 1 % (Keddy et al. 2007).

In August 2008, a new cholera epidemic was reported in Zimbabwe, which affected all 10 provinces and 56 of the 62 districts. This is the largest ever recorded outbreak of cholera in Zimbabwe. Over 7 months, more than 90,000 suspected cholera cases were reported, with more than 4,000 of these patients died. Nelson opined that these values were likely underestimates, because during the crisis reporting clinics were largely on strike, communication was severed by stolen telephone lines, and deaths in the bush devalue as fast as the currency (Nelson 2009). This epidemic brought rates of mortality similar to those witnessed as a consequence of cholera infections a hundred years ago and the Zimbabwean Government declared the outbreak a national emergency.

Nigeria is in one of the three major current cholera foci in the world (Piarroux and Faucher 2012). In 2009, outbreaks began in Nigeria and other countries at the Lake Chad basin (Quilici et al. 2010) with the first reports coming from Maiduguri, a city in the far northeast of the country. Subsequently, outbreaks were reported from distant locales in Northern and Western Nigeria, and in 2010 a severe outbreak, which started in the Northern Nigeria spreading through the country, was projected as the worst outbreak in Nigeria since 1991. This outbreak was marked with highest case fatality (Adagbada et al. 2012), what could be in part due to changes in *V. cholerae* infectivity even though the organism remains largely unknown. It can be hypothesized that an index strain has been disseminated cross-country by human travel. Marin et al. (2013) performed a comprehensive characterization of representative *V. cholerae* strains from sequential outbreaks in Nigeria and reported that recent cholera outbreaks in Nigeria are driven by atypical El Tor strains. The occurrence of cholera outbreaks in the African continent is dealt with in greater detail in another chapter in this book.

During the 2002 cholera outbreak in Chandigarh, India, *V. cholerae* O1 Ogawa was isolated from 18 % of the hand-pump water samples (Kaistha et al. 2005). Remote areas such as Andaman and Nicobar Islands were free from cholera for many years. The first cholera outbreak was recorded during early 2000 due to the spread of *V. cholerae* O1 from the main land (Shah et al. 2002). In 2002, cholera was identified due to El Tor vibrios among Nicobarese tribe in 16 villages with an attack rate of 12.8 % and a case fatality ratio of 1.3 % (Sugunan et al. 2004). Concomitant infections by *V. cholerae* O1 and O139 serogroups were reported in 2000 from a large cholera outbreak in Ahmedabad, India (Chakraborty et al. 2001).

During 2004–2005, cholera caused by the Inaba serotype was recorded in 15 states of India, mostly associated in the form of outbreaks (Dutta et al. 2006). In Delhi, the serotype switchover from Ogawa to Inaba has started in 2004 and 88 % of the strains were identified as Inaba during 2005 (Sharma et al. 2007). Among children below 5 years of age, the incidence of cholera in Delhi was 33 %. Cholera caused by the Inaba serotype was also reported from other parts of India such as

Kolkata, Orissa, Andaman and Nicobar Islands (Dutta et al. 2006; Raychoudhuri et al. 2007; Pal et al. 2006; Sugunan et al. 2007).

These Inaba strains had unique PFGE (pulsotype H1) and ribotype (RIV) profiles that were not recorded before. After its first appearance in July 2004, the Inaba serotype completely replaced the dominant Ogawa serotype from May 2005 in Kolkata (Raychoudhuri et al. 2007). These Kolkata Inaba strains belonged to a new ribotype as well as PFGE clone, identical to the Delhi strains and had a CTX prophage with two RS elements. Similar results were obtained with Inaba strains isolated in Trivandrum, southern India, except for ribotyping, which showed that the Inaba and Ogawa strains were similar (Mohapatra et al. 2007).

Based on the spatial patterns and exploratory spatial data analysis, the risk factors for cholera were associated with environmental niches (Ali et al. 2001). Environmental studies conducted during 2004 in Mathbaria and Matlab, Bangladesh, revealed that both *V. cholerae* O1 and O139 serogroups occurred predominantly as viable but non-culturable state (Alam et al. 2006). However, culturable cells were also detected in the biofilms, which were considered as additional reservoirs of toxigenic *V. cholerae* in the aquatic environments during interepidemic seasons. Isolation of *V. cholerae* O1 from the aquatic environments of Bangladesh through selective enrichment using antibiotics has re-emphasized the hypothesis that the humans act as reservoirs of this pathogen during interepidemic periods and spreading occurs through contaminated water (Faruque et al. 2006).

The cholera toxin producing *V. cholerae* non-O1 strains were isolated from seafood in Taiwan (Wong et al. 1992). Turtles and their breeding environment are the major reservoirs of *V. cholerae* and responsible for many outbreaks of cholera in Sichuan Province and Guangzhou area, China during 2003–2005 (Liu et al. 2006; Zhang et al. 2007). In an investigation it was shown that turtles and other seafood harbored toxigenic *V. cholerae* O139 (Chang et al. 2007). In Zhejiang Province, the incidence of O1 serogroup of *V. cholerae* was found to be high (9 %) in turtles and cholera epidemics in this region might be associated with consumption of contaminated turtles (Lü et al. 2006).

Resurgence of *V. cholerae* O139 in the beginning of twenty-first century was reported in many Asian countries including Pakistan (2000–2001), India (1997, 2001), and Bangladesh (2002), mostly affecting the older age groups (Jabeen and Hasan 2003; Sundaram et al. 2002; Agarwal et al. 2003; Faruque et al. 2003b; Sinha et al. 2002). *Vibrio cholerae* O1 and O139 consecutively appeared during cholera outbreaks (2002–2003) near Karachi (Siddiqui et al. 2006). This study has also revealed that children less than 2 years of age were the most affected age group with O1 (49 %) than O139 (21 %).

Following the Iraq war, the communicable disease control program was disturbed, resulting in cholera epidemics in several districts of Basrah, Iraq, in 2003 (Valenciano et al. 2003). Cholera outbreak struck Kabul, Afghanistan, in 2005 and spread nationwide. The health authorities gave importance to the disease control program that included proper management and treatment supported by partner agencies that kept the mortality rate well below 0.1 % (Kakar et al. 2008). A limited cholera outbreak occurred in Iran in the summer of 2005 and out of 1,150 patients, 11 people died (Ataei et al. 2005; Azizi and Azizi 2010). In 2007 there was an epidemic of cholera in Iraq with 4,667 cases and bacteriological testing confirmed that the outbreak was caused *by V. cholerae* O1, biotype El Tor, serotype Inaba (Khwaif et al. 2010). Another study reported the isolation of Ogawa serotype from this outbreak (Saleh et al. 2011).

8.1 Haitian Outbreak

Haiti has recently battled the world's largest cholera epidemic in half a century. On, January 12, 2010, a powerful earthquake devastated the capital city of Haiti along with southern towns as the epicenter was 16 miles west of the capital city of Port-au-Prince. Ten months after the devastating earthquake, the first case of cholera was reported from the town of Mirebalais, about 62 miles north of Port-au-Prince, Haiti for the first time in nearly a century. The first hospitalized cases of cholera occurred in Mirebalais on October 17, 2010 (Ivers and Walton 2012). This deadly outbreak has killed around 8,000 Haitians, and infected over 600,000 to date. By the first 10 weeks of the epidemic, cholera spread to all of Haiti's 10 departments or provinces.

Suspected cases of cholera have since been reported in Bolivia, Brazil, Chile, Colombia, Nicaragua, Panama, Peru, and Venezuela. Confirmed imported cases have been reported in Florida. Compared with Haiti's experience, the epidemic has been less severe in Dominican Republic. Transmission was limited, but sustained and continued at low levels. One large outbreak affected guests at a wedding in January 2011, including some visitors from Venezuela and the United States. From October 21, 2010, through July 30, 2011, a total of 14,598 suspected cases of cholera were reported; 256 persons died (of these, cases in 92 patients *V. cholerae* O1 was laboratory confirmed) (Tappero and Tauxe 2011). In late June 2012, Cuba confirmed three deaths and 53 cases of cholera in Manzanillo, in 2013 with 51 cases in Havana. The case fatality rate (CFR) was initially high in some locales (4.6 %), but within three months of the start of the epidemic CFR declined to the WHO target of <1.0 %. The CDC notes that 23 cases occurred in the U.S.; 22 were associated with travel to Haiti, one with consumption of food products from that country.

To understand the evolutionary origin of *V. cholerae* isolated in Haiti, several research groups in different parts of the world studied the Haitian cholera outbreak independently. The Harvard Cholera Group compared the entire genome sequences of the Haitian strain with two strains from Bangladesh and one isolated in South America including sequences from 23 different strains of *V. cholerae* available online in the public domain (Chin et al. 2011). A nearly identical relationship was observed between the Haitian isolates and the variant seventh pandemic El Tor O1 strains that are predominant in South Asia. No relationship was observed between the South American isolates (indicating that this strain is not related to the early-1990s cholera epidemic in South America) or with the African strains isolated between 1970 and 1998. The study of Mutreja et al. (2011) indicated that the Haitian strains were all identical and most closely related to strains of *V. cholerae* from the Indian subcontinent and distinct from strains of *V. cholerae* isolated in Africa, Bahrain, Germany, Indonesia, Vietnam, Malaysia, and South America. Another study considering the genetic diversity of a total of 187 individual isolates of *V. cholerae* O1 picked from the 16 stool samples from St. Marc hospital at Haiti showed minimal diversity, consistent with a single point source for the 2010 Haiti epidemic (Ali et al. 2011). Separate study on population genetics of *V cholerae* strains from Nepal in 2010 suggested strong epidemiological link with the Haitian outbreak (Hendriksen et al. 2011). Another comparative genomics of *V. cholerae* strains from Haiti, Asia and Africa using phylogenies for whole genome sequences and core genome single-nucleotide polymorphisms showed that the Haiti outbreak strain is genetically related to strains originating in India and Cameroon (Reimer et al. 2011). However, this study concluded that a definitive genetic origin for the outbreak in Haiti remains speculative due to the lack of identical genetic match among sequenced contemporary isolates (Reimer et al. 2011).

Interestingly, the nucleotide sequence of the *ctxB* (the gene for the B subunit of cholera toxin) of the Haitian strains was found to have a unique mutation at the 58th nucleotide position indicating three coding mutations of *ctxB* gene as opposed to only two seen in typical classical strains of *V. cholerae* O1 or in the El Tor variants (Nair et al. 2006). Retrospective analysis of *V. cholerae* strains from Kolkata, India showed that the Haitian type *ctxB* first appeared in Kolkata during April, 2006 and 93.3 % strains during 2011 carried the new allele (Naha et al. 2012). This genetic polymorphism of the *ctxB* gene was also observed in strains of *V. cholerae* O1 isolated from Orissa, India, and from the West African countries of Nigeria and Cameroon (Choi et al. 2010; Kumar et al. 2009; Quilici et al. 2010). However, the core genome of the Haitian strains resembled more closely the one found in the South Asian strains and to a lesser extent the one found in the African strains, which once again points to a South Asian origin of the Haitian strains. Whole genome sequence analysis of *V. cholerae* strain isolated from the Haitian cholera outbreak revealed a novel single-nucleotide polymorphism (SNP) at nucleotide position 266 (amino acid 89) of the *tcpA* gene uniquely associated with this variant (Chin et al. 2011; Grim et al. 2010; Talkington et al. 2011). A newly developed PCR study showed that Haitian *tcpA* first appeared in Kolkata during October, 2003, and interestingly soon after its appearance; this new variant *tcpA* displaced the canonical El Tor *tcpA* completely in the following years (Ghosh et al. 2014). The bioinformatical analysis showed that among the three different mutations present in 89th position at different alleles of TcpA, only Asparagine to Serine which is present in the Haitian *tcpA* allele is positively selected. Moreover, this particular mutation is the result of a purine–purine transition, which is evolutionarily preferred. It should be noted, however, that acquisition of Haitian *ctxB* and *tcpA* do not always occur in tandem and Haitian variant strain may be result of the sequential event in the evolution of Indian subcontinent strain (Ghosh et al. 2014). Furthermore, Haitian strains showed (i) change in satellite phage RS1 (*rstB*); (ii) mutation in *rtxA* (Repeat in toxin) involved in cytotoxin activity; (iii) mutation in *gyrase A*, and (iv) change in the number of repeat regions at the protomer region of CT. Among these, two variations seem to be unique for the Haitian strains (P. Ghosh and AK Mukhopadhyay, Unpublished).

8.2 Evolution of the El Tor Variants and Its Impact

Classical and El Tor strains of *V. cholerae* are closely related but are not directly derived from each other (Karaolis et al. 2001) and are believed to have evolved from separate lineages (Kaper et al. 1982, 1995). Although the classical and El Tor biotypes have different lineages, hybrids between the classical and El Tor biotypes resulting from genetic exchange between different bacterial lineages also exist in nature (Chakraborty et al. 2000; Mukhopadhyay et al. 2001). Since the beginning of the seventh pandemic, El Tor strains have gradually displaced the classical strains as the cause of cholera and both the biotypes had coexisted for at least over a decade following the emergence of the El Tor biotype in 1961. In Bangladesh, the classical biotype apparently disappeared in 1973, but re-emerged in 1982 (Samadi et al. 1983a, b; Siddique et al. 1991) and co-circulated with the El Tor biotype for at least a decade (the last isolation was reported in 1992) (Siddique et al. 1991). Curiously, the transient reappearance of O1 classical strains was observed only in Bangladesh. Classical strains are now believed to be extinct; hence, the source of the *rstR*^{Cla} and *ctxB1* alleles and their mode of transfer to El Tor strains in Bangladesh remains a mystery. The existence of classical strains in aquatic environments of Bangladesh was reported during the early 1990s, thereby supporting the notion that they were not completely replaced in that country (Siddique et al. 1991; Faruque et al. 1993).

Study from Matlab, Bangladesh first reported the existence of naturally occurring atypical El Tor variants among clinical strains of *V. cholerae* O1 isolated between 1991 and 1994 (Nair et al. 2002). Certain strains could not be biotyped as either classical or El Tor, and were designated as Matlab (MT) variants (Nair et al. 2002). Mozambique, a cholera-endemic country in East Africa, reported a large and extended cholera outbreak in 2004. The involved *V. cholerae* strains displayed phenotypic characteristics of the El Tor biotype. Moreover, the results of *rstR* and *ctxB* genotyping were consistent with the classical biotype (Ansaruzzaman et al. 2004; Das et al. 2007). The Mozambique variants contained, in the small chromosome, two tandem copies of the prophage whose sequence was almost identical to that of the typical CTXΦ^{Cla} (Lee et al. 2006; Faruque et al. 2007; Das et al. 2007). Notably, this was the first report of atypical El Tor strains harboring CTXΦ^{Cla} in Africa. This is against the background that the classical strains of *V. cholerae* O1 never entered into the African continent during the seventh pandemic of cholera.

Retrospective analysis from Kolkata led to the detection of variant *V. cholerae* O1 strains isolated in 1992 from clinical cases with identical traits to 2004

Mozambique variant O1 strains (Chatterjee et al. 2009). It was proposed that some of the 1992 Kolkata O1 strains might have acted as progenitors for Mozambique variant O1 strains. Similar strains carrying tandem copies of $CTX\Phi^{Cla}$ in the small chromosome have also been isolated in samples taken between 1995 and 2004 in Vietnam (Nguyen et al. 2009). Unlike the Mozambique variants, some of these strains have an additional $CTX\Phi^{Cla}$ in the large chromosome (Nguyen et al. 2009).

Studies attempting to examine the chronology of appearance of variants of El Tor strains in Kolkata indicated that classical type *ctxB* emerged in 1990, although El Tor type *ctxB* was still present in almost equal numbers during that year. During 1991, a unique event took place when the classical type became predominant, along with strains having both classical and El Tor type *ctxB*. In 1994, isolation of strains with El Tor *ctxB* became rare, and the major *ctxB* allele was of the classical type. *V. cholerae* O1 strains from 1995 onward were found to carry classical type *ctxB*, which totally replaced the El Tor type *ctxB* allele (Raychoudhuri et al. 2009). These types of El Tor variant strains producing classical toxin were isolated in Bangladesh after 2001 (Nair et al. 2006). Later on, these El Tor variant strains were isolated from different outbreaks throughout Asia and Africa including Zanzibar Island (Safa et al. 2008; Naha et al. 2013). Comparative analysis among different group of strains showed that *V. cholerae* O1 El Tor variant strains produced much more cholera toxin than did prototype El Tor strains. The amount of cholera toxin produced by El Tor variant strains both in vitro and in vivo was more or less equivalent to that produced by classical strains (Ghosh-Banerjee et al. 2010; Naha et al. 2013). Fig. 1 shows the chronology of appearance of variants of El Tor strains over two decades in Kolkata.

Vibrio cholerae strains of the recent devastating cholera outbreak in Haiti contained a unique mutation at the 58th nucleotide of *ctxB* gene. Analysis of the Kolkata strains showed that the Haitian *ctxB* first appeared in Kolkata during April, 2006 and 93.3 % strains isolated in Kolkata during 2011 carried the new allele (Naha et al. 2012). Haitian *V. cholerae* strains also contained a novel mutation at the 64th amino acid position of the matured TcpA subunit. Analysis of the Kolkata strains showed that Haitian variant *tcpA* first appeared in Kolkata during 2003 and after that all the El Tor *tcpA* was replaced by this new allele of *tcpA* (Ghosh et al. 2014). These findings indicated that Haitian *ctxB* and *tcpA* alleles might have originated in Kolkata and then spread to the neighboring regions. It must be emphasized, however, that the Haitian strains have certain minor traits not found in collections from other parts of the world, which is consistent with the microevolution that takes place continuously within the El Tor biotype as it moves from continent to continent and even country to country.

Using comparative genomic studies of different variants of *V. cholerae* strains isolated in recent time, Grim et al. (2010) concluded that the unique combination of characteristics of the genome of newly variant *V. cholerae* provides the bacterium with a competitive ecological edge and greater infectivity over that of other pathogenic clones of *V. cholerae*. Historically, El Tor strains of *V. cholerae* are considered to have an improved environmental fitness based on the observation that they have displaced classical strains. In turn, classical strains of *V. cholerae* are believed to produce a more severe form of the disease, cholera (Kaper et al. 1995; Faruque et al. 1998). However, it is unknown how the classical CT affects the pathogenicity of atypical El Tor strains. Given the fact that CT is directly responsible for the major clinical signs of the disease, genetic changes in the CT genes could alter the clinical manifestation of cholera (Safa et al. 2010). Comparative genomic studies also provided evidence of an amalgamation of environmental fitness of El Tor strains and greater infectivity of classical strains, i.e., a "mixing and matching," through recombination and lateral gene transfer, resulting in the genesis of new variants of *V. cholerae* with expanded ecological persistence, infectivity, and dispersion. The success of a clone is a combination of its ability to adapt to changing environmental conditions as a stable inhabitant, evidenced by conservation of the El Tor genomic backbone, and its ability to transmit progeny through human populations (Grim et al. 2010). WHO reported that *V. cholerae* El Tor variant caused more severe episodes of cholera with higher case fatality rates (WHO 2008b). From a study in Bakerganj, Bangladesh, it was reported that higher proportion of severe dehydration was observed in 2006 after the appearance of El Tor variant strains (Siddique et al. 2010). These new *V. cholerae* O1 El Tor variant strains not only replaced the *V. cholerae* O1 El Tor prototype strains, but also turned out to be genetically stable and spread rapidly even to remote islands in the east African continent. Moreover, the severity of the disease appears to be intensifying, and recent cholera outbreaks in various places, including Zimbabwe and Haiti, have followed a protracted pattern (Kanungo et al. 2010; Piarroux et al. 2011). An active comprehensive surveillance system should be in place in order to track the dissemination of the *V. cholerae* O1 El Tor variant strains in the population using latest molecular diagnostic assays, as these strains possess the potential and foundation for a new pandemic.

8.3 Lessons from the Haitian Epidemic

Cholera's unexpected emergence in the Americas and the Caribbean islands after 100 years of absence are tragic reminders about the speed at which infectious diseases can be transmitted globally even to other nonendemic countries. The bacteria becomes more hostile when it reaches an immunologically naïve population as happened in Haiti. Although we are passing through the twenty-first century, cholera still remains an epidemic or endemic disease in much of the developing world. New epidemic strains are likely to develop, evolve, and spread. *V cholerae* cannot be eradicated as it is a part of the normal flora and ecology of the surface water of our planet (Sack et al. 2004). Cholera always teaches us the hard lessons that no one should lack access to basic clean water and sanitation (Guerrant 2006). The Haitian epidemic shows that as long as cholera exists anywhere in the world, many who drink untreated water and live in areas of poor sanitation are at risk. The epidemic also shows how cholera can emerge where it is least expected. An understanding of the ecology of the organism should help to limit the times that human beings come into contact with this super-pathogen. Therefore, the ability to detect and confirm cholera needs to be broadly available. Recently developed molecular tools should be used for tracking the emergence and dissemination of the new variants of *V. cholerae* isolates. Implementing a coordinated, integrated, multidisciplinary approach is the only effective way to prevent and contain outbreaks among vulnerable populations living in high-risk areas. Prevention, preparedness, and response depend upon an effective and holistic surveillance system and are linked and interdependent. Although the real worldwide burden of cholera is still unknown, and will not be known until the notification of suspected and confirmed cases becomes mandatory. Denial of cholera incidence is so rampant that in this modern age of information most authorities guess that WHO figures include less than 10 % of cholera cases—probably as low as 1 % (Christopher 2009).

References

Adagbada AO, Adesida SA, Nwaokorie FO, Niemogha MT, Coker AO (2012) Cholera epidemiology in Nigeria: an overview. Pan Afr Med J 12:59

Agrawal G, Jalgaonkar SV, Jagtap PM, Kamlakar UP, Deogade NG (2003) Emergence and re-emergence of *Vibrio cholerae* O139: an epidemiological study during 1993–2002 at Nagpur, Central India. Indian J Med Sci 57:155–157

Al-Abbassi AM, Ahmed S, Al-Hadithi T (2005) Cholera epidemic in Baghdad during 1999: clinical and bacteriological profile of hospitalized cases. East Mediterr Health J 11:6–13

Alam M, Sultana M, Nair GB et al (2006) Toxigenic *Vibrio cholerae* in the aquatic environment of Mathbaria, Bangladesh. Appl Environ Microbiol 72:2849–2855

Albert MJ, Siddique AK, Islam MS et al (1993) Large outbreak of clinical cholera due to *Vibrio cholerae* non-O1 in Bangladesh. Lancet 341:704

Ali M, Emch M, Yunus M, Sack RB (2001) Are the environmental niches of *Vibrio cholerae* O139 different from those of *Vibrio cholerae* O1 El Tor? Int J Infect Dis 5:214–249

Ali A, Chen Y, Johnson JA et al (2011) Recent clonal origin of cholera in Haiti. Emerg Infect Dis 17:699–701

Alm RA, Manning PA (1990) Biotype-specific probe for *Vibrio cholerae* serogroup O1. J Clin Microbiol 28:823–824

Ansaruzzaman M, Bhuiyan NA, Nair GB et al (2004) Mozambique Cholera Vaccine Demonstration Project Coordination Group. cholera in Mozambique, variant of *Vibrio cholerae*. Emerg Infect Dis 10:2057–2059

Ataei RA, Tavana A, Ghorbani GH (2005) An analysis of recent cholera epidemic in Iran. J Mil Med 7:49–56

Azizi MH, Azizi F (2010) History of cholera outbreaks in Iran during the 19th and 20th centuries Middle East. J Dig Dis 2:51–55

Baine, WB, Zampieri A, Mazzotti M et al (1974) Epidemiology of cholera in Italy in 1973. Lancet ii:1370–1375

Barrett TJ, Blake PA (1981) Epidemiological usefulness of changes in hemolytic activity of *Vibrio cholerae* biotype El Tor during the seventh pandemic. J Clin Microbiol 13:126–129

Barua D (1972) The global epidemiology of cholera in recent years. Proc R Soc Med 65:423–428

Barua D (1992) History of cholera. In: Barua D, Greenough WB III (eds) Cholera. Plenum Press, New York, pp 1–35

Barua D, Burrows W (1974) Cholera. WB Saunders, Philadelphia

Basu A, Mukhopadhyay AK, Sharma C et al (1998) Heterogeneity in the organization of the CTX genetic element in strains of *Vibrio cholerae* O139 Bengal isolated from Calcutta, India and Dhaka, Bangladesh and its possible link to the dissimilar incidence of O139 cholera in the two locales. Microbiol Pathog 24:175–183

Bhattacharya SK, Bhattacharya MK, Nair GB et al (1993) Clinical profile of acute diarrhoea cases infected with the new epidemic strain of *Vibrio cholerae* O139: designation of the disease as cholera. J Infect 27:11–15

Bhattacharya S, Black R, Bourgeois L et al (2009) The cholera crisis in Africa. Science 32:885

Bockemühl J, Schröter G (1975) The El Tor cholera epidemic in Togo (West Africa) 1970–1972. Tropenmed Parasitol 26:312–322

Boiro MY, Lama N, Barry M, Diallo R, Morillon M (1999) Cholera in Guinea: the 1994–1995 epidemic. Med Trop (Mars) 59:303–306

Bompangue D, Giraudoux P, Handschumacher P et al (2008) Lakes as source of cholera outbreaks, Democratic Republic of Congo. Emerg Infect Dis 14:798–800

Bompangue D, Giraudoux P, Piarroux M et al (2009) Cholera epidemics, war and disasters around Goma and Lake Kivu: an eight-year survey. PLoS Negl Trop Dis 3:e436

Cameron DN, Khambaty FM, Wachsmuth K, Tauxe R, Barret TJ (1994) Molecular characterization of *Vibrio cholerae* O1 strains by pulsed-field gel electrophoresis. J Clin Microbiol 32:1685–1690

Centers for Disease Control and Prevention (CDC) (1993) Imported cholera associated with a newly described toxigenic *Vibrio cholerae* O139 strain—California, 1993. Morb Mortal Wkly Rep 42:501–503

Chakraborty S, Mukhopadhyay AK, Bhadra RK et al (2000) Virulence genes in environmental strains of *Vibrio cholerae*. Appl Environ Microbiol 66:4022–4028

Chakraborty S, Deokule JS, Garg P et al (2001) Concomitant infection of enterotoxigenic *Escherichia coli* in an outbreak of cholera caused by *Vibrio cholerae* O1 and O139 in Ahmadabad, India. J Clin Microbiol 39:3241–3246

Chang ZR, Zhang J, Wang DC et al (2007) Identification and molecular study on *Vibrio cholerae* in sea products. Zhonghua Yu Fang Yi Xue Za Zhi 41:304–306 (In Chinese)

Chatterjee S, Patra T, Ghosh K et al (2009) *Vibrio cholerae* O1 clinical strains of 1992 at Kolkata with progenitor traits of 2004 Mozambique variant. J Med Microbiol 58:239–247

Chin C, Sorenson J, Harris JB et al (2011) The origin of the Haitian cholera outbreak strain. N Engl J Med 364:33–42

Choi SY, Lee JH, Jeon YS et al (2010) Multilocus variable-number tandem repeat analysis of *Vibrio cholerae* O1 El Tor strains harbouring classical toxin B. J Med Microbiol 59:763–769

Christopher H (2009) Cholera forcing: the myth of the good epidemic and the coming of good water. Am J Public Health 99:1946–1954

Cohen J, Schwartz T, Klasmer R, Pridan D, Ghalayini H, Davies AM (1971) Epidemiological aspects of cholera El Tor outbreak in a non-endemic area. Lancet **ii:** 86–89

Colombo MM, Francisco M, Ferreira BD, Rubino S, Cappuccinelli P (1993) The early stage of the recurrent cholera epidemic in Luanda. Angola Eur J Epidemiol 9:563–565

Coppo A, Colombo M, Pazzani C et al (1995) *Vibrio cholerae* in the horn of Africa: epidemiology, plasmids, tetracycline resistance gene amplification, and comparison between O1 and non-O1 strains. Am J Trop Med Hyg 53:351–359

Dalsgaard A, Nielsen GL, Echeverria P et al (1995) *Vibrio cholerae* O139 in Denmark. Lancet 345:1637–1638

Dao S, Konaté I, Oumar AA et al (2009) Cholera epidemics in Mali between 1995 and 2004. Sante Publique 21:263–269

Darbari BS, Tiwari HL, Agarwal S (1982) Pattern of cholera in Raipur: a twelve year appraisal. J Indian Assoc Commun Dis 5:83–87

Das B, Halder K, Pal P, Bhadra RK (2007) Small chromosomal integration site of classical CTX prophage in Mozambique *Vibrio cholerae* O1 biotype El Tor strain. Arch Microbiol 188:677–683

Datta KK, Singh J (1990) Epidemiological profile of outbreaks of cholera in India during 1975–1989. J Commun Dis 22:151–159

Davis MB, Moyer KE, Boyd EF, Waldor MK (2000) CTX prophages in classical biotype *Vibrio cholerae*: functional phage genes but dysfunctional phage genomes. J Bacteriol 182:992–998

de Magny GC, Thiaw W, Kumar V (2012) Cholera outbreak in Senegal in 2005: was climate a factor? PLoS One 7:e44577

Dhamodaran S, Ananthan S, Kuganantham P (1995) A retrospective analysis of the Madras epidemic of non-O1 *Vibrio cholerae* new serogroup O139 Bengal. Indian J Med Res 101:94–97

Dutta B, Ghosh R, Sharma NC et al (2006) Spread of cholera with newer clones of *Vibrio cholerae* O1 El Tor, serotype Inaba, in India. J Clin Microbiol 44:3391–3393

Dziejman M, Balon E, Boyd D, Fraser CM, Heidelberg JF, Mekalanos JJ (2002) Comparative genomic analysis of *Vibrio cholerae* genes that correlate with cholera endemic and pandemic disease. Proc Natl Acad Sci USA 99:1556–1561

Faruque, SM., Saha MN, Asadulghani PK (2000) Genomic diversity among *Vibrio cholerae* O139 strains isolated in Bangladesh and India between 1992 and 1998. 184:279–284

Faruque SM, Alim ARMA, Rahman MM, Siddique AK, Sack RB, Albert MJ (1993) Clonal relationships among classical *Vibrio cholerae* O1 strains isolated between 1961 and 1992 in Bangladesh. J Clin Microbiol 31:2513–2516

Faruque AS, Fuchs GJ, Albert MJ (1996) Changing epidemiology of cholera due to *Vibrio cholerae* O1 and O139 Bengal in Dhaka, Bangladesh. Epidemiol Infect 116:258–275

Faruque SM, Ahmed KM, Siddique AK et al (1997a) Molecular analysis of toxigenic *Vibrio cholerae* O139 Bengal strains isolated in Bangladesh between 1993 and 1996: evidence for emergence of a new clone of the Bengal vibrios. J Clin Microbiol 35:2299–2306

Faruque SM, Ahmed KM, Alim ARMA et al (1997b) Emergence of a new clone of toxigenic *Vibrio cholerae* O1 biotype El Tor displacing *V. cholerae* O139 Bengal in Bangladesh. J Clin Microbiol 35:624–630

Faruque SM, Albert MJ, Mekalanos JJ (1998) Epidemiology, genetics, and ecology of toxigenic *Vibrio cholerae*. Microbiol Mol Biol Rev 62:1301–1314

Faruque SM, Siddique AK, Saha MN et al (1999) Molecular characterization of a new ribotype of *Vibrio cholerae* O139 Bengal associated with an outbreak of cholera in Bangladesh. J Clin Microbiol 37:1313–1318

Faruque SM, Chowdhury N, Kamruzzaman M et al (2003a) Reemergence of epidemic *Vibrio cholerae* O139, Bangladesh. Emerg Infect Dis 9:1116–1122

Faruque SM, Sack DA, Sack RB et al (2003b) Emergence and evolution of *Vibrio cholerae* O139. Proc Natl Acad Sci USA 100:1304–1309

Faruque SM, Islam MJ, Ahmad QS et al (2006) An improved technique for isolation of environmental *Vibrio cholerae* with epidemic potential: monitoring the emergence of a multiple-antibiotic-resistant epidemic strain in Bangladesh. J Infect Dis 193:1029–1036

Faruque SM, Tam VC, Chowdhury N et al (2007) Genomic analysis of the Mozambique strain of *Vibrio cholerae* O1 reveals the origin of El Tor strains carrying classical CTX prophage. Proc Natl Acad Sci U S A 104:5151–5156

Finkelstein RA (1996) Cholera, *Vibrio cholerae* O1 and O139, and Other pathogenic vibrios. Med Microbiol (4th edn), Edited by Baron S. Galveston (TX) USA, Chap. 24, 104:14–27

Finkelstein RA, Burks F, Zupan A, Dallas WS, Jacob CO, Ludwig DS (1987) Epitopes of the cholera family of enterotoxins. Rev Infect Dis 9:544–561

Freitas FS, Momen H, Salles CA (2002) The zymovars of *Vibrio cholerae*: multilocus enzyme electrophoresis of *Vibrio cholerae*. Memórias do Instituto Oswaldo Cruz 97(4):511–516

Gaffga NH, Tauxe RV, Mintz ED (2007) Cholera: a new homeland in Africa? Am J Trop Med Hyg 77:705–713

Garza DR, Thompson CC, Loureiro ECB et al (2012) Genome-wide study of the defective sucrose fermenter strain of *Vibrio cholerae* from the Latin American cholera epidemic. PLoS One 7(5):e37283

Ghosh-Banerjee J, Senoh M, Takahashi T et al (2010) Cholera toxin production by El Tor variant of *Vibrio cholerae* O1 as compared to prototype El Tor and classical biotypes. J Clin Microbiol 48:4283–4286

Ghosh P, Naha A, Basak S et al (2014) Haitian Variant *tcpA* in *Vibrio cholerae* O1 El Tor strains of Kolkata, India. J Clin Microbiol [Epub ahead of print] PMID:24371245

Goma Epidemiology Group (1995) Public health impact of Rwandan refugee crisis: what happened in Goma, Zaire, in July, 1994. Lancet 345: 339–344

Goodgame RW, Greenough WB III (1975) Cholera in Africa: a message for the West. Ann Intern Med 82:101–106

Grim CJ, Hasan NA, Taviani E et al (2010) Genome sequence of hybrid *Vibrio cholerae* O1 MJ-1236, B33, and CIRS101 and comparative genomics with *V. cholerae*. J Bacteriol 192:3524–3533

Guechi Z, Mered B (1978–1979) Some aspects of the evolution of cholera in Algeria from 1971 to 1975. Arch Inst Pasteur Alger 53:241–246

Guerrant RL (2006) Cholera: still teaching hard lessons. N Engl J Med 354:2500–2502

Guthmann JP (1995) Epidemic cholera in Latin America: spread and routes of transmission. J Trop Med Hyg 98:419–427

Hendriksen, RS, Price LB, Schupp JM et al (2011) Population Genetics of *Vibrio cholerae* from Nepal in 2010: Evidence on the Origin of the Haitian Outbreak. m Bio 2:doi: 10.1128/mBio.00157-11

Huq MI, Sanyal SC, Samadi AR, Monsur KA (1983) Comparative behaviour of classical and El Tor biotypes of *Vibrio cholerae* O1 isolated in Bangladesh during 1982. J Diarrhoeal Dis Res 1:5–9

Isaäcson M, Clarke KR, Ellacombe GH et al (1974) The recent cholera outbreak in the South African gold mining industry: a preliminary report. S Aft Med J 48:2557–2560

Ivers LC, Walton DA (2012) The "first" case of cholera in Haiti: lessons for global health. Am J Trop Med Hyg 86:36–38

Jabeen K, Hasan R (2003) Re-emergence of *Vibrio cholerae* O139 in Pakistan: report from a tertiary care hospital. J Pak Med Assoc 53:335–338

John TJ (1996) Emerging and re-emerging bacterial pathogens in India. Indian J Med Res 103:4–18

Kaistha N, Mehta M, Gautam V, Gupta V (2005) Outbreak of cholera in and around Chandigarh during two successive years (2002, 2003). Indian J Med Res 122:404–407

Kakar F, Ahmadzai AH, Habib N, Taqdeer A, Hartman AF (2008) A successful response to an outbreak of cholera in Afghanistan. Trop Doct 38:17–20

Kamal AM (1974) The seventh pandemic of cholera. In: Barua D, Burrows W (eds) Cholera. W. B. Saunders, Philadelphia, pp 1–14

Kanungo S, Sah BK, Lopez AL et al (2010) Cholera in India: an analysis of reports, 1997–2006. Bull World Health Organ 88:185–191

Kaper JB, Bradford HB, Roberts NC et al (1982) Molecular epidemiology of *Vibrio cholerae* in the US Gulf Coast. Clin Microbiol 16:129–134

Kaper JB, Morris JGJR, Levine MM (1995) Cholera. Clin Microbiol Rev 8:48–86

Karaolis DKR, Lan R, Kaper JB (2001) Comparison of *Vibrio cholerae* pathogenicity islands in sixth and seventh pandemic strains. Infect Immun 69:1947–1952

Keasler SP, Hall RH (1993) Detecting and biotyping *Vibrio cholerae* O1 with multiplex polymerase chain reaction. Lancet 341:1661

Keddy KH, Nadan S, Govind C et al (2007) Evidence for a clonally different origin of the two cholera epidemics of 2001–2002 and 1980–1987 in South Africa. J Med Microbiol 56:1644–1650

Khan MU, Samadi AR, Huq MI, Yunus M, Eusof A (1984) Simultaneous classical and El Tor cholera in Bangladesh. J Diarrhoeal Dis Res 2:13–18

Khwaif JM, Hayyawi AH, Yousif TI (2010) Cholera outbreak in Baghdad in 2007: an epidemiological study. East Mediterr Health J 16:584–589

Kumar P, Jain M, Goel AK et al (2009) A large cholera outbreak due to a new cholera toxin variant of the *Vibrio cholerae* O1 El Tor biotype in Orissa, Eastern India. J Med Microbiol 58:234–238

Kurazono T, Yamada F, Yamaguchi M et al (1994) The first report of traveler's diarrhea associated with a newly described toxigenic *Vibrio cholerae* O139 strain in Japan. Kansenshogaku Zasshi 68:8–12

Küstner HGV, Du Plessis G (1991) The cholera epidemic in South Africa, 1980–1987. Epidemiological features. S Afr Med J 7:539–544

Küstner HG, Gibson IH, Carmichael TR et al (1981) The spread of cholera in South Africa. S Afr Med J 60:87–90

Lam C, Octavia S, Reeves P, Wang L, Lan R (2010) Evolution of seventh cholera pandemic and origin of 1991 epidemic, Latin America. Emerg Infect Dis 16:1130–1132

Lee JH, Han KH, Choi SY et al (2006) Mozambique Cholera Vaccine Demonstration Project Coordination Group. Multilocus sequence typing (MLST) analysis of *Vibrio cholerae* O1 El Tor isolates from Mozambique that harbour the classical CTX prophage. J Med Microbiol 55(Pt 2):165–170

Lin W, Fulner KJ, Clayton R et al (1999) Identification of a *Vibrio cholerae* RTX toxin gene cluster that is tightly linked to the cholera toxin prophage. Proc Natl Acad Sci USA 96:1071–1076

Liu HL, Zhang JY, Feng ZH et al (2006) Application of pulsed-field gel electrophoresis typing in tracing and carrying out surveillance programs on O139 cholera outbreaks. Zhonghua Liu Xing Bing Xue Za Zhi 27:102–106 (In Chinese)

Longini IM Jr, Yunus M, Zaman K, Siddique AK, Sack RB, Nizam A (2002) Epidemic and endemic cholera trends over a 33-year period in Bangladesh. J Infect Dis 186:246–251

Lü HK, Chen EF, Xie SY et al (2006) Investigation on *Vibrio cholerae* carried in aquatic products of littoral areas, Zhejiang Province. Zhonghua Yu Fang Yi Xue Za Zhi 40:336–338 (In Chinese)

Mackowiak PA, Huq I (1974) Rapid method of determining cholera Vibrio biotype. Appl Microbiol 28:586–588

Mahalanabis D, Faruque AS, Albert MJ et al (1994) An epidemic of cholera due to *Vibrio cholerae* O139 in Dhaka, Bangladesh: clinical and epidemiological features. Epidemiol Infect 112:463–471

Mahon BE, Mintz ED, Greene KD et al (1996) Reported cholera in the United States, 1992–1994: a reflection of global changes in cholera epidemiology. JAMA 276:307–312

Marin MA, Thompson CC, Freitas FS, Fonseca EL, Aboderin AO et al (2013) Cholera outbreaks in Nigeria are associated with multidrug resistant atypical El Tor and non-O1/non-O139 *Vibrio cholerae*. PLoS Negl Trop Dis 7(2):e2049

Mitra R, Basu A, Dutta D et al (1996) Resurgence of *Vibrio cholerae* O139 Bengal with altered antibiogram in Calcutta, India. Lancet 348:1181

Mohapatra SS, Ramachandran D, Mantri CK, Singh DV (2007) Characterization of the genetic background of *Vibrio cholerae* O1 biotype El Tor serotype Inaba strains isolated in Trivandrum, southern India. J Med Microbiol 56:260–265

Moren A, Stefanaggi S, Antona D et al (1991) Practical field epidemiology to investigate a cholera outbreak in a Mozambican refugee camp in Malawi, 1988. J Trop Med Hyg 94:1–7

Mugoya I, Kariuki S, Galgalo T et al (2008) Rapid spread of *Vibrio cholerae* O1 throughout Kenya, 2005. Am J Trop Med Hyg 78:527–533

Mukerjee S (1963) Bacteriophage typing of cholera. Bull WHO 28:337–345

Mukhopadhyay AK, Garg S, Mitra R et al (1996) Temporal shifts in traits of *Vibrio cholera* strains isolated from hospitalized patients in Calcutta: a 3-year (1993 to 1995) analysis. J Clin Microbiol 34:2537–2543

Mukhopadhyay AK, Basu A, Garg P et al (1998) Molecular epidemiology of reemergent *Vibrio cholerae* O139 Bengal in India. J Clin Microbiol 36:2149–2152

Mukhopadhyay AK, Chakraborty S, Shimada T et al (2001) Characterization of VPI pathogenicity island and CTX# prophage in environmental strains of *Vibrio cholerae*. J Bacteriol 183:4737–4746

Mutreja A, Kim D, Thomson N et al (2011) Evidence for several waves of global transmission in the seventh cholera pandemic. Nature 477:462–465

Naha A, Pazhani GP, Ganguly M et al (2012) Development and evaluation of a PCR assay for tracking the emergence and dissemination of Haitian variant *ctxB* in *Vibrio cholerae* O1 strains isolated from Kolkata, India. J Clin Microbiol 50:1733–1736

Naha A, Chowdhury G, Ghosh-Banerjee J et al (2013) Molecular characterization of high-level-cholera-toxin-producing El Tor variant *Vibrio cholerae* in the Zanzibar Archipelago of Tanzania. J Clin Microbiol 51:1040–1045

Nair GB, Ramamurthy T, Bhattacharya SK et al (1994) Spread of *Vibrio cholerae* O139 Bengal in India. J Infect Dis 169:1029–1034

Nair GB, Faruque SM, Bhuiyan NA, Kamruzzaman M, Siddique AK, Sack DA (2002) New variants of *Vibrio cholerae* O1 biotype El Tor with attributes of the classical biotype from hospitalized patients with acute diarrhea in Bangladesh. J Clin Microbiol 40:3296–3299

Nair GB, Qadri F, Holmgren J et al (2006) Cholera Due to Altered El Tor Strains of *Vibrio cholerae* O1 in Bangladesh. J Clin Microbiol 44:4211–4213

Nair GB, Mukhopadhyay AK, Safa A, Takeda Y (2008) Emerging hybrid variants of *Vibrio cholerae* O1. In: Faruque SM, Nair GB (eds) *Vibrio cholerae*: genomics and molecular biology. Horizon Scientific Press, Norwich, pp 179–190

Narkevich MI, Onischenko GG, Lomov JM, Moskvitina EA, Podosinnikova LS, Medinsky GM (1993) The seventh pandemic of cholera in the USSR, 1961-89. Bull World Health Organ 71:189–196

Nelson E (2009) Beyond cholera-the Zimbabwe health crisis. Lancet Infect Dis 10:587–588

Nguyen BM, Lee JH, Cuong NT et al (2009) Cholera outbreaks caused by an altered *Vibrio cholerae* O1 El Tor biotype strain producing classical cholera toxin B in Vietnam in 2007 to 2008. J Clin Microbiol 47:1568–1571

O'Shea WA, Finnan S, Reen FJ, Morrissey JP, O'Gara F, Boyd EF (2004) The Vibrio seventh pandemic island-II is a 26.9 kb genomic island present in *Vibrio cholerae* El Tor and O139 serogroup isolates that shows homology to a 43.4 kb genomic island in *V. vulnificus*. Microbiol 150:4053–4063

Olsvik O, Wahlberg J, Petterson B et al (1993) Use of automated sequencing of polymerase chain reaction-generated amplicons to identify three types of cholera toxin subunit B in *Vibrio cholerae* O1 strains. J Clin Microbiol 31:22–25

Onyemelukwe GC, Lawande RV (1991) Serotype variation in *Vibrio cholerae* El Tor diarrhoea in northern Nigeria. Cent Afr J Med 37:186–189

Pal BB, Khuntia HK, Samal SK, Das SS, Chhotray GP (2006) Emergence of *Vibrio cholerae* O1 biotype El Tor serotype Inaba causing outbreaks of cholera in Orissa, India. Jpn J Infect Dis 59:266–269

Pan American Health Organization (1991) Cholera situation in the Americas. Epidemiol Bull 12:1–4

Pavlov AV (1976) Principals of cholera control. Kiev, pp 149–151 (in Russian)

Piarroux R, Faucher B (2012) Cholera epidemics in 2010: respective roles of environment, strain changes, and human-driven dissemination. Clinical microbiology and infection: the official publication of the European Society of Clinical Microbiology and Infectious Diseases, vol 18. pp 231–238

Piarroux R, Barrais R, Faucher B et al (2011) Understanding the cholera epidemic, Haiti. Emerg Infect Dis 17:1161–1167

Pollitzer R (1959) Cholera. With a chapter on World incidence. WHO, Geneva

Quilici ML, Massenet D, Gake B, Bwalki B, Olson DM (2010) *Vibrio cholerae* O1 variant with reduced susceptibility to ciprofloxacin, Western Africa. Emerg Infect Dis 16:1804–1805

Rader AE, Murphy JR (1988) Nucleotide sequences and comparison of the hemolysin determinants of *Vibrio cholerae* El Tor RV79(Hly+) and RV79(Hly-) and classical 569B(Hly-). Infect Immun 56:1414–1419

Ramamurthy T, Garg S, Sharma R et al (1993) Emergence of a novel strain of *Vibrio cholerae* with epidemic potential in southern and eastern India. Lancet 341:703–704

Ramos F, Lins-Lainson ZC, Silva EL et al (1997) Cholera in North Brazil: on the occurence of strains of *Vibrio cholerae* O1 which fail to ferment sucrose during routine plating on thiosulphate - Citrate - Bile Salt - Sucrose Agar (TCBS). A New Problem in Diagnosis and Control? Latin Am Microbiol 39:141–144

Raychoudhuri A, Chatterjee S, Pazhani GP et al (2007) Molecular characterization of recent *Vibrio cholerae* O1, El Tor, Inaba strains isolated from hospitalized patients in Kolkata. India J Infect 55:431–438

Raychoudhuri A, Mukhopadhyay AK, Ramamurthy, Nandy RK, Takeda Y, Nair GB (2008) Biotyping of *Vibrio cholerae* O1: time to redefine the scheme. Ind J Med Res 128:695–698

Raychoudhuri A, Patra T, Ghosh K et al (2009) Classical *ctxB* in *Vibrio cholerae* O1, Kolkata, India. Emerg Infect Dis 15:131–132

Raychoudhuri A, Mukherjee P, Ramamurthy T et al (2010) Genetic analysis of CTX prophages with special reference to *ctxB* and *rstR* alleles of *Vibrio cholerae* O139 strains isolated from Kolkata over a decade. FEMS Microbiol Lett 303:107–115

Reeves PR, Lan R (1998) Cholera in the 1990s. Br Med Bull 54:611–623

Reimer AR, Van Domselaar G, Stroika S et al (2011) Comparative genomics of *Vibrio cholerae* from Haiti, Asia, and Africa. Emerg Infect Dis 17:2113–2121

Sack RB, Siddique AK, Longini IM Jr et al (2003) A 4-year study of the epidemiology of *Vibrio cholerae* in four rural areas of Bangladesh. J Infect Dis 187:96–101

Sack DA, Sack RB, Nair GB, Siddique AK (2004) Cholera. Lancet 363:223–233

Safa A, Sultana J, Cam PD, Mwansa JC, Kong RYC (2008) *Vibrio cholerae* O1 hybrid El Tor strains, Asia and Africa. Emerg Infect Dis 14:987–988

Safa A, Nair GB, Kong RYC (2010) Evolution of new variants of *Vibrio cholerae* O1.Trends Microbiol 18: 46–54

Saleh TH, Sabbah MA, Jasem KA, Hammad ZN (2011) Identification of virulence factors in *Vibrio cholerae* isolated from Iraq during the 2007–2009 outbreak. Can J Microbiol 57:1024–1031

Samadi AR, Chowdhury MK, Huq MI, Khan MU (1983a) Seasonality of classical and El Tor cholera in Dhaka, Bangladesh: 17-year trends. Trans R Soc Trop Med Hyg 77:853–856

Samadi AR, Shahid N, Eusuf A (1983b) Classical *Vibrio cholerae* biotype displaces El Tor in Bangladesh. Lancet i:805–807

Seas C, Miranda J, Gil AI, Leon-Barua R, Patz J, Huq A (2000) New insights on the emergence of cholera in Latin America during 1991: the Peruvian experience. Am J Trop Med Hyg 62:513–517

Sergiev VM et al (1981) Zurnal mikrobiolii 3:3–8 (in Russian)

Shah WA, Shahina M, Ali N (2002) First report of *Vibrio cholerae* infection from Andaman and Nicobar, India. J Commun Dis 34:270–275

Sharma C, Maiti S, Mukhopadhyay AK et al (1997a) Unique organization of the CTX genetic element in *Vibrio cholerae* O139 strains which reemerged in Calcutta, India, in September 1996. J Clin Microbiol 35:3348–3350

Sharma C, Nair GB, Mukhopadhyay AK (1997b) Molecular characterization of *Vibrio cholerae* O1 biotype El Tor strains isolated between 1992 and 1995 in Calcutta, India: evidence for the emergence of a new clone of the El Tor biotype. J Infect Dis 175:1134–1141

Sharma NC, Mandal PK, Dhillon R, Jain M (2007) Changing profile of *Vibrio cholerae* O1, O139 in Delhi and its periphery (2003–2005). Indian J Med Res 125:633–640

Sheikh A, Khan A, Malik T, Fisher-Hoch SP (1997) Cholera in a developing megacity; Karachi, Pakistan. Epidemiol Infect 119:287–292

Shimada T, Nair GB, BC Deb et al (1993) Outbreak of *Vibrio cholerae* non-O1 in India and Bangladesh. Lancet 341:1347

Shimada T, Arakawa E, Itoh K et al (1994) Extended serotyping scheme for *Vibrio cholerae*. Curr Microbiol 28:175–178
Siddique AK, Baqui AH, Eusof A et al (1991) Survival of classic cholera in Bangladesh. Lancet 337:1125–1127
Siddique AK, Zaman K, Baqui AH et al (1992) Cholera epidemics in Bangladesh: 1985–1991. J Diarrhoeal Dis Res 10:79–86
Siddique AK, Salam A, Islam MS et al (1995) Why treatment centres failed to prevent cholera deaths among Rwandan refugees in Goma, Zaire. Lancet 345:359–361
Siddique AK, Nair GB, Alam M (2010) El Tor cholera with severe disease: a new threat to Asia and beyond. Epidemiol Infect 138:347–352
Siddiqui FJ, Bhutto NS, von Seidlein L et al (2006) Consecutive outbreaks of *Vibrio cholerae* O139 and *V. cholerae* O1 cholera in a fishing village near Karachi, Pakistan. Trans R Soc Trop Med Hyg 100:476–482
Simanjuntak CH, Larasati W, Arjoso S et al (2001) Cholera in Indonesia in 1993–1999. Am J Trop Med Hyg 65:788–797
Singh J, Bora D, Sachdeva V (1997) *Vibrio cholerae* O1 and O139 in less than five years old children hospitalised for watery diarrhoea in Delhi, 1993. J Diarrhoeal Dis Res 15:3–6
Sinha S, Chakraborty R, De K et al (2002) Escalating association of *Vibrio cholerae* O139 with cholera outbreaks in India. J Clin Microbiol 40:2635–2637
Sugunan AP, Ghosh AR, Roy S, Gupte MD, Sehgal SC (2004) A cholera epidemic among the Nicobarese tribe of Nancowry, Andaman, and Nicobar, India. Am J Trop Med Hyg 71:822–827
Sugunan AP, Roy S, Shahina M et al (2007) Emergence of *Vibrio cholerae* O1 Inaba in Andaman and Nicobar Islands, India. J Public Health 29:308–309
Sundaram SP, Revathi J, Sarkar BL et al (2002) Bacteriological profile of cholera in Tamil Nadu (1980–2001). Indian J Med Res 116:258–263
Swerdlow DL, Isaäcson M (1994) The epidemiology of cholera in Africa. In: *Vibrio cholerae* and cholera: molecular to global perspective. ASM Press, Washington, pp 297–307
Talkington D, Bopp C, Tarr C et al (2011) Characterization of toxigenic *Vibrio cholerae* from Haiti, 2010–2011. Emerg Infect Dis 17:2122–2129
Tanamal ST (1959) Notes on paracholera in Sulawesi (Celebes). Am J Trop Med Hyg 8:72–78
Tappero JW and Tauxe RV (2011) Lessons Learned during Public Health Response to Cholera Epidemic in Haiti and the Dominican Republic. 17:2087–2093
Tauxe RV, Blake PA (1992) Epidemic cholera in Latin America. JAMA 267:1388–1390
Tauxe RV, Seminario L, Tapia R, Libel M (1994) The Latin American epidemic. In: Wachsmuth I, Blake P, Olsvik O (eds) *Vibrio cholerae* and cholera: molecular to global perspectives. American Society for Microbiology Press, Washington, pp 321–344
Valenciano M, Coulombier D, Lopes Cardozo B (2003) Challenges for communicable disease surveillance and control in southern Iraq, April–June 2003. JAMA 290:654–658
Wachsmuth IK, Evins GE, Fields PI et al (1993) The molecular epidemiology of cholera in Latin America. J Infect Dis 167:621–626
Waldor MK, Rubin EJ, Pearson GDN, Kimsey H, Mekalanos JJ (1997) Regulation, replication, and integration functions of the *Vibrio cholerae* CTXΦ are encoded by region RS2. Mol Microbiol 24:917–926
Wong HC, Ting SH, Shieh WR (1992) Incidence of toxigenic vibrios in foods available in Taiwan. J Appl Bacteriol 73:197–202
World Health Organization (1991) Cholera in Africa. Wkly Epidemiol Rec 66:305–311
World Health Organization (1996) Cholera in 1995. Wkly Epidemiol Rec 71:157–164
World Health Organization (2006) Cholera, 2005. Wkly Epidemiol Rec 81: 297–308
World Health Organization (2008a) Cholera 2007. Wkly Epidemiol Rec 83:269–284
World Health Organization (2008b) Cholera country profile: Senegal, p 2
World Health Organization (2012) Cholera, 2011. Wkly Epidemiol Rec 87:289 –304
Yala F, Dodin A, Diana Y (1982) Role of inter-human infection during the cholera epidemic in the People's Republic of the Congo (1978–1979). Bull Soc Pathol Exot Filiales 75:345–351

Yamai S, Okitsu T, Shimada T, Katsube Y (1997) Distribution of serogroups of *Vibrio cholerae* non-O1 non-O139 with specific reference to their ability to produce cholera toxin, and addition of novel serogroups. Kansenshogaku Zasshi 71:1037–1045

Yamasaki S, Nair GB, Bhattachary SK et al (1997) Cryptic appearance of a new clone of *Vibrio cholerae* O1 biotype El Tor in Calcutta. India. Microbiol Immunol 41:1–6

Yoon SS, Mekalanos JJ (2006) 2, 3-Butanediol synthesis and the emergence of the *Vibrio cholerae* El Tor biotype. Infect Immun 74:6547–6556

Zhang J, Chang ZR, Zhong HJ et al (2007) Investigation on status of pollution of *Vibrio cholerae* in seafood and aquatic products in 12 provinces of China in 2005. Zhonghua Yu Fang Yi Xue Za Zhi. 41:208–211 (In Chinese)

Cholera Outbreaks in India

Thandavarayan Ramamurthy and Naresh C. Sharma

Abstract Cholera is a global health problem as several thousands of cases and deaths occur each year. The unique epidemiologic attribute of the disease is its propensity to occur as outbreaks that may flare-up into epidemics, if not controlled. The causative bacterial pathogen *Vibrio cholerae* prevails in the environment and infects humans whenever there is a breakdown in the public health component. The Indian subcontinent is vulnerable to this disease due its vast coastlines with areas of poor sanitation, unsafe drinking water, and overcrowding. Recently, it was shown that climatic conditions also play a major role in the persistence and spread of cholera. Constant change in the biotypes and serotypes of *V. cholerae* are also important aspects that changes virulence and survival of the pathogen. Such continuous changes increase the infection ability of the pathogen affecting the susceptible population including the children. The short-term carrier status of *V. cholerae* has been studied well at community level and this facet significantly contributes to the recurrence of cholera. Several molecular tools recognized altering clonality of *V. cholerae* in relation with the advent of a serogroup or serotype. Rapid identification systems were formulated for the timely detection of the pathogen so as to identify and control the outbreak and institute proper treatment of the patients. The antimicrobials used in the past are no longer useful in the treatment of cholera as *V. cholerae* has acquired several mechanisms for multiple antimicrobial resistance. This upsurge in antimicrobial resistance directly influences the management of the disease. This chapter provides an overview of cholera prevalence in India, possible sources of infection, and molecular epidemiology along with antimicrobial resistance of *V. cholerae*.

T. Ramamurthy
National Institute of Cholera and Enteric Diseases, Kolkata, India
e-mail: tramu@vsnl.net

N. C. Sharma (✉)
Maharishi Valmiki Infectious Diseases Hospital, Kingsway Camp, Delhi 110009, India
e-mail: sharmanc1@rediffmail.com; mvidh.idsp@gmail.com

Current Topics in Microbiology and Immunology (2014) 379: 49–85
DOI: 10.1007/82_2014_368

Published Online: 16 May 2014

Contents

1 Introduction

Cholera is known to exist in the Indian subcontinent since centuries. There is some description of this disease in Indian ancient medical literature (Sushruta). Presence of this disease has been recorded on 64 occasions by the independent authorities between the years 1503 and 1817 and the reports were restricted in Goa at the beginning, after the immigration of Portuguese settlers in 1502 (Pollitzer 1959). Pilgrimages and movement of troops contributed to the spread of disease during ancient period. Proper recording of the disease started in 1786 with establishment of Hospital board in Madras (now, Chennai) and Calcutta (now, Kolkata) (Pollitzer 1959). Intensive research on cholera commenced during the British rule, mainly to control the disease rather than on the basics of the pathogen. From late 1950s, there have been many advances in every aspect of the disease and the causative pathogen *Vibrio cholerae*.

In this chapter, we will not elaborate much on the history of cholera and investigations carried out during pre-independence era as other authors have extensively reviewed the early historical aspects (De 1961; Barua 1992). This chapter covers the major investigations on cholera carried out on outbreaks and other related aspects.

2 Early Works on Cholera

The world has witnessed seven cholera pandemics that may have started from the Indian subcontinent since 1817. The involvement of type/subspecies remained unknown for the first five pandemics till the identification of the pathogen in the laboratory by Robert Koch in 1884 during the fifth pandemic (1881–1896). The large cholera epidemics in early 1880s had subsided in Egypt but were very active in India. Using this opportunity, Koch visited Kolkata and other parts of India to continue his research from late 1883 to May 1884 (Howard-Jones 1984). On January 7, 1884, Koch had successfully isolated the bacillus in pure culture. One month later, he described that the bacillus was not straight like other bacilli, but was a little bent, like a "comma". His finding became very important and gained clinical significance when he pointed out that the bacillus was always found in patients with cholera but never in those with diarrhea from other causes. Koch also described that the bacillus was relatively rare in early infection, but were extensively present in the characteristic "rice water stools" of acute cholera patients. Unfortunately, Koch was unable to reproduce the disease in animals and justified his findings that the human bacillus was not suitable in animal models (Sack 1992).

Many cholera vaccine trials were conducted in Kolkata and other cholera endemic areas. During fifth cholera pandemic in the nineteenth century, most of the Asian and European countries were affected. During this time, Waldemar Mordecai Wolff Haffkine, a Russian scientist focused his research on developing an injectable cholera vaccine. In 1892, he produced an attenuated form of the bacillus (*V. cholerae*). Risking his own life, on July 18, 1892, Haffkine performed the first human test on himself. In 1894, he vaccinated 116 of 200 people living in a cholera prone slum of Kolkata. All the vaccinated people were protected from cholera in the subsequent cholera season. In 1894–1895, he had vaccinated about 20,000 subjects in Assam tea gardens and in this investigation, mortality among nonvaccinated group ranged from 22 to 45 %, whereas the highest rate among the vaccinated individuals was only 2 % (Lutzkerand and Jochnowitz 1987). Due to infection from malaria, he could not continue his research. He returned back to India in 1896 and resumed cholera vaccine trial with 30,000 people in 7 months. His vaccine saved thousands of lives in Russia and India.

Bengal is known as the "homeland of cholera," as the disease affected many people from ancient times (Macpherson 1866; MacNamara 1876). The year 1817 was marked in the history of cholera, as there was a large epidemic in Kolkata (MacNamara 1876). Literature review published by Macpherson (1872) showed that cholera existed in other parts of India before 1817. Old literatures have shown that Kolkata was not free from cholera for a single year between 1841 and 1959 (De 1961). The number of cases of cholera notified annually in Kolkata varied from 1846 to 9529 (Swaroop and Pollitzer 1955). Early epidemiological investigation conducted in Kolkata revealed 111 cholera deaths, of which 66 (59 %) occurred in persons living close to water tanks (Simpson 1888). In one such observation, Koch (1884) isolated "comma bacillus" from Kolkata tank waters.

Further studies indicated that when the tanks and ponds near the cholera affected areas were closed down, the incidence rate declined (De 1961).

The sixth pandemic is believed to be caused by *V. cholerae* O1 classical biotype and has caused many outbreaks till 1961 (Barua 1992). In 1961, the seventh pandemic started from Sulawesi, Indonesia, and soon spread to the Indian sub-continent. Cholera reached Chennai in March 1964, and thereafter to Kolkata during April in the same year. Almost a year later it appeared in Delhi and by 1965 classical biotype was replaced by El Tor through out the country (Mukherjee 1964; Sharma 1975).

3 Incidence and Changing Patterns of *V. cholerae*

Research works carried out for more than five decades show that the incidence patterns of *V. cholerae* is constantly changing. In early 1980s, Dr. Fayrer systematically studied cholera epidemics in Calcutta Medical College, which showed that an average mortality was more than 200,000 per year. In 1885, he presented the data at the fourth International Conference on Cholera, a forerunner of the World Health Organization (Hawgood 2001). In many States, the classical biotype was replaced by El Tor vibrios around 1965. In cholera-free States, the El Tor biotype had spread and become endemic foci of the infection. Incidence of classical vibrios was reported during 1968–1970 in Assam, Kolkata, Orissa (now, Odisha), Tripura, and Maharashtra. This biotype was recorded in healthy carriers in Kolkata during 1967 (CRC 1970).

We searched Pubmed for information on cholera outbreaks from 2007 to 2013 and recorded 38 reports published in India. It was found that the number of cases reported to Central Bureau of Health Intelligence (CBHI), Government of India was much low. We also did analysis on CBHI and Intergrated Disease Surveillance Program (IDSP), Government of India public database domains (http://www.cbhidghs.nic.in and http://www.idsp.nic.in, respectively). Cholera control is now a part of IDSP in India. To understand the true disease burden, IDSP was initiated including cholera as one of the priority diseases. IDSP has been implemented in 600 districts across the country and this has made district level facilities to detect *V. cholerae* and report outbreaks. From 2003 to 2012 number of cholera cases reported to CBHI has been increasing (Table 1). As shown in Table 2, prevalence of cholera has also been increasing in several Sates/Union Territories.

Meta analysis on annual incidence of cholera from 1997 to 2006 showed that the disease was constantly recorded in West Bengal followed by Maharashtra and Odisha. In addition, there were 68 outbreaks in 18 of 35 states and union territories affecting more than 220,000 cases (Kanungo et al. 2010). During 2004–2005, cholera caused by the serotype Inaba was recorded in 15 states of India, with 7 outbreaks. Based on the collection of *V. cholerae* O1/O139 strains for phage typing, Sarkar et al. (2012) reported that most of the strains were regularly received from Andhra Pradesh, Delhi, Goa, Gujarat, Karnataka, Madhya Pradesh,

Table 1 Cholera Cases and Deaths reported by States and Union Territories in India

Year	No. of cases	No. of deaths	CFR
2003	2893	2	0.07
2004	4695	7	0.15
2005	3155	6	0.19
2006	1939	3	0.15
2007	2635	3	0.11
2008	2680	1	0.04
2009	3482	12	0.34
2010	5786	52	0.89
2011	3679	23	0.62
2012	6093	51	0.83
Total	37037	160	0.43

Data from the Central Bureau of Health Intelligence
Source Central Bureau of Health Intelligence (CBHI), Government of India http://www.cbhidghs.nic.in along with corrected figure of Delhi

Table 2 Statewise distribution of cholera cases and deaths reported to IDSP, during 2010–2012*

	2010		2011		2012	
States	Cases	Deaths	Cases	Deaths	Cases	Deaths
Assam	114	1	841	7	531	9
Andhra Pradesh	0	0	0	0	23	0
Chhatisgarh	0	0	152	1	579	1
Gujarat	401	2	114	0	604	5
Haryana	15	0	5	0	188	0
Himachal Pradesh	40	1	0	0	0	0
J & K	2229	3	0	0	238	0
Karnatka	41	2	333	2	1232	3
Kerala	0	0	76	6	36	2
Madhya Pradesh	2	0	1	0	0	0
Maharashtra	208	0	164	1	426	1
Odisha	784	39	0	0	77	5
Punjab	171	0	384	0	758	20
Rajasthan	791	0	211	1	35	0
Tamilnadu	135	1	210	4	145	2
Uttra Khand	0	0	27	0	0	0
West Bengal	90	3	651	1	751	3
Chandigarh	0	0	5	0	11	0
Delhi	756	0	505	0	454	0
Puducherry	9	0	0	0	5	0
Total	5786	52	3679	23	6093	51
Outbreaks	33		59		93	

**Source* Integrated Disease Surveillance Program (IDSP) Government of India (http://www.idsp.nic.in) alongwith corrected figures of Delhi

Maharashtra, Punjab, Rajasthan, Tamil Nadu, and West Bengal. This information indirectly specifies the perennial nature of cholera in these States. Recurrence of cholera outbreaks was also reported in 11 States in multiple years (Verma et al. 2012).

3.1 Southern Region

During 1971–1984, *V. cholerae* O1 Ogawa (9.5 %) was detected from 4 outbreaks in Hyderabad (Rathna et al. 1988). In these outbreaks, both classical (31.3 %) and El Tor biotypes (68.7 %) were identified. A switch from classical to El Tor cholera was observed during 1975 and this trend continued for few more years (Rathna et al. 1988). Non-toxigenic (NT) *V. cholerae* O1 belonging to the El Tor Inaba was isolated during an outbreak in Warangal, Andhra Pradesh. This NT *V. cholerae* did not produce cholera toxin (CT) or hybridize with DNA probes specific for *ctx, zot*, or *ace* genes (Saha et al. 1996). This was the first report on NT *V. cholerae* O1 being associated with a cluster of cholera cases. In Tamil Nadu, *V. cholerae* was isolated from 1,008 of 3,496 stool samples (28.8 %) collected between 1992 and 1995 (Sundaram et al. 1998). During November to December 1992, 363 of the 370 isolates (98 %) were *V. cholerae* belonging to serogroups O139. This epidemic predominantly affected adults (91 %). Both *V. cholerae* O1 and O139 serogroups were sometimes isolated from the same locality. From January 1993 onwards, the rate of isolation of *V. cholerae* O139 declined, and in 1995, *V. cholerae* E1 Tor was isolated from most of the cases (85.6 %).

Between 1980 and 2001, 26,502 stool specimens from cholera suspected patients were processed for the presence of *V. cholerae* at the King Institute of Preventive Medicine, Chennai (Sundaram et al. 2002). Among these, 6,035 (22.8 %) yielded *V. cholerae.* Majority of the strains belong to serogroups O1 (67 %) followed by O139 (25.3 %) and non-O1, non-O139 serogroups (7.4 %). Twelve specimens were rough strains of *V. cholerae.* All the *V. cholerae* O1 isolates were of biotype El Tor and the predominant serotype was Ogawa (95.9 %). After the initial explosive epidemic caused by O139 serogroup in late 1992–1993, occurrence of O139 declined in this region and reemerged in 1997. However, during 1995–1996, O1 was the dominant serogroup (Sundaram et al. 2002).

From May to June 1996, a large El Tor cholera outbreak occurred in Alleppey and Palghat districts of Kerala (Radhakutty et al. 1997). Of the 575 patients hospitalized in Alleppey, 30 deaths occurred with a case fatality rate (CFR) of 5.2 % while in Palghat, of the 638 diarrhea patients, 30 (4.7 %) deaths were recorded. In Mysore, incidence of cholera among children was reported during 1997 (Hanumanthappa and Rajagopal 2000). Of the 565 samples of acute diarrheal stools from children collected from November 1996 to October 1997, 289 (51.1 %) cases were positive for *V. cholerae.* Out of these, 277 (95.8 %) were *V. cholerae* O1 Ogawa, 7 (2.4 %) were O139, and 5 (1.7 %) were non-O1 non-O139. Almost

8 years after its appearance in India, the O139 serogroup was recorded in 2000 in Manipal, Karnataka (Ballal et al. 2001). In Vellore, O1 Ogawa serotype was replaced by the Inaba serotype with altered antimicrobial susceptibility patterns (Jesudasson 2006). In 2000, spread of Inaba serotype was also reported in Kerala (Mohapatra et al. 2007).

3.2 Andaman and Nicobar Islands

The seventh pandemic cholera caused by the El Tor vibrios has reached Andaman and Nicobar Islands in October 2002, after 40 years of its first appearance in Indonesia during early 1960s. This outbreak affected the Nicobarese tribe in 16 of the 45 inhabited villages of Nancowry group of islands with an attack rate of 12.8 % with CFR of 1.3 % (Shah et al. 2002; Roy et al. 2005). The Nancowry and Kolkata isolates exhibited similar phenotypic and genetic features. In 2006, emergence of Inaba serotype was first reported in this island (Sugunan et al. 2007).

3.3 Western Region

The 1985 cholera outbreak in Bombay (now, Mumbai) affected mostly children (Mehta et al. 1986). Epidemic of cholera occurred in Solapur during July–September with peak incidence in August 1988 (Fule et al. 1990). The epidemiological data collected from 1986–1988 showed that cholera was widely prevalent in this region. *V. cholerae* O1 Ogawa (66.2 %) and Inaba (26.2 %) serotypes were responsible for an outbreak of cholera in Goa during July–September, 1988 (Verenkar et al. 1994). Studies conducted between 1989 and 1992 in Loni area, Ahmednagar, a district of Maharashtra showed incidence of cholera was very high from November to December and the Ogawa serotype was predominant (Jain and Basutkar 1994). In Nagpur, *V. cholerae* serogroup O1 predominated in 1991 (94.7 %) and 1992 (86.4 %) but significantly declined during the following year (10.7 %). The O139 serogroup that emerged in 1993 accounted for 89.3 % of the total vibrios isolated from diarrheal cases (Agarwal et al. 1994).

Concurrent occurrence of O1 and O139 vibrios was recorded in Yavatmal during 1993 and 1994 with variations in relative and absolute prevalence of each serotype (Ingole et al. 1997). In Aurangabad, *V. cholerae* O139 was isolated during 1998 and 2000 with intermittent appearance of O1 Inaba in 1999 (Bajaj et al. 2001). The arid zone of Bikaner in Rajasthan State was generally unaffected by cholera. The first outbreak was reported in this region during 1987 (Joshi et al. 1988; Soni et al. 1989). In 1999 outbreak, 64 *V. cholerae* O1 El Tor Ogawa strains were isolated from 475 stool samples (13.5 %) (Gupta et al. 1999a). Further outbreaks in this region were reported in 2002 (Gupta et al. 2002). Concomitant infectionConcomitant infection of enterotoxigenic *Escherichia coli* was identified in an outbreak of cholera caused by *V. cholerae* O1 and O139 in Ahmedabad, Gujarat (Chakraborty et al. 2001).

3.4 Eastern Region

Reappearance of classical *V. cholerae* was reported in Kolkata during early 1970s (Neogy and Chatterjee 1970). A large outbreak occurred during 1971 in Samudragar, Burdwan District in West Bengal, mostly among refugees from Bangladesh. Carrier status of El Tor vibrios, poor hygiene and disposal of dead bodies in river Mari Ganga and use of this river water for many purposes were the stated reasons for this outbreak (CRC 1972). Sporadic cases of acute diarrhea occurred in rural areas of northeast India throughout the year, with occasional outbreaks. In July–September 1978, an outbreak of gastroenteritis (4,469 reported cases) occurred in various villages in the central district of Manipur including Imphal with CFR of >20 % (Sircar et al. 1990). *V. cholerae* O1 was positive in 45.7 % of fecal and 47.6 % of river water samples. Outbreaks of acute diarrhea in 3 districts of Manipur state were investigated during 1985 (Singh et al. 1986; Gupta et al. 1990). In this outbreak, the overall attack rate (AR) and CFR were 0.2 % and 0.9 %, respectively. Hospital records revealed that 58.8 % of cases occurred among older children above 5 years of age.

Between May and July 1994, an unusual occurrence of severe dehydrating watery diarrhea cases and deaths were reported from Aizwal town, the capital of Mizoram (Sengupta et al. 2000). In this finding, *V. cholerae* El Tor was isolated from 50 % of hospitalized cases. In October 2002, an outbreak occurred in Assam with AR and CFR of 11.6 % and 0.8 %, respectively (Phukan et al. 2004). *V. cholerae* O1 Ogawa was isolated in 63 % of hospitalized patients. An outbreak of acute diarrhea occurred in Dhalai and North Tripura district, Tripura during May 2004. In this outbreak, the AR and CFR was 18.8 % and 6.9/1000, respectively (Gupta et al. 2004). *V. cholerae* O1, Ogawa was isolated in 40 % of hospitalized tribal patients and from water samples. Poor sanitation, use of contaminated surface water along with low literacy, lack of personal hygiene, frequent movements, and ineffective antibacterial treatment were the factors associated with persistence and spread of the pathogen.

The isolation rates of *V. cholerae* among patients admitted at the Infectious Diseases Hospital (IDH) in Kolkata with acute diarrhea during 1989–1990 were 78 and 85.1 %, respectively, with the domination of Inaba serotype in 1989 and Ogawa in 1990 (Ramamurthy et al. 1992a). *V. cholerae* O1 isolated from Kolkata at different times were analyzed to investigate the changes among the O1 strains isolated before, during and after the advent of the O139 serogroup (Mukhopadhyay et al. 1995). In this study, *V. cholerae* O1 isolated after the O139 epidemic in Kolkata were multidrug-resistant as compared to the O1 strains isolated before the advent of O139.

The O139 serogroup that dominated during 1993 in Kolkata was replaced by El Tor O1 in 1994–1995. The isolation rate of the O139 serogroup in 1994–1995 was below 9 % (Mukhopadhyay et al. 1996). In September 1997, an outbreak of diarrhea was reported from Malda with 56 % isolation rate of *V. cholerae* O1 Ogawa (Bhattacharya et al. 2000). Three of the five drinking water samples were

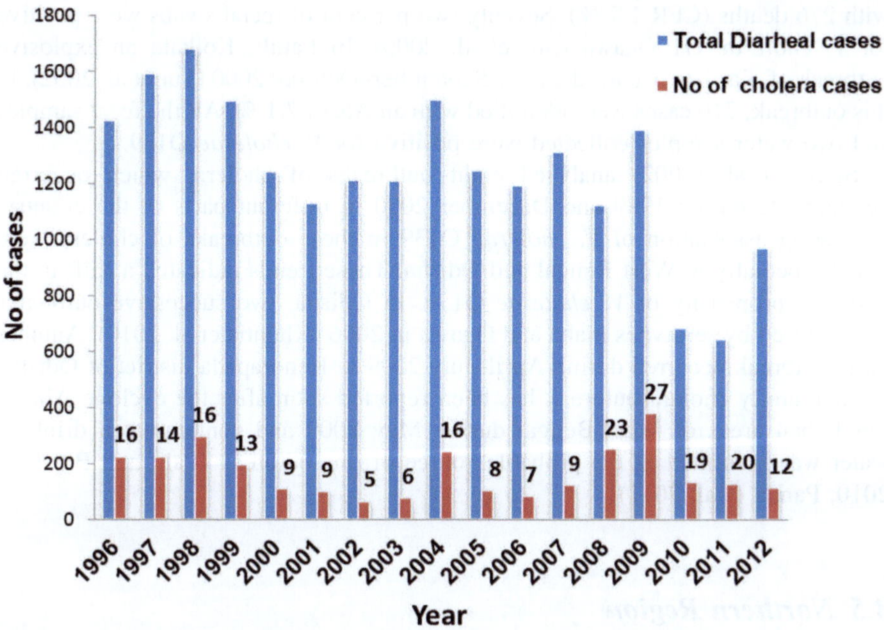

Fig. 1 Number of microbiologically confirmed cholera cases among acute gastroenteritis cases admitted in the Infectious Diseases Hospital, Kolkata from 1996 to 2012. Number above the bar indicates percentage of cholera cases

also positive for this serogroup. Outbreak of cholera was reported again in this region during July–August 1998, with an attack rate of 34/1,000 (Gupta et al. 1999b). *V. cholerae* O1 Ogawa was isolated from most of the cases (53 %). The prevalence of *V. cholerae* among the cholera patients admitted in the IDH, Kolkata showed no drastic change between the years 1996 and 2012 (Fig. 1).

An epidemiological study was carried out to find out the etiological agent for diarrheal disorders in the cyclone and flood affected areas of Odisha during October 1999 (Chhotray et al. 2002). Of the 107 rectal swabs analyzed, 72.3 % were positive for *V. cholerae* O1 Ogawa, 7.2 % for O139. Early bacteriological and epidemiological investigations have revealed the dominance of *V. cholerae* O1 among the hospitalized patients from cyclone-affected areas. Drinking water scarcity and poor sanitation are responsible for these outbreaks. *V. cholerae* O139 had not been reported earlier in south Odisha till 2000 (Samal et al. 2001). During May–June 2000, 194 patients with watery diarrhea were admitted to the IDH in Berhampur, Odisha. *V. cholerae* strains were isolated from 20 out of 94 samples, of these, 2 were found to be O1 Ogawa and 18 were confirmed as O139.

Floods resulting from overflowing of the two main rivers during July 1998 (Sur et al. 2000) induced an epidemic of cholera in the district of Malda, West Bengal. Within two weeks of its onset, cholera spread throughout the district. During the period between August and October 1998, 16,590 cases were reported with 276 deaths (CFR 1.7 %). Seventy two per cent of rectal swabs were positive for *V. cholerae* O1 Ogawa (Sur et al. 2000). In Patuli, Kolkata an explosive outbreak of diarrhea occurred during September–October 2000 (Sur et al. 2002). In this outbreak, 710 cases were identified with an AR of 7.1 %. All the fecal samples and two water samples collected were positive for *V. cholerae* O139.

Sinha et al. (2002) analyzed eight outbreaks of cholera, which occurred between December 1999 and December 2000 in different parts of the country. Escalating association of *V. cholerae* O139 in these outbreaks of cholera were noted especially in West Bengal and Odisha. These trends indicated a shift in the outbreak propensity of *V. cholerae* O139. In Odisha, two successive outbreaks were caused by serotypes Inaba and Ogawa in 2006 (Khuntia et al. 2010). Another large outbreak occurred during April–July 2009 in Kendrapada district of Odisha. A community cholera outbreak has been reported soon after the cyclone Alia in Sunderban areas of West Bengal during May 2009 and contaminated drinking water was identified as the probable source of this outbreak (Palit and Batabyal 2010; Panda et al. 2011).

3.5 Northern Region

An epidemic of classical cholera was detected in southeastern districts of Madhya Pradesh in 1970 (Sehgal et al. 1972). Following its first detection in 1965, a large outbreak of El Tor cholera occurred in Delhi during 1988 (Datta et al. 1993). Cholera cases reported from July to August 1988 was 5–10 times more than the previous years (Khanna et al. 1990). Civil lines and Shahadara zones were the most affected areas, recording 86 and 56 cases/100,000, respectively. The data on moving average showed the endemicity of cholera in Delhi with an increasing trend (Datta et al. 1993). The common risk factors identified with these outbreaks were lower socioeconomic status, poor personal hygiene, drinking water, and food storage practices.

From 1965 through 1993, no cases of cholera or carriers of *V. cholerae* were detected in Delhi (Singh et al. 1996a). Six hundred and fifty eight rectal swabs collected from possible contacts were negative for *V. cholerae*. This study suggested that transmission of cholera might also occur in winter months. In 1993, substitution of O1 for O139 serogroup was recorded in Delhi from the cholera cases admitted in the IDH (Singh et al. 1996b). Of the 1,528 laboratory confirmed cholera cases, 46 and 54 % were caused by serotype O1 and O139, respectively.

Between May 1992 and November 1994, changing trends in the isolation of *V. cholerae* O1 and O139 were recorded in Delhi (Rudra et al. 1997). In 1992, 50 of the 125 strains (40 %) were positive for *V. cholerae* O1 predominantly by Ogawa. In 1993, 44 (43.6 %) strains were positive for O139 and the rest belonged to the O1 serogroup. The IDH-based surveillance study conducted in Delhi during 1995 showed that out of 4,082 admitted cases with acute diarrhea, 2004 (49 %) and 4 (0.1 %) were positive for *V. cholerae* O1 and O139, respectively (Singh et al. 1998).

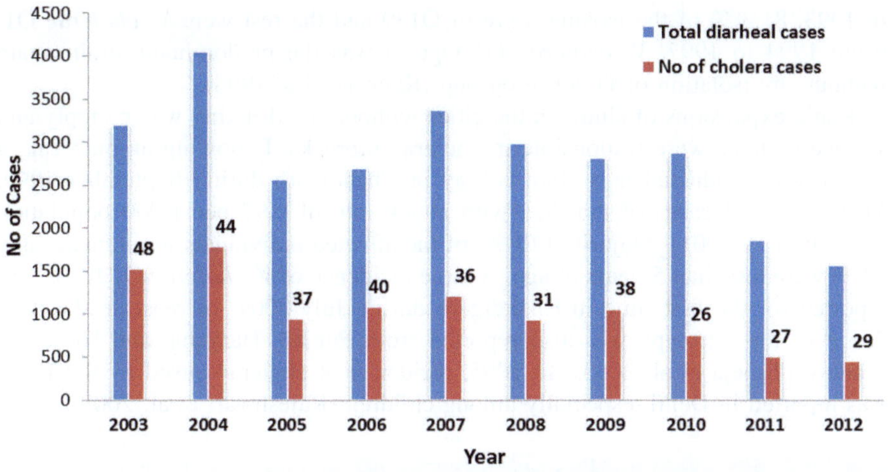

Fig. 2 Number of microbiologically confirmed cholera cases among acute gastroenteritis cases admitted in the Maharishi Valmiki Infectious Diseases Hospital, Delhi from 2003 to 2012. Number above the bar indicates percentage of cholera cases

Multiple cases were recorded in 4 % of the affected families. Among 29,196 stool samples/rectal swabs collected in Delhi during April 1992–December 2000, 11,091 were positive for *V. cholerae* O1 (80.7 %), 1,943 (14 %) for O139, and 696 (5 %) for non-O1 and non-O139 (Das and Gupta 2005). From Delhi and its surrounding areas, 3,213 stool specimens were screened between 1998 and 2002. From these stool specimens, 431 (13.4 %) were found positive for *V. cholerae*, of which, 423 were O1, 2 belonged to O139, and 6 to non-O1 non-O139 serogroups (Mohanty et al. 2004). During 2003–2012, cholera scenario at the IDH in Delhi shows the prevalence rate of cholera was 26–48 % (Fig. 2).

Outbreaks of cholera were recorded in Raipur in 1970, 1975, 1977, and from 1979 to 1981 (Darbari et al. 1982). Change in the prevalence of *V. cholerae* from classical Inaba in 1970 to El Tor Ogawa was recorded in 1974. Serotype shift from Ogawa to Inaba was recorded in 1977 but it again reverted to El Tor Ogawa, which caused larger outbreaks during 1979–1981. Bhopal district of Madhya Pradesh was considered as cholera-free area till 1988. In an outbreak of gastroenteritis in Berasia block of Bhopal district, *V. cholerae* O1 Inaba and Ogawa were isolated from 17.6 % of stool samples (Patnaik et al. 1989). Extreme insanitary conditions, large aggregation of people and probably consumption of contaminated ice candies were found to be responsible for this outbreak. During June–July 1994, an outbreak of *V. cholerae* O1 occurred in remote villages of Rohru Tehsil, in Shimla district, Himachal Pradesh (Bora et al. 1997). The AR during this outbreak was 16.4 % in 7 villages. Of the 10,427 diarrheal stool specimens collected from Punjab and other northern regions, the isolation rates of *V. cholerae* was 2, 2.6, 6.7, 7.1, 0.9, and 2.6 % in the respective years from 1992 to 1997 (Kaur and Lal 1998). Till 1992, *V. cholerae* O1 Ogawa was predominantly found in this study.

In 1993, 81.3 % of the isolates were of O139 and the rest were *V. cholerae* O1. From 1994 to 1997, *V. cholerae* O1 Ogawa was the predominant strain again without any isolation of O139 serogroup (Kaur and Lal 1998).

Rapid expansions of slums in the cities without any drinking water supply and sewage systems were responsible in cholera outbreaks. Following an outbreak, a survey was conducted in a slum colony in Chandigarh during September 1999. There were 14 cases of diarrhea with attack rate of 9.97 per 1,000 population (Thakur et al. 2001). Majority (70 %) of the affected individuals was females and 62 % were less than 5 years of age. A large incidence of *V. cholerae* O1 Inaba was reported for the first time in Chandigarh during July 2004. Increase in the incidence of this serotype was also reported from Punjab, Haryana, and Himachal Pradesh (Taneja et al. 2005). In 2005, incidence of cholera caused by the Inaba was reported in Delhi, especially among children (Rajeshwari et al. 2008).

4 Emergence of *V. cholerae* Serogroup O139

Till 1992, the toxigenic *V. cholerae* belonging to O1 was the only serogroup responsible for pandemic cholera. A novel serogroup of *V. cholerae,* which did not react with the then existing 138 somatic (O) antisera against *V. cholerae* was first isolated in October 1992 in Chennai (Ramamurthy et al. 1993a). This newly emerged strain of *V. cholerae* was identified as serogroup O139 and a synonym Bengal was added to mark its origin. The O139 strain spread rapidly through the Indian subcontinent and in many parts of Asia. In addition, cases of cholera among travelers in North America and the Middle East were also reported. Genetically, *V. cholerae* O139 is very closely related to the El Tor strains. The appearance of *V. cholerae* O139 may well herald the beginning of the eighth pandemic of cholera. Retrospective analysis of strains collected from the Communicable Diseases Hospital, Madras, from January to September 1992 showed the prevalence of O139 serogroups during pre-epidemic period (Dhamodaran et al. 1995). This information has shown that the emergence of this serogroup was around January 1992 from Chennai. During 1993, when the O139 incidence took place in Kolkata, the total admission of cholera patients at the IDH exceeded more than 44,500 (Bhattacharya et al. 1994).

In the subsequent years, spread of O139 infection in the form of outbreaks was reported in January 1993 in Kolkata (Bhattacharya et al. 1994), Odisha (Niyogi et al. 1994), Haryana (Sabherwal and Sikka 1994), Delhi (Sachdeva et al. 1995), Pondicherry (Vijayalakshmi et al. 1994), Ludhiana (Prabhakar et al. 1994), and Maharashtra (Narang et al. 1994; Jalgaonkar and Fule 1994). From November 1992 to July 1993, 95.6 % of 916 *V. cholerae* isolates submitted to the National Institute of Cholera and Enteric Diseases from 28 locations in India were confirmed as serogroup O139 (Nair et al. 1994a). Up to July 1993, *V. cholerae* O139 had been isolated from 13 Indian states and an union territory.

Clinically, the O139 serogroup seemed to be more virulent than the El Tor vibrios. The amount of CT present in stool samples of patients infected with the O139 serogroup was higher than that found in stools of patients infected with O1 El Tor indicating the potential severity of O139 infection (Nair et al. 1994b). The clinical features and blood and stool biochemical parameters of O139 infected patients were indistinguishable from those in typical cholera caused by the O1 serogroup; except for 44.3 % cases infected by O139 had abdominal cramps. In view of the above, Bhattacharya et al. (1993) designated the disease caused by *V. cholerae* O139 as cholera. Studies conducted in Ambajogai, Maharashtra also showed that the clinical features were more severe in patients infected with the serogroup O139 than O1 or the other non-O1, non-O139 serogroups (Kamble et al. 2000). Occasionally, the O139 infected cholera patients had significantly higher percentage of fever than the O1 infected cases (Singh et al. 1997).

With the passage of time, the O1 serogroup of the El Tor biotype again reappeared and displaced the O139 serogroup on the Indian subcontinent, and there was a feeling among cholera workers that the appearance of this new serogroup was an exceptional event. The resurgence of the O139 serogroup in 1996 and the coexistence of both the O1 and O139 serogroups in many cholera endemic areas in India and elsewhere suggested that the O139 serogroup had come to stay as a permanent entity in the future. During the re-emergence phase, Gomber et al. (1995) reported a large outbreak of cholera from North India caused by *V. cholerae* O139. Forty-one out of 391 patients with acute diarrhea during a 2-month-period (May–July 1993) were mainly (73 %) infected by *V. cholerae* O139.

From the surveillance results of Kolkata, it was shown that *V. cholerae* O139 dominated as the causative agent of cholera during 1992–1993 and 1996–1997, while the O1 strains dominated during the rest of the period (Basu et al. 2000a). Reappearance of *V. cholerae* serogroup O139 was also recorded in Yavatmal in 1998 (Ambhore et al. 2000), Nagpur (Agrawal et al. 2003), and Rohtak in 2001 (Gupta et al. 2005). From early 2000s, the O139 serogroup started disappearing from many parts of India.

5 Reemergence of El Tor *V. cholerae*

After its brief replacement in many parts of India by O139 serogroup during 1992, the O1 El Tor appeared in the subsequent years. A large El Tor cholera outbreak was recorded in Nagpur between June and October 2003 (Mishra et al. 2004). Reappearance of *V. cholerae* O1 and its concurrent prevalence with O139 were reported in Vellore (Jasudason et al. 1994). During June–July 1994, predominance of O1 than the O139 serogroup was recorded in Yavatmal (Fule et al. 1995).

6 Age Group Studies

In many previous findings, it was shown that cholera affects the adult population more often than the young children. The etiology of acute diarrhea investigated in 245 children less than 3 years of age showed that cholera was rare in pediatric cases in southern India (Mohandas et al. 1987). Outbreak investigations in Hyderabad showed that 67 % were less than 30 years of age with no significant difference in the incidence among females (51.4 %) and males (48.6 %) (Rathna et al. 1988). WHO has recommended that cholera should be suspected in children above the age of 2 years. To confirm this aspect, Bhattacharya et al. (1992) investigated children aged <2 years in endemic regions with diarrhea admitted in the IDH, Kolkata. In this study, of the 181 cases, 56 (31 %) were culture confirmed for cholera and the remaining had non-cholera diarrhea. This study conclusively proved that cholera can occur in children lesser than 2 years. Investigations carried out in North India during 1993 demonstrated that 1.5–12 year age groups was most affected with high incidence of O139 serogroup (73 %) than O1 (27 %) (Gomber et al. 1995). Cholera in neonates either with *V. cholerae* O139 or O1 serogroups has also been reported (Amin et al. 1995; Uppal et al. 1999; Sethi and Sethi 2001).

During a cholera outbreak in Bombay in 1985, it was found that children were the most affected age group (Mehta et al. 1986). A 5-year study (1982–1986) conducted in Delhi among diarrheal children less than 12 years showed that the overall isolation rate of *V. cholerae* O1 was 31.7 % (Aggarwal et al. 1989). Among cholera cases, 23.4 % occurred in the age group less than 2 years, 41.4 % in 2–5 years, and 35.1 % in more than 5–12 years. Infection occurred more often in males in all the age groups (Aggarwal et al. 1989). Studies conducted during an outbreak in Aizwal, Mizoram in 1994 showed that cholera affected mostly the grown-up children and adults (52.9 %) than younger children below 5 years of age (Sengupta et al. 2000).

In Delhi, cholera infection was more common (74 %) among children less than 15 years of age (Khanna et al. 1990). During the 1988 cholera outbreak, the highest incidence rate was observed in children in the age group of 1–4 years (Datta et al. 1993). Studies conducted among hospitalized cases in 1993 indicated that the *V. cholerae* O1 and O139 serogroups infected different age groups. Observations made by Amin et al. (1995) showed that out of 28 children <2 years, 11 (39.3 %) were culture positive for *V. cholerae* and the youngest child in this study was a 3 month old.

About 60 % of the *V. cholerae* O1 cases were children from Delhi with age less than 10 years and 40 % of them were infected with O139 (Singh et al. 1996b). Children excreting both *V. cholerae* O1 and O139 serogroups were rare (1.4 %) (Singh et al. 1997). The occurrence of cholera in children between 1 and 10 years age group was reported from Delhi (Singh et al. 1998) and Aurangabad (Slathia and Bansal 1999; Bajaj et al. 2001). Like children in the older age group, onset of acute diarrhea with watery/rice watery stools with or without excessive vomiting and/or rapid development of severe dehydration should be considered as typical symptoms of cholera in younger children.

7 Seasonal Patterns

In the endemic regions, cholera follows specific seasonal patterns with a major peak during summer and a minor peak in monsoon. Role of temperature during a particular season, rainfall, and humidity are considered as important factors. Using the cholera incidence data from 1907 to 1957, several analyses were made to find the correlation between the weather factors and incidence of cholera in Kolkata (Rogers 1926, 1957; Russell 1927; De 1961; CRC 1976, 1977). During this period, epidemics occurred during summer and monsoon seasons. The same trend was observed in Delhi with cholera cases occurred during May–September (summer and monsoon months) (Aggarwal et al. 1989). The period from January to March (winter) was generally completely free from cholera (Singh et al. 1998). Retrospective analysis on the seasonality of cholera was tracked over a 5-year period from January 1998 to December 2002 in Delhi (Mohanty et al. 2004). The number of cholera cases was high from May to June, followed by July–August. Except in 2002, the cholera cases were recorded during April in all the years. During 1977–1978, along with a major peak in May–June, a small peak during September–October was recorded in Kolkata. The observed change may be attributed to the local climate, sanitary conditions, food habits, and cholera control measures (CRC 1978).

In Hyderabad, the cholera outbreaks showed a protracted pattern with a peak during monsoon (May–August). The severity of the cholera was found to be related to the average rainfall during the year leading to the sewage stagnation in the downhill of Hyderabad (Rathna et al. 1988). Prevalence of cholera in West Bengal was correlated with several ecological factors. In a mathematical modeling, relative humidity and heavy rainfall were identified as major climatic conditions for *V. cholerae* infection (Rajendran et al. 2011). Monsoon season (June/July–October) seems favorable for cholera infection in Chandigarh and Odisha (Chander et al. 2009; Pal et al. 2010).

8 Incidence of Cholera-Related with Water and Food

Most of the cholera outbreaks are associated with poor water supply and/or secondary contamination of the stored water in the households. Some of the studies revealed sewage contamination of drinking water supply in many parts of India (Thakur et al. 2001). During an epidemic investigation, drinking water sources tested in Shimla were fit for human consumption (Bhardwaj et al. 1993). Rapid expansion of slum areas in the cities is one of the reasons for outbreaks. Water sample collected from a hand pump was positive for *V. cholerae* O1 Ogawa during an outbreak investigation conducted at Chandigarh in September 1999 (Taneja et al. 2003). In Patuli near Kolkata, a large outbreak of cholera was controlled after initiation of extensive chlorination of all the major water resources (Sur et al. 2002).

Studies conducted in Varanasi showed that an estimated 200 million liters or more of untreated human sewage is discharged daily into the river Ganges (Hamner et al. 2006). River water monitoring over 12 years has demonstrated fecal coliform counts up to 10^8 MPN (most probable number) per 100 ml and biological oxygen demand levels averaging over 40 mg/l. A questionnaire-based survey conducted among resident users of the river Ganges in Varanasi revealed that the overall rate of waterborne/enteric disease incidence, including cholera was about 66 % (Hamner et al. 2006). Logistic regression analysis revealed significant associations between water-borne/enteric disease occurrence and the use of the river for bathing, laundry, washing eating utensils, and brushing teeth. Thirty-three cases of cholera were identified among families exposed to washing clothes or bathing in the Ganges while no cholera cases occurred in unexposed families.

Foodborne cholera is rarely reported in India. In one case-control investigation, milk product was found to be associated with a small cholera outbreak in Odisha during 2005 (Das et al. 2009a). Repeated exposure of *V. cholerae* in vitro to chlorine induced resistance and formation of atypical and rough vibrios (Ganguly et al. 1966). Further studies revealed that these rough forms of *V. cholerae* are highly resistant to chlorine. The incidence of rough forms of *V. cholerae* from the patients and aquatic environments and their chlorine resistance are not studied in detail.

Based on the annual cholera incidence in Kolkata from 1998–2006 and the chlorophyll concentrations measured through satellite during corresponding years, demonstrated that it is possible to predict epidemic cholera in coastal areas (Constantin de Magny et al. 2008). This investigation confirms that the environmental factors are useful in forecasting epidemics of cholera and give health workers enough time to make plans, spread cautions, and recommendations to the public in a timely manner.

Outbreak investigations conducted in Odisha have shown the association of several water bodies including rivers, streams, ponds, and wells with cholera infection in the adjacent population who used the water for several purposes (Khuntia et al. 2008; Das et al. 2009b; Pal et al. 2010). Several surveys conducted in West Bengal during 2004–2008 showed that the use of pond waters were responsible for five cholera outbreaks with 277 cases (Mukherjee et al. 2011). Many cholera outbreaks in West Bengal and Gujarat were related due to leakage in the municipal water pipe lines (Bhunia et al. 2009; Shah et al. 2012). Surveillance of *V. cholerae* O1 in water samples from Kolkata urban areas during cholera outbreaks showed its presence in about 17 % of the samples, which is more than the samples collected from non-outbreak affected areas (5.2 %) (Batabyal et al. 2012). *V. cholerae* O1 was also reported from environmental waters in Chandigarh (Mishra et al. 2011) or stored waters in Kolkata and Tamil Nadu (Palit et al. 2012; Sekar et al. 2012).

9 Cholera at the Community Level

Contact or healthy carriers may play an important role in the spread and maintenance of the infection in the cholera endemic areas. In Kolkata, during the cholera epidemics in 1956, 45 % of culture-positive subjects had a history of direct or indirect contact with cases of cholera, 41 % gave no history but taken food or drink outside their homes (De et al. 1957). In addition, 67 % of culture positive cases of cholera had the habit of using service-privies and 78 % shared lavatories with a number of other families (De et al. 1957).

In many community-based studies, both classical and El Tor vibrios were identified among asymptomatic carriers. *V. cholerae* isolated from these carriers expressed its virulence in the animal models (Sinha et al. 1969) indicating their importance and role in the transmission of cholera. Studies conducted during 1968 inter-epidemic cholera period in Kolkata showed 6.2 % carriers of *V. cholerae* O1 in households, of which 52.4 and 38.1 % were identified as El Tor and classical vibrios, respectively. Interestingly, 9.5 % of the carriers had both the biotypes (CRC 1971).

In order to prevent and control diarrheal illness, the defecation habits of 172 adults before and after cholera epidemic in New Delhi was investigated (Murthy et al. 1990). Intensive educational activities were undertaken during the epidemic and a community latrine facility was constructed in the study area. A statistically significant relationship with age was observed, while literacy was not found to exert a statistically significant effect. Cost and distance were the main reasons cited for nonutilization of latrines. Most children were refrained from using the public latrines.

To determine the extent of *V. cholerae* O139 infection among healthy contacts and other suspected vehicles of transmission at the intrafamilial level, an extensive study was conducted in Kolkata (Sengupta et al. 1995). In this study, a total of 27 families of hospitalized patients (index case families) suffering from acute watery diarrhea and 14 neighborhood families were bacteriologically screened for 4 consecutive days. *V. cholerae* O139 was isolated from feces of 14.6 % of healthy contacts in index case families as compared to none in neighborhood families. In addition, the pathogen was recovered from 3.7 % of hand washings of contacts of index cases and also from stored drinking water (8.0 %), open well water (28.6 %), flies (3.8 %), and pond water (25.0 %) used by the index case families and none from neighborhood families. The large numbers of asymptomatic infected persons indicate an epidemiological similarity of O139 to that of O1 serogroup. The organisms may be carried on hands and may act as a potential source of infection to other inmates through contamination of stored drinking water, open wells, etc. Such studies are very important in formulating strategies for intervention of transmission of cholera at the community level.

To investigate an outbreak of cholera in Delhi during 1991, a hybrid design using a retrospective case-control method superimposed on a population-based cross-sectional study was made (Tilak et al. 1997). A total of 9 cholera confirmed cases were identified using population-based survey and compared with 33 controls from the same population. The cholera incidence rate was 0.71 % and showed a significant rising trend with age. Two of the food handlers, working in the same mess from where cases had occurred, were found positive for *V. cholerae* O1 Ogawa.

Diarrheal surveillance was conducted (2003–2004) to measure the burden of cholera, describe its epidemiology, and search for potential risk factors that could be addressed by public health strategies in an urban site in Kolkata (Sur et al. 2005). From 62,329 individuals under surveillance, 3,284 diarrheal episodes were detected. Of the 126 (4 %) culture-confirmed cholera cases, 19 (15 %) were children less than 2 years of age. Risk factors for cholera included a household member with cholera during the period of surveillance, young age, and lower educational level. This study has shown a substantial burden of cholera in an impoverished urban population with risk factors not easily amenable to intervention.

10 Molecular Epidemiology of Cholera

Molecular epidemiology is becoming a useful discipline as several informations can be generated specially on the strain origin, mode of spread, and its virulence features. While identifying the progenitor strains for *V. cholerae* O139, Pajni et al. (1995) found some of the O1 strains had neither classical nor E1 Tor in their biotype attributes. The *ctx* restriction fragment length polymorphism (RFLP) and outer membrane protein profiles displayed by these strains were identical with those exhibited by O139 strains but were different from classical and El Tor biotypes. All the O139 and the two O1 strains carried an identical number of *ctx* in their chromosomes. In the pulsed-field gel electrophoresis (PFGE) of the *Not*I and *Sfi*I enzymes digested genome of *V. cholerae* O139 strains collected from different parts of India were identified as single clone and its genome size was estimated as 2.2 Mb (Bhadra et al. 1995). In addition, *ctx* RFLP analysis suggested that O139 strains are genetically close to *V. cholerae* O1 biotype El Tor, but different from the classical vibrios. Using restriction enzymes, which cleave a single site in either the core region or in the direct repeat sequence (RS) of the CTX genetic element, it was shown that most of the O139 have two copies of the *ctx* in tandem connected by two RSs. The organization of the virulence gene cassettes in different O139 strains showed genetic heterogeneity and had two copies of the CTX genetic element.

Sharma et al. (1997a) studied the RFLP of the rRNA gene and CTX genetic element in *V. cholerae* O139, which appeared again in Kolkata in September 1996. The resurged strains were indistinguishable from the earlier ones in the ribotyping, but the structure of the CTX genetic element was unique. Molecular studies were conducted with clinical strains of *V. cholerae* O1 isolated in Kolkata before, during, and after the *V. cholerae* O139 Bengal outbreak to find out if the O1 strains of the post-O139 period were different from those that existed before (Sharma et al. 1997b). Comparison of the RFLP of the rRNA genes by ribotyping and the CTX genetic element revealed that all most all the pre-O139 strains belonged to a single known ribotype, whereas majority of the post-O139 strains belonged to a new ribotype. Most of the pre-O139 strains harbored two or more copies of CTX in tandem and also a "free" RS1 element away from CTX, whereas the post-O139 strains had a single copy of CTX without RS1 element. CTX occupied different chromosomal locations in pre and post-O139 strains. This investigation showed that El Tor strains, which displaced *V. cholerae* O139 in Kolkata, belonged to a new clone with a continuous genetic reassortment.

Comparison of the phenotypic traits of representative O139 strains from Kolkata and Dhaka isolated between December 1996 and April 1997 showed similar phenotypic traits with an exception that Dhaka strains were susceptible to streptomycin while Kolkata strains were resistant (Basu et al. 1998). The Dhaka and Kolkata O139 strains displayed identical ribotypes but showed remarkable differences in the structure and organization of the CTX genetic element. In the Dhaka O139 strains, two copies of the CTX element were arranged in tandem and this resembled the pattern displayed by the 1992 epidemic strains of O139. On the other hand, the Kolkata O139 strains carried three copies of the CTX genetic element arranged in tandem and a new *Hind*III site replaced the conserved *Bgl*II restriction site in the RS1 element. The two copies of the CTX elements were connected by two RSs, whereas in the reemerged O139 strains had three such elements connected by a single RS (Khetawat et al. 1999). Ribotyping and *ctx* RFLP showed clonal diversity among the O139 strains isolated during 1992–1993 and 1996–1997 with respect to its structure, organization, and location of the CTX prophages (Basu et al. 2000a).

Phenotypically, the re-emerged O139 strains during August 1996 were susceptible to SXT but the ribotyping patterns were identical to those exhibited by strains of O139 isolated in 1992 (Mukhopadhyay et al. 1996). The RFLP of *ctxA* identified three clones of *V. cholerae* O139 in different parts of India. RFLP of the rRNA and the *ctx* genes along with the antimicrobial-resistant profile of *V. cholerae* O1 and O139 associated with mixed infection were examined to determine their relatedness (Sharma et al. 1998). The results of this study also demonstrated that although the phenotypic profiles were the same, genetically they are different.

The ribotyping patterns of strains isolated from different parts of India during 1996–1997 were identical and were similar to that of 1994 strains from Kolkata (Bag et al. 1998). Likewise, majority of the strains examined by PFGE showed identical profile to that exhibited by the new clone of O1. The RFLP of CTX genetic element of these strains also matched with the new clone of O1, which emerged after the outbreak of *V. cholerae* O139 in Kolkata. The intron-encoded enzyme *Ceu*I provides an excellent tool for examining the organization of genomes in related bacterial species. Studies conducted with *V. cholerae* strains belonging to different biotypes and serotypes revealed different *Ceu*I RFLP profiles (Nandi et al. 1997). Several genetic markers, including virulence determinant genes were identified at different positions in the genomes of O139 and classical O1 strains (Khetawat et al. 1998). The endonuclease I-*Ceu*I had 10 sites in the genomes of re-emerged O139 strains, compared to 9 in the genomes of old O139 strains. This variation in the number of *rrn* operons within a serogroup has not been identified in other organisms (Khetawat et al. 1999).

Phylogentic analysis of the *Not*I PFGE profiles of NT *V. cholerae* O1 associated with a cluster of cases of cholera in Warangal, Andhra Pradesh showed that these strains formed a tight cluster with more than 80 % similarity (Pal et al. 1999). Interestingly, the NT *V. cholerae* O1 cluster was more closely related to *V. cholerae* O139 than classical and El Tor biotypes of *V. cholerae* O1. This indicates closer genetic relationships between NT *V. cholerae* O1 and O139 Bengal that were isolated during the same period.

The CTX prophage arrangement in classical biotype strains of *V. cholerae* O1 isolated between 1970 and 1979 showed clonal diversity (Basu et al. 2000b). This clonal variation was further substantiated by other typing methods. Molecular characterization by ribotyping, RFLP, and PFGE results indicated that the reappeared Inaba strains during 1998–1999 in Kolkata were similar to the Ogawa strains but were different from the earlier Inaba strains isolated in 1989 (Garg et al. 2000a). In addition, antibiograms of the Inaba strains were also similar to that of the *V. cholerae* Ogawa strains.

In the variable number of tandem repeat (VNTR) analysis, 64 novel alleles distributed among 51 sequence types from *V. cholerae* O139 strains (Garg et al. 2003). Lateral gene transfer (LGT) events produced three times the number of nucleotide changes compared to mutation. In contrast to the traditional concept of epidemic spread of a homogeneous clone, the establishment of variant alleles generated by LGT during the rapid expansion of O139 clonal population is a paradigm in infections and epidemics. A study was performed to compare the genetic relatedness of the patient and environmental strains of *V. cholerae* to determine clonal relationships (Sinha et al. 2001). DNA fingerprinting of the strains showed considerable diversity among toxigenic clinical and non-toxigenic environmental O1 Ogawa strains and between the O1 and non-O1, non-O139 isolates. *V. cholerae* O1 strains from clinical and environmental sources belonged to two different clones. Characterization of a *V. cholerae* O139 strain isolated from a diarrheal patient in Alleppey, Kerala in 2000 showed a distinct genotype with unique ribotype designated B-VII compared to O139 strains isolated from other parts of India (Bhanumathi et al. 2002). Genetic recombination or mutations in the conserved *rrn* operon and variations in CTXΦ are constantly occurring in the genomes of *V. cholerae*. Using the VNTR typing tool, Ghosh et al. (2008) have shown that O1 and O139 strains isolated in different parts of India during 1992–2007 formed four large groups, two with O1 and the other two with O139. The O139 strains isolated from Kerala in 2002 had different copy numbers of CTXΦ and multiple ribotypes, including B-I and B-II, and new ribotypes designated B-VIIIa, B-VIIIb, and B-IX (Fazil et al. 2011).

Ribotyping results of *V. cholerae* O1 strains isolated from Ahmedabad outbreak during 2000 exhibited a pattern identical to that of the prevailing O1 clone in areas where cholera is endemic. All the O139 strains were identical to the B-II clone of *V. cholerae* O139 strains that prevailed during previous year in India (Chakraborty et al. 2001). PFGE analysis of the *V. cholerae* O139 strains showed identical patterns, but these differed from the PFGE patterns of O139 isolates reported during 1992–1997 in Kolkata. Genotypic diversity among *V. cholerae* has been attributed to several reasons. Natural calamities such as heavy rainfall may support the spread of mixed genotypes in a population (Goel and Jiang 2011). In 2004, the substituted Inaba strains were identified as ribotype R-IV and H-1 pulsotype that is very close to the pattern exhibited by Ogawa strains isolated during the same period in Kolkata (Raychoudhuri et al. 2007). During 2002–2008, several outbreak strains of *V. cholerae* O1 from Punjab and Haryana were screened for clonality using PFGE and ribotying (Taneja et al. 2012). The PFGE generated 15 pulsotypes, of which four matched the previously designated pulsotypes and there were 11 new pulsotypes. In these outbreaks, ribotype IV was the most predominant followed by R-III. This ribotype IV was not isolated after 2003 and became the most predominant one from 2004 onwards.

V. cholerae O1 strains harbor integrative conjugative elements (ICEs), which are self-transmissible mobile elements, able to integrate into the host bacterial chromosome and to transfer by conjugation (Wozniak and Waldor 2010). The SXT/R391 family of ICEs are recently acquired by this pathogen especially after the emergence of the serogroup O139 in Chennai. These ICEs confer resistance to chloramphenicol, streptomycin, SXT, and are used in the identification of clonality of *V. cholerae* O1/O139. The ICEVchInd5 was consistently detected in *V. cholerae* O1 clinical strains isolated in Wardha, Maharashtra for more than 10 years from 1994 to 2005. However, the other molecular methods identified that these strains belong to different types (Ceccarelli et al. 2011). Thus, the utility of any molecular tool depends on the experimental purpose and the target genes.

11 Diagnosis of Cholera and Toxigenic *V. cholerae*

Rapid diagnosis of cholera has become very important as the disease affects large populations in a short time. Conventional culture techniques require 2–3 days for confirmation of the isolates. Many immunological and molecular biology-based techniques are now established for the detection of pathogens. The genes encoding CT (*ctx*) has been targeted for the rapid diagnosis of cholera or for the toxigenic strains of *V. cholerae.* A highly sensitive sandwich enzyme-linked immunosorbent assay (ELISA) using polystyrene beads has been evaluated for the detection of free CT present in cholera stool specimens (Ramamurthy et al. 1992b). This assay system was useful even with stool specimens from which *V. cholerae* cannot be isolated due to delayed processing for culture or patients treated with antibiotics (Ramamurthy et al. 1990).

A PCR-based assay was designed for the detection of toxigenic *V. cholerae* that harbors the *ctx* (Shirai et al. 1991). Three combined methods such as PCR, CT beads-ELISA, and culture methods were simultaneously tested for the detection of toxigenic *V. cholerae* from the stool specimens (Ramamurthy et al. 1993b). PCR provided a more sensitive and specific assay for rapid diagnosis of cholera than culture methods.

Sack and Barua (1964) established a fluorescent-antibody technique for the diagnosis of cholera. A monoclonal antibody-based rapid immunodiagnostic kits, BengalScreen, a coagglutination test, and Bengal DFA, a direct fluorescent-antibody test were used for the detection of *V. cholerae* O139 in clinical and environmental samples (Hasan et al. 1995). The assay time varied from 5 to 20 min. The Bengal DFA, being more sensitive than BengalScreen, requires only one reagent and less than 20 min for detection and enumeration of *V. cholerae* O139 with 100 % specificity. Compared to the conventional tests, the field testing of both BengalScreen and Bengal DFA with stool specimens demonstrated a high sensitivity and specificity. BengalScreen results were unequivocally positive when water samples contained at least 2.0×10^3 CFU/ml, whereas Bengal DFA demonstrated positive reaction when the water sample contained at least 1.5×10^2 CFU/ml.

PCR-RFLP with *ori* (encoding the origin of replication) sequence was formulated for the rapid identification and differentiation of *V. cholerae* O1 biotypes and *Vibrio mimicus* strains (Saha et al. 2006). In this assay, a point mutation in the *ori*CIVC sequence of the classical biotype of O1 serogroup led to the loss of a *Bgl*II site, which was utilized for differentiation from El Tor vibrios. Interestingly, the PCR assay amplified the *ori* segment, designated as *ori*CIVM, from *V. mimicus* strains also. The *Bgl*II RFLP between *ori*CIVM and *ori*CIVC sequences differentiated these two species. Several multiplex PCR were also designed for the detection of virulence genes such as *rtxA, tcpA, ctxA*, *hlyA*, and *sto* (Kumar et al. 2010). Crystal VC was found to be useful (66.7 %) for the rapid detection cholera in an outbreak in Secunderabad during May 2009 (Sinha et al. 2012). However, this method was less sensitive compared with a real-time PCR, which detected presence of *V. cholerae* in all the samples. In a hospital-based study, the sensitivity and specificity of the Crystal VC dipsticks were about 92 and 73 %, respectively (Mukherjee et al. 2010).

12 Emergence of Antimicrobial Resistance

Antimicrobials have been used for the treatment of cholera and other diarrheal diseases, as this method is effective during initial stages of the infection and plays a role in reducing stool volume. Drug-resistance in *V. cholerae* caused problems in the management of cholera. The effectiveness of tetracycline in the treatment of cholera was first demonstrated in Kolkata (Carpenter et al. 1964). Chemoprophylaxis field trials with doxycycline (vibramycin), and sulfadoxine were performed in Kolkata to observe their effectiveness in the transmission of *V. cholerae* among family contacts of cholera patients (CRC 1974; Deb et al. 1976). A single dose of 300 mg of doxycycline effectively reduced the number of carriers among contacts of cholera patients for 5 days (Sengupta et al. 1978). Clinical trials were also conducted to examine the effect of Ibuprofen (brufen) with cholera and other diarrheal patients in Kolkata as this drug possess anti-inflammatory analgesic and anti-rheumatic property. This study showed no significant difference between groups treated with brufen and placebo (De et al. 1974). In a controlled clinical trial of minocycline and tetracycline, it was observed that there was no difference in the volume and duration of diarrhea between the two treated groups (Guha-Mazumdar et al. 1974).

In the rabbit model, efficacy of ciprofloxacin, norfloxacin, and tetracycline were tested for prevention of colonization of *V. cholerae* O1 (Chakrabarti et al. 1993). Like tetracycline, norfloxacin and ciprofloxacin inhibited the colonization of *V. cholerae* O1 in the rabbit intestine. In a double blind, randomized clinical trial conducted in Kolkata with 37 adults with culture positive cholera patients, norfloxacin was found superior to sulfamethoxazole-trimethoprim (SXT) in reducing stool output, duration of diarrhea, fluid requirements, and excretion of vibrios (Bhattacharya et al. 1990). The efficacy of varying regimens of norfloxacin and doxycycline were compared for the treatment of cholera caused by *V. cholerae* O139 Bengal in an open randomized controlled clinical trial with 160 adults with acute watery diarrhea and severe dehydration (Dutta et al. 1996). These clinical trials have shown that multidose norfloxacin treatment significantly reduced stool output, duration of diarrhea, and fluid requirement compared with the other regimens.

Considering the emergence of multidrug resistant *V. cholerae* to the commonly used drugs, several new antimicrobials were tested for the efficient treatment of cholera. In Kolkata, azithromycin was tested for the treatment of cholera in children (Bhattacharya et al. 2003). Patients who received azithromycin had significantly less stool output, shorter duration of diarrhea, and lower fluid intake compared with patients who received erythromycin.

Use of antimicrobials as a prophylactic measure has also been reported during diarrheal outbreaks. However, the patients do not follow the recommended treatment regime. Generally, excess use of antimicrobials in the treatment of cholera enhances the development of resistance in many vibrios. Major works carried out on this aspect includes surveillance of drug-resistance among clinical strains of *V. cholerae* and their mechanism of resistance. Intestopan was effective against *V. cholerae* even at low concentrations and resistant strains to this drug were detected in 1970 (Sasmal and Ganguly 1971). The resistant strains to intestopan were found to be less virulent due to changed synthesis of biopolymers.

V. cholerae strains isolated during 1972 were susceptible to chloramphenicol and streptomycin (CRC 1973). The efficacy of SXT was found superior to tetracycline and chloramphenicol in 175 bacteriologically confirmed cases of cholera admitted in the IDH, Delhi (Dutta et al. 1978). SXT showed greater in vitro inhibition and earlier eradication from the intestinal tract. The antimicrobials such as furazolidone and SXT were also used for the treatment of cholera cases for many years in India. These drugs are commonly advocated in the treatment of cholera in children. However, studies conducted in 1987 in Vellore showed that *V. cholerae* O1 was resistant to trimethoprim and this feature was genetically transferable (Jesudason and John 1990; Jesudason and Saaya 1997).

Investigations conducted during a cholera outbreak in Goa during 1988 showed that *V. cholerae* O1 was susceptible to chloramphenicol, gentamicin, and nalidixic acid (Verenkar et al. 1994). Similarly, *V. cholerae* O1 strains isolated in Bombay during 1990 were mostly susceptible to gentamicin, nalidixic acid, kanamycin, SXT, and chloramphenicol (Saraswathi and Deodhar 1990). *V. cholerae* strains are generally susceptible to tetracycline and this drug is used for the treatment of cholera for many years. Intermittent appearance of tetracycline-resistant strains was reported in Loni area near Delhi (Jain et al. 1992). Tetracycline resistance among *V. cholerae* was also detected in Bombay (Saraswathi and Deodhar 1990), Vellore (Jesudasan 2006) and Assam (Borkakoty et al. 2012). In Kolkata, majority of the *V. cholerae* strains were found to be resistant to furazolidone (95.7 %), SXT (83 %), and tetracycline (63.1 %) (Ramamurthy et al. 1992a).

In the classical microbial taxonomy, sensitivity for 2, 4-diamino-6, 7-diiso-propylpteridine (O/129) was used to differentiate vibrios from aeromonads. Studies conducted in Kolkata with consecutive isolates of *V. cholerae* recovered from cholera patients showed resistance for 10 and 150 μg of O/129, respectively (Ramamurthy et al. 1992c). Additionally, all the O/129-resistant strains of *V. cholerae* were multiply resistant to different antimicrobials especially to SXT.

V. cholerae O1 isolated from 1994 Mizoram outbreak was uniformly resistant to furazolidone and SXT (Sengupta et al. 2000). Emergence of furazolidone and SXT-resistant strains of *V. cholerae* O1 in other eastern parts were reported subsequently (Niyogi et al. 1995). When *V. cholerae* O139 appeared again in Kolkata during 1996, there was change in the antimicrobial-resistant pattern especially to nalidixic acid and SXT (Mitra et al. 1996). In Pondicherry, 51 % of the *V. cholerae* O139 strains were susceptible to cefotaxime and majority of the strains were resistant to furazolidone, ampicillin, and SXT (Vijayalakshmi et al. 1997). Studies conducted in Punjab and other northern regions showed that *V. cholerae* strains were susceptible to tetracycline, gentamycin, neomycin, norfloxacin, and furazolidine (Kaur and Lal 1998).

In Delhi and other places, the re-emerged *V. cholerae* O139 in 2000 were susceptible to SXT compared to those that appeared in 1992–1993. Resistance to nalidixic acid and furazolidone was constantly high in *V. cholerae* O1 and O139 but they were uniformly susceptible to chloramphenicol, tetracycline, amikacin, and norfloxacin (Das and Gupta 2005). Studies conducted in Tamil Nadu from 1980 to 2001 showed that almost all the *V. cholerae* strains were susceptible to chloramphenicol, tetracycline, gentamicin, and ciprofloxacin (Sundaram et al. 2002). However, 97 % of the O1 strains and 48.9 % of the O139 strains isolated in this study were resistant to SXT.

Due to the emergence of resistant strains to commonly used antimicrobials, fluoroquinolones became an alternative choice in the late 1990s for the treatment of cholera. Emergence of fluoroquinolone-resistant *V. cholerae* that also exhibited multidrug resistance is of great significance in the epidemiology and control of cholera. Mukhopadhyay et al. (1998) first reported emergence of fluoroquinolone resistance among *V. cholerae* non-O1, non-O139 strains in Kolkata. In the subsequent years, ciprofloxacin-resistant strains of *V. cholerae* O1 were identified

(Garg et al. 2001). However, the O139 strains isolated almost during the same period remained susceptible to ciprofloxacin. Studies on antimicrobial resistance conducted between 1997 and 1999 in Vellore have shown that few O1 and all the O139 strains were susceptible to nalidixic acid and norfloxacin (Jesudason et al. 2002). This could be due to longer exposure of *V. cholerae* to quinolones. Mutations in the *gyrA,* and *parC* genes and proton motive force-dependent efflux were described for the first time in quinolone resistance in *V. cholerae* (Baranwal et al. 2002). *V. cholerae* resistant to fluoroquinolones were isolated during the 2002 cholera epidemic in and around Hubli (Krishna et al. 2006). The non-O1, non-O139 serogroups in this investigation were resistant to norfloxacin (55.9 %) and ciprofloxacin (47.1 %). However, only 12.5 % of the O1 serogroup strains were resistant to both norfloxacin and ciprofloxacin. The O139 strains isolated during the same period were susceptible to fluoroquinolones, but resistant to other antimicrobials.

In Kolkata, about 46 % of the *V. cholerae* O1 Ogawa strains isolated during 2003 showed reduced susceptibility to ciprofloxacin. Genetically, these strains were identical to the ones isolated during previous years (Chatterjee et al. 2007). Many of the *V. cholerae* O1 strains associated with cholera outbreaks in various parts of India from 2006 to 2009 were increasingly resistant to fluoroquinolones (Pal et al. 2010, 2013; Balaji et al. 2013). The resistance trend of *V. cholerae* O1 toward chloramphenicol, streptomycin, ampicillin, furazolidone, SXT, and nalidixic acid continued in India during 2004–2009 (Kingston et al. 2009; Goel and Jiang 2010; Pal et al. 2013). *V. cholerae* O1 strains isolated from outbreaks in Belgundi area, Belgaum during June 2010 and Odisha in 2009 showed unusually resistance to cephalosporins or tetracycline (Roy et al. 2012; Kumar et al. 2012). Presence of bla_{NDM-1} gene that encode resistance to third-generation cephalosporins was reported from water samples collected in New Delhi (Walsh et al. 2011) and a stool specimen from Pondicherry (Mandal et al. 2012).

To investigate the changing trends in multidrug resistance (MDR) among different serogroups of *V. cholerae,* software-assisted cluster analysis was made (Ramamurthy et al. 2000). Most of the MDR strains exhibited fluctuating trends as the resistance profile diverged each year. About 120 different resistance profiles exhibited by *V. cholerae* O1, O139, and non-O1, non-O139 serogroups were analyzed by cluster combination method. During 1993 and 1994, 53 % of *V. cholerae* O139 and 82 % of *V. cholerae* O1 serogroups exhibited several new resistance patterns. The frequency of new patterns among *V. cholerae* non-O1, non-O139 was constantly high (33–47 %) from 1995 to 1997. With few exceptions, preponderance of the resistance profiles was generally not confined to any serogroup. The cluster analysis showed dissemination of some of the resistance patterns commonly found in *V. cholerae* belonging to different serogroups to the O139 in the succeeding years (Ramamurthy et al. 2000).

A 6 year study (1992–1997) was conducted on antimicrobial susceptibility patterns of *V. cholerae* strains isolated from cholera patients admitted to the IDH, Kolkata (Garg et al. 2000b). Of the 840 *V. cholerae* strains, the O1 and O139 serogroups showed increased ampicillin resistance from 1992 to 1997. Resistance to furazolidone and streptomycin was constantly high among *V. cholerae* O1 with gradual increase in other drugs such as ciprofloxacin, SXT, neomycin, and nalidixic acid. *V. cholerae* O1 and O139 strains exhibited similar susceptibility patterns toward furazolidone and streptomycin. However, after initial increase in resistance to chloramphenicol and SXT, all the O139 strains became susceptible to these two drugs from 1995. Both *V. cholerae* O1 and O139 remained largely susceptible to gentamicin and tetracycline. *V. cholerae* non-O1, non-O139 strains on the other hand exhibited high levels of resistance to virtually every class of antimicrobial agents, especially from 1995. Kruskal-Wallis one-way analysis showed that *V. cholerae* O1 serogroup exhibited significant yearly increase in resistance to nine antibiotics followed by non-O1 non-O139 and O139 strains. Interesting observation encountered in this study was the spread of some of the resistance patterns commonly found among *V. cholerae* non-O1 non-O139 or O1 serogroups to the O139 serogroup and vice versa in the succeeding years. *V. cholerae* O139 strains isolated from the environments of Varanasi were also resistant to SXT, streptomycin, and to the O/129 compound (Bhanumathi et al. 2003).

Of the several mechanisms studied, integron-mediated drug resistance has been considered as important factor in *V. cholerae*. These mobile genetic elements help in the acquiring resistance to different antimicrobials. Studies on integrons were first made with clinical strains of *V. cholerae* belonging to non-O1, non-O139 strains (Thungapathra et al. 2002). The resistance gene cassettes identified in class 1 integrons harboring *V. cholerae* include *dfrA1*, *dfrA15*, *dfrA5*, and *dfrA12* for trimethoprim; *aac(6′)-Ib* for amikacin and tobramycin; *aadA1* and *aadA2* for streptomycin and spectinomycin; and *ereA2* for erythromycin resistance. This was the first report on the presence of *dfrA5*, *dfrA12*, *aac(6′)-Ib,* and *ereA2* cassettes in class 1 integron of *V. cholerae*. In 14 plasmid-bearing strains, class 1 integron was identified either on chromosomes, on plasmids, or on both. Besides class 1 integron and plasmids, a conjugative transposon element, SXT was suspected for multiple antibiotic resistance among *V. cholerae* strains (Thungapathra et al. 2002). Amita et al. (2003) examined the distribution of class 1 integron and SXT elements in *V. cholerae* O1 El Tor strains, isolated in Kolkata before and after the O139 outbreak in 1992. Class 1 integrons, with *aadA1* gene cassette, was detected in some of the pre-O139 strains but the SXT element was found in most of the post-O139 strains. In a study conducted in Kolkata, *V. cholerae* strains revealed the importance of integrons (Shi et al. 2006). Several O1, O139, and non-O1, non-O139 strains were found to contain class 1 integron harboring genes *aadA1, aadA2* (encoding resistance to streptomycin and spectinomycin), *blaP1* (resistance to beta-lactams), *aar-3* (resistance to rifampicin), *aacA4* (resistance to kanamycin and gentamicin), and *dfrA1* and *dfrA15* (resistance to trimethoprim).

13 Modes of Transmission and Intervention Studies

Cholera is known to be one of the important waterborne diseases. Early studies conducted in Kolkata reported prevalence of *V. cholerae* in Hooghly river water (Panja and Ghosh 1947). Clinical observations made in Kolkata have shown that consumption of untreated river water was the cause of cholera among boatman and also due to poor water supply in the city (De 1961). Works of Dastidar and Narayanaswami (1968) is the first report on occurrence of chitinase in vibrios. Subsequent to this finding, many investigators worked on the adherence of *V. cholerae* in chitin of marine zooplankton and possible transmission of vibrios to humans. The El Tor vibrios survived in sewage-irrigated or sewage-freshened fruits and vegetables for considerable number of days and hence these foodstuffs may act as a potential vehicle of cholera (Prescott and Bhattacharjee 1969).

During cholera outbreaks, it is possible to isolate *V. cholerae* from stagnant and stored waters in the households (Godbole and Wagle 1970). Studies on mode of transmission of *V. cholerae* within the families of cholera patients indicated that carrier rate of this pathogen varied from 5.5 to 9.8 % (CRC 1976; Niyogi et al. 1979). Studies conducted in Kolkata showed insignificant role of water in transmission of cholera at the community level (CRC 1977, 1978). Finger wash samples collected from the positive index cases yielded culture positive in 5.9 % of the samples (CRC 1979; Niyogi et al. 1979). Leftover food, stored water, and open well water showed culture positive results with 8.9, 8.9, and 18.2 %, respectively (CRC 1979). In a cholera outbreak investigation in Delhi, the role of carriers in outbreak of cholera has also been highlighted (Tilak et al. 1997). The food handlers were found positive for *V. cholerae* O1 Ogawa and treatment of carriers promptly abated the outbreak.

Studies were undertaken to determine whether simple intervention measures could effectively prevent the transmission of infection of *V. cholerae* in communities of lower socioeconomic status. The rate of detection of cholera carriers was much lower as compared to control group among houses provided with narrow pitcher pots. Similar reduction was also found in houses where water has been chlorinated (Deb et al. 1986). A study conducted in Delhi showed that house fly collected from a low socioeconomic area, where an outbreak of cholera had occurred was positive for *V. cholerae* (Fotedar 2001). This finding suggests that houseflies may act as mechanical vectors for the dissemination of the pathogen.

The priorities for cholera control is still continuing in the form of many public health interventions through improved drinking water, sanitation, surveillance, and access to health-care facilities. Current safe oral vaccines may lower the number of infections and could thus represent an effective intervention measure to control antibiotic resistance in cholera. Recently, a cluster-randomized, placebo-controlled trial of a two-dose regimen of killed whole cell oral cholera vaccine conducted in Kolkata showed the protective efficacy of 66 % during 3 years (Sur et al. 2011).

References

Aggarwal P, Khanna KK, Kumari S (1989) Cholera gastroenteritis amongst children in Delhi. Indian J Pediatr 56:93–96

Agarwal V, Biswas M, Chande CA, Pathak AA, Saoji AM (1994) Changing bacteriological profile of cholera in Nagpur, 1991–93. Indian J Med Res 100:93–94

Agrawal G, Jalgaonkar SV, Jagtap PM, Kamlakar UP, Deogade NG (2003) Emergence and re-emergence of *Vibrio cholerae* O139: an epidemiological study during 1993–2002 at Nagpur, Central India. Indian J Med Sci 57:155–157

Ambhore NA, Ingole KV, Fule RP (2000) Reappearance of *Vibrio cholerae* serogroup O139 in Yavatmal during June-August-1998. Indian J Med Sci 54:63–64

Amin V, Patwari AK, Kumar G, Anand VK, Diwan N, Peshin S (1995) Clinical profile of cholera in young children-a hospital based report. Indian Pediatr 32:755–761

Amita, Chowdhury SR, Thungapathra M, Ramamurthy T, Nair GB, Ghosh A (2003) Class I integrons and SXT elements in El Tor strains isolated before and after 1992 *Vibrio cholerae* O139 outbreak, Calcutta, India. Emerg Infect Dis 9:500–502

Bag PK, Maiti S, Sharma C et al (1998) Rapid spread of the new clone of *Vibrio cholerae* O1 biotype El Tor in cholera endemic areas in India. Epidemiol Infect 21:245–251

Bajaj JK, Baradker VP, Joshi SG, Damle AS, Kayararte RP, Deshmukh AB (2001) Epidemiology of cholera-a five-year study. J Commun Dis 33:282–285

Balaji K, Okonjo PA, Thenmozhi R, Karutha Pandian S (2013) Virulence and multidrug resistance patterns of *Vibrio cholerae* O1 isolates from diarrheal outbreaks of South India during 2006–2009. Microb Drug Resist 19:198–203

Ballal M, Nandanan B, Shivananda PG (2001) Emergence of *Vibrio cholerae* O139 in Manipal-coastal Karnataka-South India. Indian J Pathol Microbiol 44:177

Baranwal S, Dey K, Ramamurthy T, Nair GB, Kundu M (2002) Role of active efflux in association with target gene mutations in fluoroquinolone resistance in clinical isolates of *Vibrio cholerae*. Antimicrob Agents Chemother 46:2676–2678

Barua D (1992) History of cholerae. In: Barua D, Greenough WB III (eds) Cholera. Plenum Publishing, New York, pp 1–55

Basu A, Mukhopadhyay AK, Sharma C et al (1998) Heterogeneity in the organization of the CTX genetic element in strains of *Vibrio cholerae* O139 Bengal isolated from Calcutta, India and Dhaka, Bangladesh and its possible link to the dissimilar incidence of O139 cholera in the two locales. Microb Pathog 24:1751–1783

Basu A, Garg P, Datta S et al (2000a) *Vibrio cholerae* O139 in Calcutta, 1992–1998: incidence, antibiograms, and genotypes. Emerg Infect Dis 6:139–147

Basu A, Mukhopadhyay AK, Garg P et al (2000b) Diversity in the arrangement of the CTX prophages in classical strains of *Vibrio cholerae* O1. FEMS Microbiol Lett 182:35–40

Batabyal P, Mookerjee S, Palit A (2012) Occurrence of toxigenic *Vibrio cholerae* in accessible water sources of cholera endemic foci in India. Jpn J Infect Dis 65:358–360

Bhadra RK, Roychoudhury S, Banerjee RK et al (1995) Cholera toxin (CTX) genetic element in *Vibrio cholerae* O139. Microbiol 141:1977–1983

Bhanumathi R, Sabeena F, Isac SR, Radhakutty G, Singh DV (2002) Characterization of a toxigenic *Vibrio cholerae* O139 strain belonging to a new ribotype and isolated from a diarrheal patient. J Clin Microbiol 40:4779–4781

Bhanumathi R, Sabeena F, Isac SR, Shukla BN, Singh DV (2003) Molecular characterization of *Vibrio cholerae* O139 Bengal isolated from water and the aquatic plant *Eichhornia crassipes* in the River Ganga, Varanasi, India. Appl Environ Microbiol 69:2389–2394

Bhardwaj AK, Thakur TS, Sharma VK, Ahluwalia SK, Vaidya NK (1993) Problems and prospects of a traditional source of potable water in hilly terrains. Indian J Public Health 37:111–113

Bhattacharya SK, Bhattacharya MK, Dutta P (1990) Double-blind, randomized, controlled clinical trial of norfloxacin for cholera. Antimicrob Agents Chemother 34:939–940

Bhattacharya SK, Datta D, Bhattacharya MK et al (1992) Cholera in young children in an endemic area. Lancet 340:1549

Bhattacharya SK, Bhattacharya MK, Nair GB et al (1993) Clinical profile of acute diarrhoea cases infected with the new epidemic strain of *Vibrio cholerae* O139: designation of the disease as cholera. J Infect 27:11–15

Bhattacharya SK, Goswami AG, Bhattacharya MK et al (1994) Epidemic of *Vibrio cholerae* O139 in Calcutta. Indian J Med Res 100:213–216

Bhattacharya MK, Ghosh S, Mukhopadhyay AK, Deb A, Bhattacharya SK (2000) Outbreak of cholera caused by *Vibrio cholerae* O1 intermediately resistant to norfloxacin at Malda, West Bengal. J Indian Med Assoc 98:389–390

Bhattacharya MK, Dutta D, Ramamurthy T, Sarkar D, Singharoy A, Bhattacharya SK (2003) Azithromycin in the treatment of cholera in children. Acta Paediatr 92:676–678

Bhunia R, Ramakrishnan R, Hutin Y, Gupte MD (2009) Cholera outbreak secondary to contaminated pipe water in an urban area, West Bengal, India, 2006. Indian J Gastroenterol 28:62–64

Bora D, Dhariwal AC, Jain DC et al (1997) *V. cholerae* O1 outbreak in remote villages of Shimla district, Himachal Pradesh, 1994. J Commun Dis 29:121–125

Borkakoty B, Biswas D, Devi U, Yadav K, Mahanta J (2012) Emergence of classical ctxB genotype 1 and tetracycline resistant strains of *Vibrio cholerae* O1 El Tor in Assam, India. Trans R Soc Trop Med Hyg 106:382–386

Carpenter CC, Sack RB, Mondal A, Mitra PP (1964) Tetracycline therapy in cholera. J Indian Med Assoc 43:309–312

Ceccarelli D, Spagnoletti M, Bacciu D et al (2011) ICEVchInd5 is prevalent in epidemic *Vibrio cholerae* O1 El Tor strains isolated in India. Int J Med Microbiol 301:318–324

Chakrabarti MK, Bhattacharya MK, Sinha AK, Chatterjee DC, Bhattacharya SK (1993) Evaluation of the efficacy of different antibiotics in inhibiting colonisation of *Vibrio cholerae* O1 in the rabbit intestine. Zentralbl Bakteriol 278:69–72

Chakraborty S, Deokule JS, Garg P et al (2001) Concomitant infection of enterotoxigenic *Escherichia coli* in an outbreak of cholera caused by *Vibrio cholerae* O1 and O139 in Ahmedabad, India. J Clin Microbiol 39:3241–3246

Chander J, Kaistha N, Gupta V et al (2009) Epidemiology and antibiograms of *Vibrio cholerae* isolates from a tertiary care hospital in Chandigarh, North India. Indian J Med Res 129:613–617

Chatterjee S, Ghosh K, Raychoudhuri A et al (2007) Phenotypic and genotypic traits and epidemiological implication of *Vibrio cholerae* O1 and O139 strains in India during 2003. J Med Microbiol 56:824–832

Chhotray GP, Pal BB, Khuntia HK et al (2002) Incidence and molecular analysis of *Vibrio cholerae* associated with cholera outbreak subsequent to the super cyclone in Orissa, India. Epidemiol Infect 128:131–138

Cholera Research Center (1970) Annual Report

Cholera Research Center (1971) Annual Report

Cholera Research Center (1972) Annual Report

Cholera Research Center (1973) Annual Report

Cholera Research Center (1974) Annual Report

Cholera Research Center (1976) Annual Report

Cholera Research Center (1977) Annual Report

Cholera Research Center (1978) Annual Report

Cholera Research Center (1979) Annual Report

Constantin de Magny G, Murtugudde R, Sapiano MRP et al (2008) Environmental signatures associated with cholera epidemics. Proc Natl Acad Sci U S A 105:17676–17681

Darbari BS, Tiwari HL, Agarwal S et al (1982) Pattern of cholera in Raipur: a twelve year appraisal. J Indian Assoc Commun Dis 5:83–87

Das S, Gupta S (2005) Diversity of *Vibrio cholerae* strains isolated in Delhi, India, during 1992–2000. J Health Popul Nutr 23:44–51

Das A, Manickam P, Hutin Y et al (2009a) Two sequential outbreaks in two villages illustrate the various modes of transmission of cholera. Epidemiol Infect 137:906–912

Das A, Manickam P, Hutin Y et al (2009b) An outbreak of cholera associated with an unprotected well in Parbatia, Orissa, Eastern India. J Health Popul Nutr 27:646–651

Dastidar SG, Narayanaswami A (1968) The occurrence of chitinase in vibrios. Indian J Med Res 56:654–658

Datta KK, Bandyopadhyay S, Khanna KK, Banerjee K (1993) Epidemiological features of cholera outbreak in Delhi in 1988. J Commun Dis 25:57–61

De SN, Bhattacharya KK, Mondal A (1957) J Indian Med Assoc xxvii:514

De SN (1961) Cholera Its Pathology and Pathogenesis. Oliver and Boyd, London

De S, Sircar BK, Sasmal D, De SP, Mondal A (1974) Ibuprofen (Brufen) in cholera and other diarrhoeas. Indian J Med Res 62:756

Deb BC, Sengupta PG, De SP, Sil J, Sikdar SN, Pal SC (1976) Effect of sulfadoxine on transmission of *Vibrio cholerae* infection among family contacts of cholera patients in Calcutta. Bull World Health Organ 54:171–176

Deb BC, Sircar BK, Sengupta PG et al (1986) Studies on the interventions to prevent El Tor cholera transmission in urban slums. Bull Wld Hlth Org 64:127–131

Dhamodaran S, Ananthan S, Kuganantham P (1995) A retrospective analysis of the Madras epidemic of non-O1 *Vibrio cholerae* new serogroup O139 Bengal. Indian J Med Res 101:94–97

Dutta JK, Santhanam S, Misra BS, Ray SN (1978) Effect of trimethoprim-sulphamethoxazole on vibrio clearance in cholera (El Tor): a comparative study. Trans R Soc Trop Med Hyg 72:40–42

Dutta D, Bhattacharya SK, Bhattacharya MK et al (1996) Efficacy of norfloxacin and doxycycline for treatment of *Vibrio cholerae* O139 infection. J Antimicrob Chemother 37:575–581

Fazil MH, Bhanumathi R, Pandey HP, Singh DV (2011) Characterization of *Vibrio cholerae* O139 belonging to multiple ribotypes and isolated from diarrhoeal patients in Kerala, Southern India. Infect Genet Evol 11:454–459

Fotedar R (2001) Vector potential of houseflies (*Musca domestica*) in the transmission of *Vibrio cholerae* in India. Acta Trop 78:31–44

Fule RP, Powar RM, Menon S, Basutkar SH, Saoji AM (1990) Cholera epidemic in Solapur during July–August, 1988. Indian J Med Res 91:24–26

Fule RP, Jalgaonkar SV, Ingole KV, Fule C (1995) Outbreak due to *Vibrio cholerae* E1 Tor and serotype O139 in Yavatmal (Maharashtra) during June–July, 1994. Indian J Med Res 101:62–63

Ganguly R, Ghosh AK, Shrivastava DL (1966) Effect of chlorine on some of the biological characters of *Vibrio cholerae*. Indian J Med Res 54:24

Garg P, Nandy RK, Chaudhury P et al (2000a) Emergence of *Vibrio cholerae* O1 biotype El Tor serotype Inaba from the prevailing O1 Ogawa serotype strains in India. J Clin Microbiol 38:4249–4253

Garg P, Chakraborty S, Basu I et al (2000b) Expanding multiple antibiotic resistance among clinical strains of *Vibrio cholerae* isolated from 1992–1997 in Calcutta, India. Epidemiol Infect 124:393–399

Garg P, Sinha S, Chakraborty R et al (2001) Emergence of fluoroquinolone-resistant strains of *Vibrio cholerae* O1 biotype El Tor among hospitalized patients with cholera in Calcutta, India. Antimicrob Agents Chemother 45:1605–1606

Garg P, Aydanian A, Smith D, Glenn JM, Nair GB, Stine OC (2003) Molecular epidemiology of O139 *Vibrio cholerae*: mutation, lateral gene transfer, and founder flush. Emerg Infect Dis 9:810–814

Ghosh R, Nair GB, Tang L et al (2008) Epidemiological study of *Vibrio cholerae* using variable number of tandem repeats. FEMS Microbiol Lett 288:196–201

Godbole SH, Wagle PM (1970) Isolation of *Vibrio cholerae* from a well water during a small outbreak of cholera. Indian J Med Sci 24:484–486

Goel AK, Jiang SC (2010) Genetic determinants of virulence, antibiogram and altered biotype among the *Vibrio cholerae* O1 isolates from different cholera outbreaks in India. Infect Genet Evol 10:815–819

Goel AK, Jiang SC (2011) Association of heavy rainfall on genotypic diversity in *V. cholerae* isolates from an outbreak in India. Int J Microbiol 2011:230597

Gomber S, Mathur M, Sharma PP (1995) Diarrhoeal outbreak of *Vibrio cholerae* O139 from north India. Acta Paediatr 84:206–207

Guha-Mazumdar DN, Sircar BK, De SP (1974) Minocycline in the treatment of cholera: comparison with tetracycline. Indian J Med Res 62:712

Gupta DN, Sen D, Saha MR et al (1990) Report of an outbreak of diarrhoeal disease caused by cholera followed by rotavirus in Manipur. Indian J Public Health 34:62–65

Gupta A, Jain S, Mahawal BS (1999a) Outbreak of cholera in arid zone of Bikaner. Indian J Med Res 110:126–127

Gupta DN, Sarkar BL, Bhattacharya MK, Sengupta PG, Bhattacharya SK (1999b) An El Tor cholera outbreak in Maldah district, West Bengal. J Commun Dis 31:49–52

Gupta RS, Meena VR, Jain DC, Datta KK (2002) Cholera outbreak in rural areas of Southern Rajasthan. J Commun Dis 34:228–229

Gupta DN, Mondal SK, Sarkar BL, Mukherjee S, Bhattacharya SK (2004) An El tor cholera outbreak amongst tribal population in Tripura. J Commun Dis 36:271–276

Gupta N, Dewan S, Saini S (2005) Resurgence of *Vibrio cholerae* O139 in Rohtak. Indian J Med Res 121:128–130

Hamner S, Tripathi A, Mishra RK et al (2006) The role of water use patterns and sewage pollution in incidence of water-borne/enteric diseases along the Ganges river in Varanasi. India. Int J Environ Health Res 16:113–132

Hanumanthappa AR, Rajagopal V (2000) Serotypes and phage types of *Vibrio cholerae* in Mysore. J Commun Dis 32:313–315

Hasan JA, Huq A, Nair GB et al (1995) Development and testing of monoclonal antibody-based rapid immunodiagnostic test kits for direct detection of *Vibrio cholerae* O139 synonym Bengal. J Clin Microbiol 33:2935–2939

Hawgood BJ (2001) Sir Joseph Fayrer MD FRS (1824–1907) Indian Medical Service: snakebite and hospitalised patients with diarrhoea. J Med Microbiol 50:268–276

Howard-Jones N (1984) Robert Koch and the cholera vibrio: a centenary. Brt Med J 288:379–381

Ingole KV, Jalgaonkar SV, Fule C, Fule RP (1997) Changing pattern of *Vibrio cholerae* serotype El Tor and O139 in Yavatmal (Maharashtra, India) during 1992 to 1994. Indian J Pathol Microbiol 40:369–371

Jain RC, Bhat BD, Basutkar SH (1992) Tetracycline resistant El Tor Vibrios in Loni area. J Assoc Physicians India 40:636

Jain RC, Basutkar SH (1994) Endemicity of cholera among rural areas of Loni, Ahmednagar district of Maharashtra. Indian J Med Res 100:95–97

Jalgaonkar SV, Fule RP (1994) Cholera outbreak due to *Vibrio cholerae* serogroup O139 in Yavatmal (Maharashtra) in March–July, 1993. Indian J Med Res 99:101–102

Jesudason MV (2006) Change in serotype and appearance of tetracycline resistance in *V. cholerae* O1 in Vellore, South India. Indian J Med Microbiol 24:152–153

Jesudason MV, John TJ (1990) Transferable trimethoprim resistance of *Vibrio cholerae* O1 encountered in southern India. Trans R Soc Trop Med Hyg 84:136–137

Jesudason MV, Samuel R, John TJ (1994) Reappearance of *Vibrio cholerae* O1 and concurrent prevalence of O1 and O139 in Vellore, South India. Lancet 344:335–336

Jesudason MV, Saaya R (1997) Resistance of *Vibrio cholerae* O1 to nalidixic acid. Indian J Med Res 105:153–154

Jesudason MV, Balaji V, Thomson CJ (2002) Quinolone susceptibility of *Vibrio cholerae* O1 and O139 isolates from Vellore. Indian J Med Res 116:96–98

Joshi KR, Chaudhary SK, Singh R, Solanki A (1988) Cholera epidemic in Kharabera Purohitana, a village of west Rajasthan. Indian J Pathol Microbiol 31:178–181

Kamble TK, More SR, Chavan SS, Kulkarni ND, Lodha NS, Kamble AS (2000) Clinical profile of non-O1 strain-O139 of *Vibrio cholerae* in the region of Ambajogai, Maharashtra. J Assoc Physicians India 48:505–506

Kanungo S, Sah BK, Lopez AL et al (2010) Cholera in India: an analysis of reports, 1997–2006. Bull World Health Organ 88:185–191

Kaur H, Lal M (1998) Typing and antibiotic susceptibility patterns of *Vibrio cholerae* during six consecutive cholera seasons in north India. Trop Gastroenterol 19:59–61

Khanna KK, Dhanvijay A, Riley LW, Sehgal S, Kumari S (1990) Cholera outbreak in Delhi-1988. J Commun Dis 22:35–38

Khetawat G, Bhadra RK, Kar S, Das J (1998) *Vibrio cholerae* O139 Bengal: combined physical and genetic map and comparative analysis with the genome of *V. cholerae* O1. J Bacteriol 180:4516–4522

Khetawat G, Bhadra RK, Nandi S, Das J (1999) Resurgent *Vibrio cholerae* O139: rearrangement of cholera toxin genetic elements and amplification of *rrn* operon. Infect Immun 67:148–154

Khuntia HK, Pal BB, Meher PK, Chhotray GP (2008) Environmental *Vibrio cholerae* O139 may be the progenitor of outbreak of cholera in coastal area of Orissa, eastern India, 2000: molecular evidence. Am J Trop Med Hyg 78:819–822

Khuntia HK, Samal SK, Kar SK, Pal BB (2010) An Ogawa cholera outbreak 6 months after the Inaba cholera outbreaks in India, 2006. J Microbiol Immunol Infect 43:133–137

Kingston JJ, Zachariah K, Tuteja U, Kumar S, Batra HV (2009) Molecular characterization of *Vibrio cholerae* isolates from cholera outbreaks in North India. J Microbiol 47:110–115

Koch R (1884) Brit Med J ii:453

Krishna BV, Patil AB, Chandrasekhar MR (2006) Fluoroquinolone-resistant *Vibrio cholerae* isolated during a cholera outbreak in India. Trans R Soc Trop Med Hyg 100:224–226

Kumar P, Peter WA, Thomas S (2010) Rapid detection of virulence-associated genes in environmental strains of *Vibrio cholerae* by multiplex PCR. Curr Microbiol 60:199–202

Kumar P, Jain M, Goel AK, Kamboj DV, Kumar O (2012) Tetracycline resistant *V. cholerae* O1 biotype El Tor serotype Ogawa with classical *ctxB* from a recent cholera outbreak in Orissa, Eastern India. J Infect Public Health 5:217–219

Lutzkerand E, Jochnowitz C (1987) Waldemar Haffkine: Pioneer of Cholera vaccine. Am Soc Microbiol News 53:366–369

Macpherson J (1866) Cholera in its home. Churchill and Sons, London

Macpherson J (1872) Annals of cholera from the earliest periods to the year 1817. Ranken, London

MacNamara C (1876) A History of Asiatic Cholera. MacMillian, London

Mandal J, Sangeetha V, Ganesan V et al (2012) Third-generation cephalosporin-resistant *Vibrio cholerae* India. Emerg Infect Dis 18:1326–1328

Mehta MN, Daruwalla DR, Prabhu SV, Deodhar L (1986) An outbreak of cholera in children from Bombay slums. J Diarrhoeal Dis Res 4:94

Mishra M, Mohammed F, Akulwar SL, Katkar VJ, Tankhiwale NS, Powar RM (2004) Re-emergence of El Tor vibrio in outbreak of cholera in and around Nagpur. Indian J Med Res 120:478–480

Mishra A, Taneja N, Sharma RK, Kumar R, Sharma NC, Sharma M (2011) Amplified fragment length polymorphism of clinical and environmental *Vibrio cholerae* from a freshwater environment in a cholera-endemic area, India. BMC Infect Dis 11:249

Mitra R, Basu A, Dutta D, Nair GB, Takeda Y (1996) Resurgence of *Vibrio cholerae* O139 Bengal with altered antibiogram in Calcutta, India. Lancet 348:1181

Mohandas V, Unni J, Mathew M et al (1987) Aetiology and clinical features of acute childhood diarrhoea in an outpatient clinic in Vellore, India. Ann Trop Paediatr 7:167–172

Mohanty S, Kapil A, Das BK (2004) Seasonality and antimicrobial resistance pattern of *Vibrio cholerae* in a tertiary care hospital of North India. Trop Doct 34:249–251

Mohapatra SS, Ramachandran D, Mantri CK, Singh DV (2007) Characterization of the genetic background of *Vibrio cholerae* O1 biotype El Tor serotype Inaba strains isolated in Trivandrum, southern India. J Med Microbiol 56:260–265

Mukherjee S (1964) Cholera El Tor in Calcutta. Brit Med J 2:546–548
Mukherjee P, Ghosh S, Ramamurthy T et al (2010) Evaluation of a rapid immuno chromatographic dipstick kit for diagnosis of cholera emphasizes its outbreak utility. Jpn J Infect Dis 63:234–238
Mukherjee R, Halder D, Saha S et al (2011) Five pond-centred outbreaks of cholera in villages of West Bengal, India: evidence for focused interventions. J Health Popul Nutr 29:421–428
Mukhopadhyay AK, Garg S, Nair GB et al (1995) Biotype traits and antibiotic susceptibility of *Vibrio cholerae* serogroup O1 before, during and after the emergence of the O139 serogroup. Epidemiol Infect 115:427–434
Mukhopadhyay AK, Garg S, Mitra R et al (1996) Temporal shifts in traits of *Vibrio cholerae* strains isolated from hospitalized patients in Calcutta: a 3-year (1993 to 1995) analysis. J Clin Microbiol 34:2537–2543
Mukhopadhyay AK, Basu I, Bhattacharya SK, Bhattacharya MK, Nair GB (1998) Emergence of fluoroquinolone resistance in strains of *Vibrio cholerae* isolated from hospitalized patients with acute diarrhea in Calcutta, India. Antimicrob Agents Chemother 42:206–207
Murthy GV, Goswami A, Narayanan S, Amar S (1990) Effect of educational intervention on defaecation habits in an Indian urban slum. J Trop Med Hyg 93:189–193
Nair GB, Ramamurthy T, Bhattacharya SK et al (1994a) Spread of *Vibrio cholerae* O139 Bengal in India. J Infect Dis 169:1029–1034
Nair GB, Shimada T, Kurazono H et al (1994b) Characterization of phenotypic, serological, and toxigenic traits of *Vibrio cholerae* O139 Bengal. J Clin Microbiol 32:2775–2779
Nandi S, Khetawat G, Sengupta S et al (1997) Rearrangements in the genomes of *Vibrio cholerae* strains belonging to different serovars and biovars. Int J Syst Bacteriol 47:858–862
Narang P, Mendiratta DK, Kannathe J, Ramnani VK, Wasekar V, Deotale V (1994) Characteristics of *Vibrio cholerae* O139 strains isolated in Sevagram (Maharashtra) during April-August 1993. Indian J Med Res 99:103–104
Neogy KN, Chatterjee BD (1970) Reappearance of classical *V. cholerae* in Calcutta during early 1970. Bull Calcutta Sch Trop Med 18:52
Niyogi GS, Deb BC, Sircar BK et al (1979) Studies on cholera carriers and their role in transmission of the infection: a preliminary report. Indian J Med Res 70:892–897
Niyogi SK, Mondal S, Sarkar BL, Garg S, Banerjee D, Dey GN (1994) Outbreak of cholera due to *Vibrio cholerae* O1 in Orissa state. Indian J Med Res 100:217–218
Niyogi SK, Sengupta PG, Bhattacharya SK, Garg S, Mukhapadhayay AK, Nair GB (1995) Emergence of furazolidone and cotrimoxazole resistant *Vibrio cholerae* O1 in eastern India. J Infect 30:265–266
Pajni S, Sharma C, Bhasin N et al (1995) Studies on the genesis of *Vibrio cholerae* O139: identification of probable progenitor strains. J Med Microbiol 42:20–25
Pal A, Saha PK, Nair GB et al (1999) Clonal analysis of non-toxigenic *Vibrio cholerae* O1 associated with an outbreak of cholera. Indian J Med Res 109:208–211
Pal BB, Khuntia HK, Samal SK, Kar SK, Patnaik B (2010) Epidemics of severe cholera caused by El Tor *Vibrio cholerae* O1 Ogawa possessing the *ctxB* gene of the classical biotype in Orissa, India. Int J Infect Dis 14:384–389
Pal BB, Khuntia HK, Samal S et al (2013) Large outbreak of cholera caused by El Tor variant *Vibrio cholerae* O1 in the eastern coast of Odisha, India during 2009. Epidemiol Infect 141:2560–2567
Palit A, Batabyal P (2010) Toxigenic *Vibrio cholerae* from environmental sources associated with the cholera outbreak after 'AILA' cyclone in West Bengal, India. Lett Appl Microbiol 51:241–243
Palit A, Batabyal P, Kanungo S, Sur D (2012) In-house contamination of potable water in urban slum of Kolkata, India: a possible transmission route of diarrhea. Water Sci Technol 66:299–303
Panda S, Pati KK, Bhattacharya MK, Koley H, Pahari S, Nair GB (2011) Rapid situation and response assessment of diarrhoea outbreak in a coastal district following tropical cyclone AILA in India. Indian J Med Res 133:395–400

Panja G, Ghosh SK (1947) Indian J Med Res xxxv:979

Patnaik SK, Shukla P, Verma P, Dixit GC, Pal D, Sharma SN (1989) Outbreak of cholera in Berasia block of Bhopal District in Madhya Pradesh. J Commun Dis 21:123–128

Phukan AC, Borah PK, Biswas D, Mahanta J (2004) A cholera epidemic in a rural area of northeast India. Trans R Soc Trop Med Hyg 98:563–566

Pollitzer R (1959) Cholera. World Health Organization, Geneva, Switzerland

Prabhakar H, Lal M, Kaur H (1994) Outbreak of gastroenteritis due to a new strain of non O group 1 *Vibrio cholerae,* in Ludhiana in May–August 1993. Indian J Med Res 99:107–108

Prescott LM, Bhattacharjee NK (1969) Viability of El Tor vibrios in common foodstuff found in an endemic cholera area. Bull World Health Organ 40:980–982

Radhakutty G, Sircar BK, Mondal SK et al (1997) Investigation of the outbreak of cholera in Alleppey and Palghat districts, South India. Indian J Med Res 106:455–457

Rajendran K, Sumi A, Bhattachariya MK et al (2011) Influence of relative humidity in *Vibrio cholerae* infection: a time series model. Indian J Med Res 133:138–145

Rajeshwari K, Gupta A, Dubey AP, Uppal B, Singh MM (2008) Diarrhoeal outbreak of *Vibrio cholerae* O1 Inaba in Delhi. Trop Doct 38:105–107

Ramamurthy T, Pal A, Nair GB, Pal SC, Takeda T, Takeda Y (1990) Experience with a toxin bead-ELISA in a cholera outbreak. Lancet ii:375–376

Ramamurthy T, Pal A, Bhattacharya MK et al (1992a) Serovar, biotype, phage type, toxigenicity & antibiotic susceptibility patterns of *Vibrio cholerae* isolated during two consecutive cholera seasons (1989–1990) in Calcutta. Indian J Med Res 95:125–129

Ramamurthy T, Bhattacharya SK, Uesaka Y et al (1992b) Evaluation of the bead enzyme-linked immunosorbent assay for detection of cholera toxin directly from stool specimens. J Clin Microbiol 30:1783–1786

Ramamurthy T, Pal A, Pal SC, Nair GB (1992c) Taxonomical implications of the emergence of high frequency of occurrence of 2,4-diamino-6,7-diisopropylpteridine-resistant strains of *Vibrio cholerae* from clinical cases of cholera in Calcutta, India. J Clin Microbiol 30:742–743

Ramamurthy T, Garg S, Sharma R et al (1993a) Emergence of novel strain of *Vibrio cholerae* with epidemic potential in southern and eastern India. Lancet 341:703–704

Ramamurthy T, Pal A, Bag PK et al (1993b) Detection of cholera toxin gene in stool specimens by polymerase chain reaction: comparison with bead enzyme-linked immunosorbent assay and culture method for laboratory diagnosis of cholera. J Clin Microbiol 31:3068–3070

Ramamurthy T, Rajendran K, Garg P et al (2000) Cluster-analysis and patterns of dissemination of multidrug resistance among clinical strains of *Vibrio cholerae* in Calcutta, India. Indian J Med Res 112:78–85

Rathna K, Khairunnisa, Rajyalakshmi K, Naidu AS (1988) Epidemiological patterns and incidence of bio-, sero- and phage types of *Vibrio cholerae* in Hyderabad, India, during 1971–1984. Acta Microbiol Hung 35:313–322

Raychoudhuri A, Chatterjee S, Pazhani GP et al (2007) Molecular characterization of recent *Vibrio cholerae* O1, El Tor, Inaba strains isolated from hospitalized patients in Kolkata, India. J Infect 55:431–438

Rogers L (1926) Proc Roy Soc Med xix:59

Rogers L (1957) Brit Med J ii:1193

Roy S, Dutta B, Ghosh AR et al (2005) Molecular tracking of the lineage of strains of *Vibrio cholerae* O1 biotype El Tor associated with a cholera outbreak in Andaman and Nicobar Islands, India. Trop Med Int Health 10:604–611

Roy S, Parande MV, Mantur BG et al (2012) Multidrug-resistant *Vibrio cholerae* O1 in Belgaum, south India. J Med Microbiol 61:1574–1579

Rudra S, Mathur M, Talwar V, Kathuria K et al (1997) Changing patterns of *Vibrio cholerae* isolation over three consecutive cholera seasons (1992–1994) in east Delhi. J Commun Dis 29:15–22

Russell AJH (1927) Trans Far East Assoc Trop Med ii:131

Sabherwal U, Sikka R (1994) Emergence of *Vibrio cholerae* serogroup O139 in Haryana in May–June 1993. Indian J Med Res 99:105–106

Sachdeva V, Khanna KK, Singh M, Singh J, Kumari S, Verghese T (1995) Widespread emergence of *Vibrio cholerae* O139 in India. Southeast Asian J Trop Med Public Health 26:342–346

Sack RB (1992) Colonization and pathology. In: Barua D, Greenough WB (eds) Cholera. Plenum Medical Book Co., New York, pp 189–197

Sack RB, Barua D (1964) The fluorescent antibody technique in the diagnosis of cholera. Indian J Med Res 52:848–854

Saha A, Deb R, Shah S et al (2006) PCR-based identification of *Vibrio cholerae* and the closely related species *Vibrio mimicus* using the large chromosomal *ori* sequence of *Vibrio cholerae*. FEMS Microbiol Lett 257:84–91

Saha PK, Koley H, Mukhopadhyay AK et al (1996) Nontoxigenic *Vibrio cholerae* O1 serotype Inaba biotype El Tor associated with a cluster of cases of cholera in southern India. J Clin Microbiol 34:1114–1117

Samal B, Ghosh SK, Mohanty SK, Patnaik K (2001) Epidemic of *Vibrio cholerae* serogroup O139 in Berhampur, Orissa. Indian J Med Res 114:10–11

Sarkar BL, Kanungo S, Nair GB (2012) How endemic is cholera in India? Indian J Med Res 135:246–248

Saraswathi K, Deodhar LP (1990) A study of *V. cholerae* strains isolated in Bombay. J Postgrad Med 36:128–130

Sasmal D, Ganguly R (1971) Studies on intestopan resistant vibrios. Indian J Med Res 59:526

Sehgal PN, Misra BS, Pal SC et al (1972) An epidemic of classical cholera in the south eastern districts of Madhya Pradesh in 1970. Indian J Med Res 60:7–14

Sekar R, Amudhan M, Sivashankar M, Mythily N, Mythreyee M (2012) An outbreak of cholera among a rural population in south India: is it time to vaccinate the children in endemic areas? Indian J Med Res 135:678–679

Sengupta PG, Sircar BK, Mandal S et al (1978) Effect of doxycyline on transmission of *Vibrio cholerae* infection amongst family contacts of cholera patients in Calcutta. Bull World Health Organ 56:323–326

Sengupta PG, Sircar BK, Mandal SK et al (1995) Epidemiology of *Vibrio cholerae* O139 with special reference to intrafamilial transmission in Calcutta. J Infect 31:45–47

Sengupta PG, Niyogi SK, Bhattacharya SK (2000) An outbreak of Eltor cholera in Aizwal town of Mizoram, India. J Commun Dis 32:207–211

Sethi NK, Sethi SK (2001) *Vibrio cholerae* diarrhoea in a three-day-old breastfed neonate. Indian J Pediatr 68:791–792

Shah WA, Shahina M, Ali N (2002) First report of *Vibrio cholerae* infection from Andaman and Nicobar, India. J Commun Dis 34:270–275

Shah HD, Shah VP, Desai AN (2012) An epidemic outbreak of *Vibrio cholerae* El Tor O1 serotype Ogawa biotype in a Lalpur town, Jamnagar, India. J Postgrad Med 58:14–18

Sharma MID (1975) Problem of Cholera in India. J Com Dis 7:79–83

Sharma C, Ghosh A, Ghosh RK, Mukhopadhyay AK, Nair GB (1998) Molecular analysis of the cholera toxin gene and antibiotic sensitivity profile of *Vibrio cholerae* O1 and O139 associated with mixed infection. Indian J Med Res 107:199–203

Sharma C, Maiti S, Mukhopadhyay AK et al (1997a) Unique organization of the CTX genetic element in *Vibrio cholerae* O139 strains which reemerged in Calcutta, India, in September 1996. J Clin Microbiol 35:3348–3350

Sharma C, Nair GB, Mukhopadhyay AK, Bhattacharya SK, Ghosh RK, Ghosh A (1997b) Molecular characterization of *Vibrio cholerae* O1 biotype El Tor strains isolated between 1992 and 1995 in Calcutta, India: evidence for the emergence of a new clone of the El Tor biotype. J Infect Dis 175:1134–1141

Shi L, Fujihara K, Sato T et al (2006) Distribution and characterization of integrons in various serogroups of *Vibrio cholerae* strains isolated from diarrhoeal patients between 1992 and 2000 in Kolkata, India. J Med Microbiol 55:575–583

Shirai H, Nishibuchi M, Ramamurthy T, Bhattacharya SK, Pal SC, Takeda Y (1991) Polymerase chain reaction for detection of the cholera enterotoxin operon of *Vibrio cholerae*. J Clin Microbiol 29:2517–2521

Simpson WJ (1888) Cholera and its fostering conditions within the endemic area. BMJ II:416

Singh YI, Singh TS, Devi U, Singh NB (1986) Cholera outbreak in Manipur. J Commun Dis 18:9–112

Singh J, Khanna KK, Dhariwal AC et al (1996a) Unusual occurrence of cholera in Delhi during January 1994: epidemiological investigations. J Diarrhoeal Dis Res 14:107–109

Singh J, Bora D, Khanna KK et al (1996b) Epidemiology and transmission of *V. cholerae* O1 and *V. cholerae* O139 infections in Delhi in 1993. J Diarrhoeal Dis Res 14:182–186

Singh J, Bora D, Sachdeva V, Sharma RS, Verghese T (1997) *Vibrio cholerae* O1 and O139 in less than five years old children hospitalised for watery diarrhoea in Delhi, 1993. J Diarrhoeal Dis Res 15:3–6

Singh J, Sachdeva V, Bhatia R, Bora D, Jain DC, Sokhey J (1998) Endemic cholera in Delhi, 1995: analysis of data from a sentinel centre. J Diarrhoeal Dis Res 16:66–73

Sinha R, Deb BC, Ghosh AK, Shrivastava DL (1969) Virulence of *Vibrio cholerae* strains isolated from carriers in the rabbit ileal loop. Indian J Med Res 57:1636

Sinha S, Chowdhury P, Chowdhury NR et al (2001) Molecular comparison of toxigenic clinical & non-toxigenic environmental strains of *Vibrio cholerae* O1 Ogawa isolated during an outbreak of cholera in south India. Indian J Med Res 114:83–89

Sinha S, Chakraborty R, De K et al (2002) Escalating association of *Vibrio cholerae* O139 with cholera outbreaks in India. J Clin Microbiol 40:2635–2637

Sinha A, Sengupta S, Ghosh S et al (2012) Evaluation of a rapid dipstick test for identifying cholera cases during the outbreak. Indian J Med Res 135:523–528

Sircar BK, Saha MR, Deb BC, Singh PK, Pal SC (1990) Effectiveness of oral rehydration salt solution (ORS) in reduction of death during cholera epidemic. Indian J Public Health 34:68–70

Slathia P, Bansal MP (1999) Incidence of *Vibrio cholerae* in different age groups and sex in Aurangabad. Province isolated during January 1994 to December 1994. Indian J Med Sci 53:349–351

Soni GS, Gupta BL, Gupta U, Joshi KR (1989) An outbreak of El Tor cholera in rural population of Barmer in Rajasthan State of India, Aug–Sep 1987. Indian J Public Health 33:77–78

Sugunan AP, Roy S, Shahina M et al (2007) Emergence of *Vibrio cholerae* O1 Inaba in Andaman & Nicobar Islands, India. J Public Health 29:308–309

Sundaram SP, Revathi J, Elango V, Shanthakumari SL (1998) Aetiology of cholera in Tamil Nadu: recent observations. Trans R Soc Trop Med Hyg 92:164–165

Sundaram SP, Revathi J, Sarkar BL, Bhattacharya SK (2002) Bacteriological profile of cholera in Tamil Nadu (1980–2001). Indian J Med Res 116:258–263

Sur D, Dutta P, Nair GB, Bhattacharya SK (2000) Severe cholera outbreak following floods in a northern district of West Bengal. Indian J Med Res 112:178–182

Sur D, Sengupta PG, Mondal SK et al (2002) A localised outbreak of *Vibrio cholerae* O139 in Kolkata, West Bengal. Indian J Med Res 115:149–152

Sur D, Deen JL, Manna B et al (2005) The burden of cholera in the slums of Kolkata, India: data from a prospective, community based study. Arch Dis Child 90:1175–1181

Sur D, Kanungo S, Sah B et al (2011) Efficacy of a low-cost, inactivated whole-cell oral cholera vaccine: results from 3 years of follow-up of a randomized, controlled trial. PLoS Negl Trop Dis 5:e1289

Swaroop S, Pollitzer R (1955) Bull World Health Organ xii:311

Taneja N, Kaur J, Sharma K et al (2003) A recent outbreak of cholera due to *Vibrio cholerae* O1 Ogawa in & around Chandigarh, North India. Indian J Med Res 117:243–246

Taneja N, Biswal M, Tarai B, Sharma M (2005) Emergence of Vibrio cholerae O1 Biotype El Tor Serotype Inaba in North India. Jpn J Infect Dis. 58:238–240

Taneja N, Sangar G, Chowdhury G et al (2012) Molecular epidemiology of *Vibrio cholerae* causing outbreaks & sporadic cholera in northern India. Indian J Med Res 136:656–663

Thakur JS, Swami HM, Dutt R, Mehta M, Gupta V (2001) Epidemiological investigation of cholera outbreak in a periurban slum colony in Chandigarh. Indian J Med Sci 55:429–433

Thungapathra M, Amita Sinha KK et al (2002) Occurrence of antibiotic resistance gene cassettes *aac(6′)-Ib*, *dfrA5*, *dfrA12*, and *ereA2* in class I integrons in non-O1, non-O139 *Vibrio cholerae* strains in India. Antimicrob Agents Chemother 46:2948–2955

Tilak VW, Bhalwar R, Ratti JS (1997) Epidemiological study of an outbreak of cholera in Delhi cantonment. Indian J Public Health 41:61–67

Uppal B, Berry N, Kakar S, Ramji S, Mathur MD (1999) *Vibrio cholerae* O1 serotype Ogawa in a neonate. Diagn Microbiol Infect Dis 33:63–64

Verenkar M, Savio R, Venkatesh N, Pinto MJ, Singh I (1994) Cholera epidemic in Goa. Indian J Pathol Microbiol 37:289–292

Verma R, Khanna P, Chawla S (2012) Cholera vaccine: new preventive tool for endemic countries. Hum Vaccin Immunother 8:682–684

Vijayalakshmi N, Rao RS, Sujatha S, Hamid A, Dutta TK, Das AK (1994) An outbreak of gastroenteritis due to *Vibrio cholerae* O139 in Pondicherry, South India. Southeast Asian J Trop Med Public Health 25:314–315

Vijayalakshmi N, Rao RS, Badrinath S (1997) Minimum inhibitory concentration (MIC) of some antibiotics against *Vibrio cholerae* O139 isolates from Pondicherry. Epidemiol Infect 119:25–28

Walsh TR, Weeks J, Livermore DM, Toleman MA (2011) Dissemination of NDM-1 positive bacteria in the New Delhi environment and its implications for human health: an environmental point prevalence study. Lancet Infect Dis 11:355–362

Wozniak RA, Waldor MK (2010) Integrative and conjugative elements: mosaic mobile genetic elements enabling dynamic lateral gene flow. Nat Rev Microbiol 8:552–563

Cholera Outbreaks in South-East Asia

Kaushik Bharati and S. K. Bhattacharya

Abstract This chapter highlights the cholera situation in South Asia and the Bay of Bengal region, the original 'homeland' of cholera. A detailed discussion of cholera outbreaks in individual countries in South-East Asia follows. The countries of the World Health Organization (WHO) SEARO (South-East Asia Region) region are discussed first, followed by discussions about the other countries in South-East Asia that do not fall within the purview of the WHO SEARO classification of the member countries of the region. Therefore, the chapter attempts to provide a comprehensive yet precise outline of the major cholera outbreaks that have occurred in the region over the years.

Contents

K. Bharati (✉)
Policy Center for Biomedical Research,
Translational Health Science and Technology Institute, 496,
Udyog Vihar Phase III, Gurgaon, Haryana 122016, India
e-mail: kaushik@thsti.res.in

S. K. Bhattacharya
Indian Council of Medical Research, New Delhi, India

Current Topics in Microbiology and Immunology (2014) 379: 87–116
DOI: 10.1007/82_2014_362

Published Online: 30 January 2014

1 Introduction

Enteric diseases represent a leading cause of death by infectious diseases in the world just after respiratory diseases and HIV/AIDS. Among them cholera remains a major public health issue. Cholera, an acute waterborne diarrhoeal disease, continues to be a significant global health threat. The currently ongoing seventh pandemic of cholera, which started in 1961, has been reported in over 50 countries and has affected over 7 million individuals. It is affecting all ages and is primarily due to unhygienic living conditions, poverty and lack of clean drinking water. Importantly, the disease remains a threat in many tropical regions of the world, specifically in the coastal parts of South Asia, Africa and Latin America. The World Health Organization (WHO) estimates that 3–5 million cholera cases occur every year, leading to 100,000–120,000 deaths due to cholera every year with an average case fatality rate of 2.25 % (range 1–10 %) (WHO 2012). Its actual mortality and morbidity is underestimated due to gross under-reporting, growing risks due to climate change, increased bacterial virulence (new variants of O1 El Tor) and emergence of antibiotic resistance, etc.

In May 2011, the World Health Assembly (WHA) recognised the re-emergence of cholera as a significant global public health problem and adapted resolution WHA 64.15, calling for the implementation of an integrated comprehensive global approach to cholera control (WHO 2011). The dismal picture of cholera in recent years is reflected by a 130 % increase in the number of cases of cholera from 2000 to 2010 (WHO 2011). Importantly, in 2010, 48 countries reported the incidence of the disease. The situation is critical in Asia where the disease is both endemic and epidemic. Despite current national and international efforts, the morbidity and mortality rates remain high and represent a significant burden in the region, both economic as well as societal (WHO 2010).

2 Cholera: Global Scenario

Cholera is a widespread and serious disease, which is still endemic in approximately 50 countries that fall under the category of developing nations. Between 2006 and 2008 an average of 200,000 suspected cases and 5,000 deaths were reported to WHO (WHO 2010). Studies reviewing unreported epidemics actually found significant under-reporting because of various reasons including stigmatisation and fear of economic losses. Importantly, a review of the Indian notification data between 1997 and 2006 showed that only 37,783 cases were reported to WHO, when 222,038 cases were actually identified (Kanungo et al. 2010). It should be noted that although 98 % of all cholera cases and 99 % of all deaths in 2009 were reported from 30 affected African countries, the disease is still endemic in most countries in South-East Asia and outbreaks are periodically reported although countries with high rates have not started reporting (Waldor et al. 2010).

The current pandemic is the seventh in line, which began in 1961 and is still ongoing. Unlike the first six, it originated in Indonesia. It devastated populations across Asia and the Middle East and eventually reached Africa in 1971. By 1973, the pandemic had spread to Italy. There were also small outbreaks of the same El Tor strain in Japan and the South Pacific in the late 1970s. In 1991, a century after cholera had been vanquished from South America, there was a fresh outbreak in Peru that spread throughout the continent, killing about 10,000 people in its wake. In 1994, there was a big outbreak among Rwandan refugee camps in the Democratic Republic of Congo that killed tens of thousands of people. In 2008, an outbreak in Zimbabwe involved almost 12,000 cases. The outbreak is believed to be the result of deteriorating infrastructure resulting from political unrest. In recent times, the Haiti outbreak is the largest outbreak to be recorded that devastated the country (Fig. 1). From the scientific front, the major discovery from this period has been the identification of the new serogroup of cholera bacteria (O139) in India (Ramamurthy et al. 1993) and Bangladesh in 1992 (Albert et al. 1993), which has since been detected in 11 countries. This discovery has raised concerns about the fear of an eighth pandemic. Recent studies using robust molecular techniques, however, place *Vibrio cholerae* O139 as a derivative of El Tor *V. cholerae* O1 (Mutreja et al. 2011).

3 Cholera in South Asia and Bay of Bengal Region

The coastal regions of South Asia, for example Bangladesh and Kolkata in the state of West Bengal in India, have a long history of cholera outbreaks and are collectively considered the native homeland of the cholera disease since the early nineteenth century. Cholera incidence data at the International Center for Diarrhoeal Disease Research in Bangladesh (ICDDR,B) is very well documented and is one of the longest and most detailed cholera datasets in the world.

Cholera seasonality in the Bengal delta region is unique in the sense that it shows two cholera outbreaks in a given annual cycle. It is believed that the spring outbreaks are the results of intrusion of coastal water in the Bay of Bengal aided through low river discharge, while the autumn cholera outbreaks are the result of flooding caused by high river discharge. Importantly, cholera incidence in this region has been historically linked to environmental and climate variables such as precipitation, floods, river level, sea surface temperature, coastal salinity, dissolved organic material and faecal contamination. Also, ponds known as *pukurs*

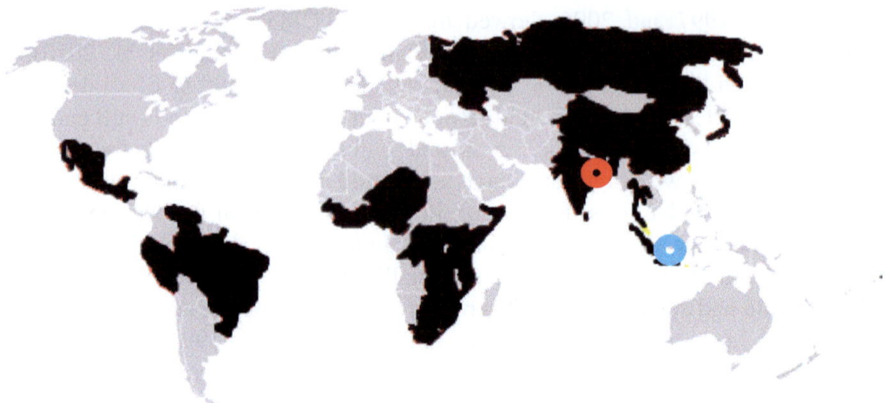

Fig. 1 Countries that have experienced cholera outbreaks during the seventh cholera pandemic. *Black shading* indicates areas where cholera outbreaks have occurred. The *red circle* (India) indicates the origin of the first six pandemics, while the *blue circle* (Indonesia) indicates the origin of the seventh pandemic (Data compiled from the WHO and CDC)

in common Bengali parlance are a source of *V. cholerae* for cholera outbreaks, as many country folk use the water not only for washing purposes but also for drinking purposes.

4 Cholera Outbreaks in Specific Countries of South-East Asia

As per the classification of the SEARO by WHO, this region is constituted by 11 countries. These include Bangladesh, India, Nepal, Sri Lanka, Bhutan, Thailand, Indonesia, Maldives, Myanmar, Timor-Leste and the Democratic People's Republic of Korea. Outbreak of cholera will be covered in these WHO Member States first before moving on to some other countries in the region, which although do not fall within the WHO classification, we feel should not be left out as some of these countries have also experienced cholera outbreaks from time to time. These include Malaysia, Singapore, Philippines, Vietnam and Laos.

4.1 Bangladesh

Bangladesh is a low-lying South Asian country with a population of over 164 million people that lies mainly within the broad delta of the Ganges and Brahmaputra rivers. Given its location, the country has often been the victim of devastating floods and cyclones. It is the most densely populated country in the world, with an estimated 1,102 people /km^2. Although the country's population growth is declining rapidly, its population is still expected to reach more than 215 million by 2040 (World Bank 2011).

Bangladesh has a gross domestic product (GDP) per capita of USD 560 (in 2008)—placing it among the least developed countries in the world. Around 40 % of the population lives below the poverty line, with approximately 20 % being considered very poor. Around 20 % of the population does not have access to safe drinking water and 64 % do not have improved sanitation (United Nations 2008). An estimated 44 % of the population over the age of 15 is still illiterate. However, despite these statistics, Bangladesh has been making steady economic progress over the past two decades, achieving economic growth rates of 4–5 % per year since 2004. During this period, Bangladesh has made impressive improvements in the health status of its population, compared to other nations in South Asia. Life expectancy at birth has risen from 55 years in 1991 to 66 years by 2008 (World Bank 2013), with inappreciable differences between male and female populations.

The three top causes of death in Bangladesh for all ages are pneumonia (14 %), respiratory failure (7.5 %) and diarrhoea (6.26 %) (WHO 2005). Diarrhoeal disease was the number one cause of hospitalisation at public health facilities in 2008, which accounted for more than 15 % of all admissions. Importantly, diarrhoeal disease due to *V. cholerae* continues to be a major problem in Bangladesh (Sack et al. 2003).

Cholera in Bangladesh occurs both as endemic disease, with seasonal peaks before and after the monsoons, and in epidemics that often take place during or following the frequent floods, droughts and cyclones that occur in the country.

As in most developing countries, Bangladesh does not have a national surveillance system that can identify cholera through laboratory diagnosis. Most of the available information on cholera has been generated by the ICDDR,B, which has conducted cholera-related research since 1960 and treats cholera patients both in its hospital in Dhaka and at its field station hospital in Matlab. Based on the available disease surveillance data of ICDDR,B and disease outbreak data, the Institute of Epidemiology, Disease Control & Research (IEDCR) estimates annual 450,000 cholera cases each year in Bangladesh. The diarrhoeal hospital of ICDDR,B estimates about 300,000 severe cholera cases requiring hospitalisation each year in the country. Importantly, for each hospitalised case there are three more cases in the community. This gives around 1,200,000 infections due to *V. cholerae* each year.

Cholera is both a rural and an urban disease in Bangladesh. It is associated with poor sanitation, contaminated water supplies—including surface water and shallow tube wells that are the main sources of drinking water in rural areas—as well as crowded living conditions, such as those found in the country's urban slums. Tube wells, until recently were considered a safe source of drinking water particularly in rural areas are now contaminated with arsenic, forcing people to revert back to using untreated surface water from *pukurs* and rivers.

Few cholera outbreaks have been reported during the past few years. However, in September 1991, a major outbreak of cholera broke out in Bangladesh, which

Table 1 1991 cholera outbreak in Bangladesh: Epidemic investigation by ECPP

Regions	No. of cases with watery diarrhoea	No. of rectal swabs collected	*V. cholerae* 01	
			Positive	Rate per 1,000 swabs
North-West	1,265	266	137	515
North-East	1,598	507	299	589
Mid-West	162	56	36	642
Total	3,025	829	472	569[a]

[a] 95 % CI: 535–603

started in the North-Western region and spread throughout most of the northern part of the country. The government epidemic surveillance between September and November 1991, reported 214,856 cases of diarrhoea with 2,620 deaths (Siddique et al. 1992). In 1985, escalation of cholera epidemics prompted the Government of Bangladesh (GOB) and the ICDDR,B to develop an Epidemic Control Preparedness Programme (ECPP). The ECPP, between 1985 and 1991, collaborated with the GOB health services in the investigation of and intervention in diarrhoeal epidemics in nearly 400 rural *upazilas* (sub-districts). During the 1991 outbreak, the ECPP physicians saw 4,018 diarrhoea patients during their epidemic investigations; 3,025 (75 %) had acute watery diarrhoea from which 829 rectal swabs were collected (Table 1). Table 1 also shows the *V. cholerae* isolation rates from each of the regions. The overall *V. cholerae* 01 isolation was 569 cases per 1,000 rectal swabs (95 % CI: 535–603).

Besides the outbreak in 1991, there were a number of outbreaks in Bangladesh between 1985 and 1990. The GOB carried out epidemic surveillance, which was supplemented by the surveillance carried out by the ECPP. There were a large number of cases in 1987 and 1988. In those years, there were severe floods that affected most of the country, particularly the northern and the middle regions, perhaps increasing the number of cases during these periods (Table 2). Importantly, Table 2 also shows the number of cases treated by the ECPP physicians and the rate of *V. cholerae* 01 isolations.

The region-wise distribution of *V. cholerae* 01 by biotype is depicted in Table 3.

In 1992, *V. cholerae* 0139 Bengal emerged in Bangladesh, which is a derivative of the El Tor biotype that was responsible for an extensive epidemic. This new serogroup has now been detected in 11 countries and warrants close surveillance. While currently there is no evidence available to gauge the significance of these developments, the possibility of a new pandemic cannot be ruled out.

Several programmes and initiatives are in place to control cholera. Following research conducted on oral rehydration solution (ORS) by the ICDDR,B, the government has established a Control of Diarrhoeal Disease (CDD) Program throughout the country. Several initiatives, both by the government as well as non-governmental organisations (NGOs) to increase awareness about the benefits of ORS has led to a significant decrease in case fatality rates due to diarrhoeal diseases, including cholera.

Table 2 Diarrhoea epidemic surveillance of outbreaks in Bangladesh: 1985–1990

Government epidemic surveillance			ECPP epidemic investigation			
Year	No. of attacks	No. of deaths	No. of cases examined	No. of rectal swabs collected	*V. cholerae* 01	
					No. of positive	Per cent
1985	47,150	4,101	4,983	296	112	37.8
1986	53,046	3,997	3,432	211	78	36.9
1987[a]	303,391	4,726	3,692	312	141	45.1
1988[a]	988,391	3,676	13,879	1,967	764	38.8
1989	43,535	1,783	1,821[b]	419	226	53.9
1990	48,916	1,309	–[b]	–	–	–

[a] Years of heavy flooding

[b] ECPP non-operational from June 1989 to December 1990

Table 3 Distribution of *V. cholerae* 01 by biotype and region: Bangladesh (September 1988–May 1989)

Regions	No. of rectal swabs collected	*V. cholerae* 01 positive		
		Classical	El Tor	Rate per 1,000 swabs
North-Western	131	0	55	442
North-Eastern	702	2	272	359
Middle Belt	1,021	1	414	339
Southern	532	164	43	375
Total	2,386	167	784	

Regarding water and sanitation, a number of large donor-supported projects are being implemented to improve population access to safe water and adequate sanitation. These projects include the construction of piped water systems and water treatment facilities in urban areas, arsenic mitigation in rural areas and decentralised initiatives to build improved sanitation facilities. The Director General of Health Services (DGHS) has a diarrhoeal case-reporting system in place from all the districts and *upazila* (sub-district) hospitals in the country, but cholera surveillance is not routinely conducted by the Government, due to the lack of systematic laboratory testing in government facilities for the disease. This is why, in an effort to build an early warning system for infectious disease outbreaks, the IEDCR has developed a sentinel site, hospital-based Priority Communicable Disease Surveillance (PCDS) system, which tracks 13 priority diseases, including acute watery diarrhoea and others. In addition, IEDCR conducts laboratory-based surveillance during cholera outbreaks, often in collaboration with ICDDR,B. Several long-term, laboratory-confirmed surveillance studies of cholera and other diarrhoeal diseases are being conducted.

Overall, cholera is both endemic and causes epidemics in Bangladesh. Case fatality due to cholera is low, but mortality is still too high in the country.

Providing access to all Bangladeshis with adequate care for cholera and the prevention of severe dehydration requires increasing household use of ORS in rural areas and slums, and the use and access of public sector health facilities for the treatment of diarrhoeal diseases by the population. Improvement in the water and sanitation facilities for the whole population is likely to take many years, during which time cholera vaccination in the high risk population could provide a short- to medium-term solution to control the disease in Bangladesh. Moreover, it should be noted that cholera is not officially reported from Bangladesh. This could have political connotations or could arise from embargoes on trade and travel. However, this mindset needs to change in order to tackle the problem in a more holistic fashion.

4.2 India

India, which comprises 28 states and seven union territories, has a total population of 1.27 billion people and approximately two-thirds of the population lives in rural areas, where only 28 % use piped drinking water and 26 % access to good sanitation (MOHFW, Govt. of India 2013). Therefore, it is but natural that cholera continues to be an important public health problem in India. Cholera cases are severely under-reported mainly because disease surveillance is incomplete, laboratory capacity, especially in peripheral health centres, is inadequate. Importantly, the ground reality is that there is a breakdown in sanitation and safe water supply, which is often not acknowledged by the authorities for fear of societal repercussions.

Over the last decade or so, a large number of cholera outbreaks have occurred in India, with the highest frequency in West Bengal and Odisha (formerly Orissa). The other states which have reported cholera outbreaks include Tamil Nadu, Karnataka, Gujarat, Andhra Pradesh, Maharashtra, Punjab, Haryana and Delhi. These outbreaks are briefly described below.

4.2.1 West Bengal

In May 2010, a cluster of diarrhoeal disease cases were reported among the inmates of a shelter-home for mentally retarded females in Parbaksi village of Howrah district in West Bengal. Of the 101 inmates, 91 (90 %) developed diarrhoea, and three patients died (case fatality: 3 %). Four of the five stool specimens were positive for *V. cholerae* O1 Ogawa. Importantly, drinking of water from the pond-connected tube well (adjusted odds ratio: 25.7; 95 % CI: 2.7–236.4) was associated with the illness. Relocation of the pond-connected tube well away from the groundwater tube well, colour-coding of the tube wells meant for drinking purposes and regular disinfection of the tube wells were recommended (Datta et al. 2012).

In March 2010, an outbreak of diarrhoeal disease was reported among workers of a jute mill in Kolkata, West Bengal. Rectal swabs were collected from the hospitalised case-patients, and the local water supply system was assessed. In total, 197 case patients were identified among 5,910 residents of the workers' colony (attack rate: 3.33 %). Of 24 stool samples, 15 were positive for *V. cholerae* O1. The outbreak started on 7 March, peaked on 11 March and ended on 16 March 2010. Compared to 120 controls, 60 cases did not differ in terms of age and socioeconomic status. Drinking water from the reservoir within the mill premises was associated with the outbreak, which had been contaminated during a strike at which time the mill was closed. The outbreak occurred almost immediately after the strike was called off and the mill reopened (Mridha et al. 2011).

The year 2009 was marked by the occurrence of the super-cyclone *Aila* that passed through West Bengal and entered Bangladesh to wreak havoc. Three independent studies were carried out that centred around this cyclone. In one study, it was observed that following *Aila*, at the end of May, a block in the Sunderbans area of West Bengal reported increased cases of diarrhoea (Bhunia and Ghosh 2011). A matched case-control study was conducted and rectal swabs and water specimens were collected. In total, 1,076 probable case patients and 14 deaths (attack rate: 44/10,000) were identified. *V. cholerae* O1 El Tor Ogawa was isolated from two of the five probable case-patients' stool specimens. The outbreak started in the fourth week of May, with two peaks in the second and fourth weeks of June, and lasted until August 2009. Compared with controls, cases were more likely to drink non-chlorinated piped water [matched odds ratio (mOR): 16; 95 % CI: 4.9–51; population attributable fraction: 58 %] and were less likely to drink chlorine-treated water (mOR: 0.06; 95 % CI: 0.02–0.18). Villagers had broken the water pipelines near their houses for easy access to water, which subsequently led to faecal contamination. Importantly, there is a need for more education efforts at the ground level with regard to hygiene and sanitation. Another study examined two subdivisions in the district of Midnapore (East) in West Bengal, immediately following the aftermath of the tropical cyclone *Aila* (Panda et al. 2011). Significantly, increased occurrence of diarrhoea was observed in June 2009 in two subdivisions, namely Haldia and Egra (OR 1.6 and 1.3 respectively; 95 % CI: 1.52–1.65 and 1.21–1.32; $p < 0.001$) considering 2007 as baseline. *V. cholerae* grew from 54 % of the stool samples (21/39; 17 *V. cholerae* O1-Ogawa and four non-O1-non-139), confirming a community outbreak of cholera. Increased rate of admission in treatment centres due to diarrhoea in the whole district coincided with the formation of cyclone and showed over two-fold rise compared to the admission recorded 6 days prior. Haldia subdivision had the highest attack rate of nine per 1,000 in the month of June, 2009 whereas for the whole district it was five per 1,000 in the same month. It may be concluded from the study that pre-*Aila* changes in the environment, *Aila* and seasonality of diarrhoea in the study district interplayed towards increased occurrence of diarrhoea. The third study supported the other two studies as it investigated the environmental sources of *V. cholerae* associated with the cholera outbreak post-*Aila* (Palit and Batabyal 2010). A total of 33 water samples (from tap, tubewell and ponds) were analysed. From them, 11

(33.3 %) samples were found to be contaminated with *V. cholerae* among which 5 (45 %) isolates were *V. cholerae* O1 biotype Ogawa. Three (36 %) *V. cholerae* isolates were found to be *ctxB* positive (2 *ctxB* Classical).

The year 2006 saw another cholera outbreak in West Bengal (Bhunia et al. 2009). In April 2006, Garulia municipality reported a cluster of diarrhoea cases. A total of 298 cases of diarrhoea were reported to various healthcare facilities (attack rate: 3.5/1,000; no deaths). The attack rate was highest among children (6.4/1,000). *V. cholerae* El Tor O1 Inaba was isolated from two of seven rectal swabs. The outbreak started on 10 April, peaked on 26 April and lasted till 6 May. Importantly, cases clustered in an area distal to leaking water pipelines. Drinking municipal water exclusively was significantly associated with the illness (OR 13; 95 % CI: 6.5–27). Out of the 12 water specimens from the affected area, 8 had faecal contamination and poor chlorine content.

In rural West Bengal, outbreaks of cholera are often centred around ponds (*pukurs*) that is a feature of the environment. Five investigations of laboratory-confirmed, pond-centred outbreaks of cholera occurred between the years 2004 and 2008 (Mukherjee et al. 2011). Case–control odds ratios were approximated with relative risks (RRs) as the incidence was low. The environment was investigated to understand how the ponds could have become contaminated and could have infected villagers. These outbreaks led to 277 cases and three deaths (median attack rate: 51/1,000 people; case fatality: 1.1 %; median age of case-patients: 22 years; median duration: 13 days; range: 6–15 days). Factors significantly ($p < 0.05$) associated with cholera in the case-control ($n = 4$) and cohort investigations ($n = 1$) included washing utensils in ponds (four outbreaks; RR range: 6–12), bathing (three outbreaks; RR range: 3.5–9.3) and exposure to pond water, including drinking (two outbreaks; RR range: 2.1–3.2), mouth washing (one outbreak; RR: 4.8) and cooking (one outbreak; RR: 3.0). Initial case-patients contaminated ponds through washing soiled clothes ($n = 4$) or defecation ($n = 1$). This study reiterates the fact that ubiquitous ponds used for many purposes transmit cholera in West Bengal and there is a need for focused health education, hygiene and sanitation in order to protect the villagers.

4.2.2 Odisha

A large outbreak of cholera occurred during April–July 2009 in the Kendrapada district of Odisha (Pal et al. 2013). A total of 41 rectal swabs and 41 water samples, collected from diarrhoeal patients and from different villages were bacteriologically analysed for the isolation of bacterial enteropathogens, antibiogram profile and detection of various toxin genes. The bacteriological analyses of rectal swabs and environmental water samples revealed the presence of *V. cholerae* O1 Ogawa biotype El Tor. The multiplex polymerase chain reaction (PCR) assay on *V. cholerae* strains revealed the presence of *ctxA* and *tcpA* genes. The mismatch amplification of mutation assay (MAMA) PCR on clinical and environmental isolates of *V. cholerae* revealed that the strains were El Tor biotype, which harboured the *ctx* gene of the classical strain. The random amplified polymorphic DNA (RAPD) PCR analysis and pulsed-field gel electrophoresis (PFGE) results indicated that the *V. cholerae* isolates belonged to the same clone. The investigation gives a warning that the El Tor variant of *V. cholerae* has spread to the coastal areas of Odisha that requires closer monitoring and surveillance.

An outbreak of cholera in Odisha in 2008 (Kumar et al. 2009) resulted in collection of 32 *V. cholerae* isolates. All the isolates belonged to serogroup O1, biotype El Tor, serotype Ogawa. Two multiplex PCR assays confirmed the presence of various toxigenic and pathogenic genes in all of the isolates, suggesting infection of isolates by classical CTXφ. The molecular diversity of *V. cholerae* isolates studied by enterobacterial repetitive intergenic consensus sequence PCR, BOX-PCR and RAPD analysis uniformly showed the clonal relationship among the outbreak *V. cholerae* O1 isolates. The results of this study suggest that cholera-causing *V. cholerae* strains are constantly evolving in epidemic areas, highlighting the potential of the emergence of more virulent strains.

An outbreak of cholera occurred in Kashipur and Dasmantpur blocks of Odisha during July–September 2007 (Pal et al. 2010). A total of 60 rectal swabs and 28 water samples collected from diarrhoea patients at different hospitals and villages were bacteriologically analysed for the identification, antibiogram and detection of toxic genes of *V. cholerae*. The outbreak was caused by *V. cholerae* O1 Ogawa biotype El Tor in both Kashipur and Dasmantpur blocks. The multiplex PCR assay revealed that all the clinical and environmental *V. cholerae* isolates were positive for the *ctxA* and *tcpA* genes, showing biotype El Tor. Interestingly, 88 % of the *ctxB* gene of the classical strain, as confirmed by MAMA-PCR assay. Importantly, this was the first report of the El Tor variant of *V. cholerae* O1 Ogawa having the *ctxB* gene of the classical strain with altered antibiogram causing epidemics of cholera in Odisha.

Two sequential outbreaks of severe diarrhoea were investigated in two neighbouring villages of Odisha in 2005 (Das et al. 2009a). The attack rates were 5.6 % (n = 62) and 5.2 % (n = 51), respectively. One death was reported in the second village (case fatality: 2 %). Consumption of milk products prepared in the household of the index case (mOR: 5.7; 95 % CI: 1.7–30] in the first village and drinking well water in the second village were associated with the illness (mOR: 4.7; 95 % CI: 1.6–19). *V. cholerae* El Tor O1 Ogawa was isolated from stool samples from both the villages. Mishandling of milk products led to the cholera outbreak in the first village, which led to sewerage contamination of a well and another outbreak in the second village. The study re-emphasises the need to prevent environmental contamination during cholera outbreaks.

In November 2003, an outbreak of severe diarrhoea was reported from Parbatia, a village in Odisha (Das et al. 2009b). There were 41 cases, with an attack rate of 4.3 %, and no deaths. Thirteen of these cases were hospitalised. A matched case-control study was conducted to identify the possible exposure variables. Descriptive epidemiology suggested clustering of cases around one public well. *V. cholerae* El Tor O1, serotype Ogawa was isolated from four of six rectal swabs. The water from the public well was associated with the outbreak (mOR: 12; 95 %

CI: 1.2–44.1). On the basis of these conclusions, access to the well was immediately barred. Importantly, the study highlights the broader use of field epidemiology methods to implement public health actions guided by epidemiologic data to control an epidemic of cholera.

4.2.3 Tamil Nadu

An outbreak of cholera occurred in Uthamapalayam village, Theni district of Tamil Nadu in May 2010 (Sekar et al. 2012). Stool and rectal swab specimens were collected from the randomly selected patients attending the Government Theni Medical College (GTMC) Hospital and various primary healthcare centres of Theni district for bacteriological investigation. Of the 66 faecal samples collected, *V. cholerae* O1 was isolated in 37 samples (56 %). All the isolates of *V. cholerae* were identified as El Tor biotype and Ogawa serotype. The samples collected from the village were found to be contaminated with El Tor *V. cholerae* O1, Ogawa serotype. During this outbreak, one death was recorded.

Cholera has been associated with rainfall and flooding events by contamination of potable water with environmental *V. cholerae*. The continuation of the epidemic in a region, however, is often due to secondary transmission of the initial outbreak strain through human excreta. A study from Chennai, Tamil Nadu reports, on the contrary, a rapid shift of genotype from one *V. cholerae* strain to another one in an epidemic region (Goel and Jiang 2011). The isolates were characterised by PCR, antibiogram and genomic fingerprinting analysis. The results showed that in spite of the similarity of toxin genes and antibiogram, the *Vibrio* isolates grouped into two different clusters based on the ERIC-PCR fingerprinting. Each cluster corresponded to a distinct peak of cholera outbreak, which occurred after separate heavy rainfall. The results suggested that the rainfall event can bring various genotypes of *V. cholerae* strains causing multiple outbreaks.

4.2.4 Karnataka

A cholera outbreak occurred in a village in Kolar district of Karnataka in early 2012 (Deepthi et al. 2013). A total of 73 cases were reported during the outbreak, with an attack rate of 17.5 %. Attack rates were similar among males and females and the highest rates were observed among the elderly (33.3 %), while the lowest rates were observed among adults (14.7 %). Importantly, most households (81 %) surveyed did not use any method of water purification, 79.7 % practiced open field defecation and 58.2 % practiced inadequate hand washing, indicating poor sanitary practices. Cases were most commonly observed in houses which did not practice any method of water purification ($p < 0.001$) and among people living below the poverty line ($p = 0.02$). Of importance, despite the high attack rate, no deaths were reported.

4.2.5 Gujarat

An outbreak of gastroenteritis broke out in Lalpur town, Jamnagar district of Gujarat on 19 December 2010 (Shah et al. 2012). Although initially 57 cases were reported, this number increased to 330 between 19 December 2010 and 2 January 2011. Nineteen patients were found to be positive for *V. cholerae* O1 (Ogawa) out of 117 stool samples. The outbreak had an attack rate of 1.88 % with no mortality. Investigations revealed that the epidemic was waterborne. Ten leakages were found in the pipelines of the affected areas of Lalpur town.

4.2.6 Andhra Pradesh

Thirty-four *V. cholerae* isolates collected from a cholera outbreak in Hyderabad, Andhra Pradesh in 2010 (Goel et al. 2011), were found to belong to serogroup O1 biotype El Tor serotype Ogawa. All the isolates were found to be PCR positive for *ctxAB*, *ompW*, *rflO1*, *rtxC* and *tcpA* genes. All the isolates but one harboured *rstR* (El Tor) allele. However, one isolate carried both *rstR* (El Tor) as well as *rstR* (Classical) alleles. Cholera toxin (*ctxB*) genotyping of the isolates confirmed the presence of altered CTB of classical biotype in all the isolates. The results of this study suggest that altered El Tor biotype *V. cholerae* with the classical cholera toxin gene are involved in cholera outbreaks in India.

4.2.7 Maharashtra

A cholera outbreak occurred in Solapur, Maharashtra in 2010 (Jain et al. 2011). A total of 41 *V. cholerae* isolates were found to belong to serogroup O1, biotype El Tor and serotype Ogawa. All the isolates harboured *rstR* (El Tor) allele indicating the presence of CTXΦ (El Tor). However, cholera toxin (*ctxB*) gene sequencing and a *ctxB* allele specific PCR of the isolates confirmed the presence of *ctxB* of classical biotype. All the isolates were PCR positive for class 1 integron and SXT elements also. Fingerprinting analysis revealed the clonal relationship among the outbreak isolates. The results suggested the involvement of multi-drug resistant *V. cholerae* El Tor biotype isolates having *ctxB* gene of classical biotype in the cholera outbreak.

4.2.8 Punjab and Haryana

In Punjab and Haryana states of northern India, during July–September 2007, six clusters of cholera outbreak were identified (Taneja et al. 2009). A total of 745 case-patients were admitted to local governmental hospitals; the attack rate was 183/1,000 population. Four deaths were reported (case-fatality rate: 0.5 %). The number of cases per cluster varied from 15 to 400, and adults were primarily affected (74 %); 20 % of patients had severe dehydration. *V. cholerae* O1 Ogawa was confirmed from stool cultures by using standard techniques. Of 53 water samples tested during the 2007 outbreak, 4 grew *V. cholerae*. Three samples were confirmed to be non-O1, non-139 strains. Only one isolate was *V. cholerae* O1, which was positive for *tcp*, *ctxA* and *ctxB* of both Classical and El Tor types. The four deaths from cholera, along with adult preponderance, high attack rate, more severe illness and six different clusters, point towards a change in the disease's epidemiology. This change may be related to circulation of the hybrid vibrios in the region.

4.2.9 Chandigarh

An outbreak of cholera occurred in Chandigarh in 2002 (Taneja et al. 2009). In this outbreak one death was reported (case-fatality rate: <0.01 %); the attack rate was 20/1,000, 58.6 % were children and only 10 % had severe dehydration.

4.2.10 Delhi

There was a cholera outbreak in Delhi in 2005 (Rajeshwari et al. 2008). *V. cholerae* O1 El Tor serotype Ogawa has been responsible for most of the cholera outbreaks in India. The 2005 outbreak in Delhi documented the occurrence of *V. cholerae* O1 Inaba as a predominant causative organism of cholera in children. All strains isolated were sensitive to gentamicin and a high level of resistance towards nalidixic acid and amoxicillin was seen. No case fatality was reported.

4.3 Nepal

Nepal, officially known as the Democratic Republic of Nepal, is a landlocked sovereign state located in South Asia. It is located in the Himalayas and bordered to the north by China, and to the south, east and west by India. It has a population of approximately 27 million, with approximately 2 million absentee workers living abroad.

Documented cholera is fairly new to Nepal. The first report of cholera was officially published in the years 1958–1960 in Kathmandu by a medical doctor visiting Nepal (Dixit et al. 2011). In November 2011, there was a small outbreak of cholera in Saptari district of eastern Nepal, which was investigated by the B.P. Koirala Institute of Health Sciences. Importantly, two people from *Tilathi* village died in this outbreak. Clinical and water samples were collected from three wards with active cases of diarrhoeal illness. Five clinical samples from symptomatic individuals without any antibiotic administration and four water samples (pond and underground) were collected for investigation. The causative agent of diarrhoeal illness was found to be *V. cholerae* O1, El Tor, Ogawa serotype, in three clinical and water samples each. Phenotypically, the isolates from the pond water samples were identical to the samples isolated from the patients. This finding suggests that the clinical isolates probably disseminated from the pond. In this context, the villagers had recently celebrated one of their important festivals, *Chhath*; the rituals for which are performed in ponds. Moreover, the habit of open defecation and use of pond water as a major source of water for drinking, cooking and bathing had a foremost role in the cholera outbreak. Importantly, the people seemed to be aware of the spread of diarrhoeal illnesses but were not motivated to use their toilets at home, thereby aggravating the problem.

There was an outbreak of diarrhoeal diseases in districts of far-western region of Nepal in early-2009 followed by a massive outbreak in Jajarkot district of mid-western region in late-2009 (Bhandari and Bhusal 2013). A descriptive study was conducted from three districts of the far-western region (Achham, Baitadi and Doti) from middle of April to September 2009 to observe the trend of morbidity. Similarly, 51 stool samples were taken from the patients for laboratory analysis. Out of the total 51 stool samples tested, 27 were diagnosed as *V. cholerae.* All the isolates were sensitive to commonly used antibiotics except Nalidixic acid and Cotrimoxazole. The highest number of cases were seen in the month of July–August.

A prospective study was carried out at Dhulikhel Hospital, Kathmandu University Teaching Hospital, Kavrepalanchok during 1 May 2004 to 31 October 2004 (Tamang et al. 2005). A total of 148 stool samples from patients with acute diarrhoea were collected for investigation. Out of the 148 stool samples, 46 cases (31 %) were found to be positive for *V. cholerae* serogroup O1, biotype El Tor and serotype Ogawa. Both sexes were equally affected. The young age group of less than 30 years was mostly affected. *Brahmin* was the most affected ethnic group. The isolates were sensitive to all the antibiotics tested except cotrimoxazole. Among the laboratory-confirmed cholera cases 30 % exhibited co-infection with other parasites among which *Giardia lamblia* and *Ascaris lumbricoides* were the most common.

Seasonal outbreaks of cholera have been reported from Kathmandu in 1995 (Ise et al. 1996). *V. cholerae*, O1 biotype El Tor Ogawa was the major causative agent of these outbreaks. The pattern of spread suggested a waterborne infection related to contaminated river water and this was confirmed by a field survey. Although the mortality rate was low, younger children were more susceptible. It has been suggested that in the Kathmandu Valley, a major problem is the old water supply infrastructure, which is prone to leakages leading to contamination of the drinking water (Sharma 2006).

A study was conducted from May 1995 to April 1996 to track cholera outbreaks (Pokhrel and Kubo 1996). One thousand one hundred seven children with acute diarrhoea receiving Oral Rehydration Therapy (ORT) at National Kanti Children's Hospital were included in the study. Stool samples were investigated, but none showed growth of *V. cholerae* 0139 synonym Bengal. In Nepal, *V. cholerae* could be isolated from June to November. From December to May, no cases of

V. cholerae were detected. Mixed infections along with *V. cholerae* were also seen in 29 % of cholera patients. *V. cholerae* O1, Hikojima types were the major isolates in the study followed by Ogawa type. *V. cholerae*, Hikojima and Ogawa serotypes were associated with mixed infection in 16.1 and 12.9 % of patients, respectively. These isolates were associated with *Shigella*, *Salmonella* and pathogenic *E. coli.*

During 1991, a substantial cholera outbreak occurred in Nepal (WHO 1992). It presented as one of the causes of a multicausal gastroenteritis epidemic which reportedly resulted in nearly 92,000 cases and 1,800 deaths. The 1991 epidemic appeared to have been more severe with a longer duration than the epidemic which occurred in 1990. The overall case-fatality rate was 2.0 %. Cholera was confirmed in 63 % of faecal specimens processed, compared with 46 % during the 1990 epidemic. Specimens from the first and last laboratory-confirmed cases were collected on 14 June and 26 September 1991, respectively. The presence of cholera was confirmed in all five developmental regions in the country and contaminated water was incriminated in sustaining the transmission.

4.4 Sri Lanka

Sri Lanka, officially the Democratic Socialist Republic of Sri Lanka, is an island country in the northern Indian Ocean off the southern coast of the Indian subcontinent in South Asia, known until 1972 as Ceylon. Sri Lanka has maritime borders with India to the north-west and the Maldives to the south-west.

In all, there has been three publications from Sri Lanka that documents the spread of El Tor in the country during the early and mid-1970s (Mendis et al. 1975, 1977; Sivagnanasundram et al. 1975). However, no abstracts are available for these. Other than these, there are no reports of any cholera outbreaks.

4.5 Thailand

Thailand, officially the Kingdom of Thailand, formerly known as Siam, is a country located at the centre of the Indochina peninsula in South-East Asia. It is bordered in the north by Myanmar and Laos, in the east by Laos and Cambodia, in the south by the Gulf of Thailand and Malaysia and in the west by the Andaman Sea and the southern extremity of Myanmar.

A study was undertaken to characterise *V. cholerae* O1 isolates from outbreaks in Thailand with special reference to genotypic variations over time (Okada et al. 2012). A total of 343 isolates of *V. cholerae* O1 from cholera outbreaks from 2007 to 2010 were investigated, and 99.4 % were found to carry the classical cholera toxin B subunit (*ctxB*) and El Tor *rstR* genes. Pulsed-field gel electrophoresis differentiated the isolates into 10 distinct pulsotypes, clustered into two major groups, A and B, with an overall similarity of 88 %. Ribotyping, multiple-locus variable-number tandem-repeat analysis (MLVA), and PCR to detect Vibrio seventh pandemic island II (VSP-II) related genes of randomly selected isolates from each pulsotype corresponded to the results obtained by PFGE. Epidemiological investigations revealed that MLVA type 2 was strongly associated with a cholera outbreak in north-eastern Thailand in 2007, while MLVA type 7 dominated the outbreaks of the southern Gulf areas in 2009 and MLVA type 4 dominated the outbreaks of the central Gulf areas during 2009–2010. Only MLVA type 16 isolates were found in a Thai–Myanmar border area in 2010, whereas those of MLVA types 26, 39 and 41 predominated this border area in 2008. Type 39 then disappeared 1–2 years later as MLVA type 41 became prevalent. Type 41 was also found to infect an outbreak area. Importantly, in the present study, MLVA provided a high-throughput genetic typing tool for understanding the in-depth epidemiology of cholera outbreaks.

A number of outbreaks of food borne cholera have occurred in Thailand over the years. Two consecutive outbreaks involved the consumption of Hainanese chicken rice, a Chinese delicacy, in north-western Thailand in April 2010 (Swaddiwudhipong et al. 2012). The two outbreaks involved persons who attended two meetings. The first outbreak involved 17 cholera cases (35.4 %) among 48 attendants and 16 cases in the community. The onset of symptoms was between 19 and 23 April 2010. People who ate the chicken rice had a higher attack rate of infection than those who did not. All 12 food handlers at the implicated food shop were screened for cholera infection by rectal swab, culture; three were culture-positive. Although the food shop was closed temporarily following the outbreak, some chicken rice was produced and served at the second meeting and caused 11 more cases (23.4 %) among 47 meeting attendants. All cholera isolates obtained from patients and food handlers were *V. cholerae* O1, biotype El Tor and serotype Ogawa. Another foodborne cholera outbreak occurred among tourists in a cruise liner sailing in South-East Asia (Boyce et al. 1995). Serum samples were collected from all passengers reporting diarrhoea. A case was defined as diarrhoeal illness with onset between 8 and 28 February 1994 and a cholera antitoxic titer more than or equal to 800. Six passengers met the case definition. Illness was associated with eating yellow rice at a buffet restaurant in Bangkok. This international outbreak demonstrates foodborne transmission of *V. cholerae* O139 Bengal, an emerging cause of epidemic cholera in Asia, to tourists from Western countries. Another foodborne outbreak of cholera occurred in July 1988 with 71 culture-confirmed cases of biotype El Tor, serotype Ogawa, which occurred in a non-endemic area in Mae Sot district, Tak Province (Swaddiwudhipong et al. 1992). Fifty-two cases had diarrhoea and 19 had asymptomatic cholera infection. No deaths were recorded. Epidemiological investigation revealed a significant association between cholera infection and the consumption of uncooked beef. The beef was possibly contaminated with *V. cholerae* O1 from an infected butcher. In yet another outbreak of foodborne cholera, which occurred in a village near Chiangmai in October 1987, 264 attendants of a funeral were affected (Swaddiwudhipong et al. 1990). All the attendants were screened for infection by bacteriological examination of their rectal swabs and were kept under diarrhoeal surveillance. Of them, 20 patients and 40 matched controls were interviewed about the details of their eating foods served at the funeral. *V. cholerae* O1, Inaba, El Tor was detected from 24 persons (9.1 %), 15 of whom suffered from mild diarrhoea and the rest 9 had inapparent infections. There were no deaths. The only significant association ($p < 0.01$; OR = 15) was found between an attack of cholera and eating *laeb-moo*—an uncooked pork preparation with Thai spices and chilli. The transmission of cholera appeared to have occurred through eating the uncooked pork presumably due to its contamination with *V. cholerae* shed by the infected butcher. As outbreaks of foodborne diseases, including cholera, have been reported frequently after the consumption of raw food in many parts of Thailand, preventive educational efforts should be directed towards modifying the traditional behaviour patterns of consuming raw food among the Thai people.

A couple of nosocomial cholera outbreaks have been reported from Thailand over the years. One study reports nosocomial cholera outbreak in a general hospital located in a Thai–Myanmar border area (Swaddiwudhipong and Peanumlom 2010). Between May and October 2007, a community outbreak of cholera with 477 cases took place in Mae Sot District, Tak Province. A 71-year-old diabetic female who had undergone craniotomy following intracerebral haemorrhage contracted nosocomial cholera with mild diarrhoea on 6 August 2007, 37 days after admission in a female ward of the Mae Sot hospital. She received a nasogastric tube-fed diet four times a day. The investigation suggested that the tube-fed diet might have been contaminated with *V. cholerae* O1 directly from an infected caregiver. Importantly, the concerned caregiver was culture-positive for cholera of the same biotype, serotype and antibiograms. Another study reports that from 30 October to 7 December 1984, an outbreak of nosocomial cholera involving 11 cases of biotype El Tor, serotype Inaba, took place in a 755-bed hospital in southern Thailand (Swaddiwudhipong and Kunasol 1989). The outbreak occurred primarily among patients admitted with severe illness. Of the 11 cases, 7 were children and 4 were adults. Most cases had mild symptoms of cholera and no case died in the outbreak. The first two cases occurred sporadically with a subsequent cluster of cases showing an explosive pattern. A case–control study found that a history of receiving liquid tube-fed diet was significantly more common among cholera cases than their matched controls, but it could not be determined how the diet was contaminated with cholera.

Outbreaks of cholera occurred twice in the same institutional home for mentally retarded persons, once in 1987 (Swaddiwudhipong and Limpakarnjanarat 1991) and again in 1992 (Jiraphongsa et al. 1994). The first outbreak in June–July 1987 was caused by *V. cholerae* O1, biotype El Tor, serotype Inaba. Of the 447 retarded inmates, 74 were found to be infected and 1 died. The second outbreak occurred between 29 July and 9 August 1992, and was due to the Ogawa strain. The clinical attack rate was 8 % of 440 children; there were two deaths.

Cholera outbreaks occurred in Thailand in 2007 (Okada et al. 2010). Isolates from the north-eastern regions were analysed. Interestingly, the outbreak strain was identified as biotype El Tor; serotype Ogawa with cholera toxin B subunit gene (*ctxB*) of the classical type and CTX prophage repressor gene of the El Tor type. The clone was genetically closely related to pulsotype H, which is predominantly found in India. It was probably subsequently introduced into Thailand quite recently.

There was a cholera outbreak in 2007 that involved mainly Myanmar migrants living in overcrowded conditions with poor sanitation in a Thai–Myanmar border district (Swaddiwudhipong et al. 2008). Both passive and active case surveillance were carried out in Mae Sot District, Tak Province since the beginning of the outbreak. Samples of various types of drinking and non-drinking water from the infected areas, communal waters and some selected foods were analysed for the presence of cholera contamination. A case–control study was conducted to determine the vehicle of cholera transmission among Myanmar migrants in one municipal community with a cluster of 72 cholera cases. Between May and October 2007, 477 cholera cases of biotype El Tor, serotype Inaba, were identified in the district. The majority of them (93.1 %) were detected by active case surveillance in the communities. None died in this outbreak. Most (84.9 %) were Myanmar migrants and the remainder were local Thai residents. Three samples of seafood illegally imported from Myanmar were positive for cholera of the same biotype and serotype. A total of 15 of 324 (4.6 %) food handlers in the district were found to carry *V. cholerae* O1. A case–control study in one municipal community revealed a significant association between infection and frequently having food purchased from one infected food handler.

An unusually high incidence of *V. cholerae* O1 infection was observed in southern Thailand between late December 1997 and March 1998. Fifty-seven *V. cholerae* O1 strains were isolated in five provinces during the outbreak and were examined (Kondo et al. 2001). They were El Tor Ogawa strains exhibiting similar antibiograms. All strains were resistant to tetracycline, which had not been reported in Thailand since 1993. All southern Thailand strains and the 1998 international traveller strain of Thai origin showed indistinguishable genetic fingerprinting patterns that were distinct from those of other test strains. The results suggest that a tetracycline-resistant clone newly emerged in late December 1997 caused the large outbreak in southern Thailand and that the variants with a slightly different antibiogram appeared during the course of the spreading epidemic.

An epidemic of a cholera-like disease occurred among Khmers in a camp in Aranyaprathet, Thailand, in May 1990 (Bagchi et al. 1993). Of 215 patients with diarrhoea, *V. cholerae* O1 was isolated from 25 (12 %) and *V. cholerae* non-O1 was isolated from 15 (7 %). Five of 15 (33 %) non-O1 *V. cholerae* isolates hybridised with two different oligonucleotide probes previously used to detect *V. cholerae* non-O1 that produces a heat-stable toxin. Importantly, this was the first description of an epidemic of diarrhoea caused by *V. cholerae* non-O1 that produces heat-stable toxin.

From September through October 1987, a cholera outbreak involving 59 cases of biotype El Tor, serotype Inaba occurred in Sunpathong district, Chiang Mai (Swaddiwudhipong et al. 1989). No cases died. A total of 27 cases were males and 32 were females. The age ranged between 4 months and 85 years, with a median of 36 years. The outbreak affected seven small communities, and showed different vehicles of infection. Six housewives and one girl were infected with cholera in the first localised outbreak. The transmission of infection appeared due to the consumption of packed food contaminated by an infected food handler. In the second localised outbreak, six young males acquired cholera after eating uncooked fish harvested from a canal contaminated with *V. cholerae*. Another outbreak of cholera with 24 culture-confirmed cases occurred among guests at a funeral held in one rural village. The source of infection was traced to uncooked pork contaminated from an infected butcher.

4.6 Indonesia

Indonesia, officially the Republic of Indonesia, is a sovereign state in South-East Asia and Oceania. Indonesia is an archipelago comprising approximately 17,508 islands. It encompasses 34 provinces with over 238 million people, making it the world's fourth most populous country. The nation's capital city is Jakarta. The country shares land borders with Papua New Guinea, East Timor and Malaysia. Other neighbouring countries include Singapore, the Philippines, Australia, Palau and the Indian territory of the Andaman and Nicobar Islands.

Indonesia has been plagued by the consumption of street food as a major health risk, particularly in its capital, Jakarta. Importantly, edible ice used in the preparation of street food has been incriminated as a major source of *V. cholerae* contamination, as two recent papers testify (Waturangi et al. 2012, 2013).

Cholera-specific surveillance in Indonesia was initiated to identify the introduction of the newly recognised *V. cholerae* non-O1, O139 serotype (Simanjuntak et al. 2001). Findings from 7 years (1993–1999) of surveillance efforts yielded regional profiles of the importance of cholera in both epidemic and sporadic diarrhoeal disease occurrence throughout the archipelago. Outbreak findings showed that *V. cholerae* O1, Ogawa serotype, was the predominant aetiology in all 17 instances of investigated epidemic transmission. Importantly, there was no instance of non-O1, O139 serotype introduction in either epidemic or sporadic disease form.

An outbreak of El Tor biotype cholera occurring in a rural village in Irian Jaya, Indonesia was evaluated for risk factors associated with death from cholera (Korthuis et al. 1998). Among those dying in the village during the epidemic, a significant association between membership in one of the five tribal groups in the village complex was associated with an elevated risk of suffering a cholera death (OR: 5.9). Interviews with members of the decedents' families revealed a very strong association (OR: 11.6) between risk of cholera death and having attended the 2-day funeral of a woman who died of cholera-like illness a few days prior to an outbreak of cholera-like diarrhoeal disease in the village complex. Importantly, recent flooding may have contributed to the creation of an environment conducive to cholera transmission.

4.7 *Other Countries Within the WHO SEARO Classification System*

The other countries within the WHO SEARO classification system, namely Bhutan, Maldives, Myanmar, Timor Leste and the Democratic People's Republic of Korea have no documented reports of cholera outbreaks from within their borders.

4.8 *South-East Asian Countries Where Cholera Outbreaks have been Reported but Which are Outside the WHO SEARO Classification System*

Below, we describe a few countries where cholera outbreaks have been reported from time to time, and which are within the confines of South-East Asia, but which are excluded from the WHO SEARO Classification System.

4.8.1 Malaysia

Malaysia is a federal constitutional monarchy in South-East Asia. It consists of thirteen states and three federal territories. It is separated by the South China Sea into two similarly sized regions, Peninsular Malaysia and Malaysian Borneo. Land borders are shared with Thailand, Indonesia and Brunei, and maritime borders exist with Singapore, Vietnam and the Philippines. The capital is Kuala Lumpur, while Putrajaya is the seat of the federal government.

Malaysia is a country that has been associated with a number of cholera outbreaks. For example, in November 2009, a cholera outbreak in Terengganu, Malaysia was caused by two El Tor *V. cholerae* variants resistant to typical antimicrobial drugs (Teh et al. 2012). Importantly, evidence of replacement of treatable *V. cholerae* infection in the region with antimicrobial-resistant strains calls for increased surveillance and prevention measures.

A cholera outbreak occurred in Kelantan, Malaysia between November and December 2009, in which a total of 20 *V. cholerae* isolates were recovered for investigation (Ang et al. 2010). All isolates were biochemically characterised as *V. cholerae* serogroup O1 Ogawa of the El Tor biotype. The isolates were found to be resistant to multiple antibiotics. However, all isolates were sensitive to ciprofloxacin, norfloxacin, chloramphenicol, gentamicin and kanamycin. Multiplex PCR analysis confirmed the biochemical identification and revealed the presence of virulence genes, viz. *ace*, *zot* and *ctxA*, in all of the isolates. Interestingly, the sequencing of the *ctxB* gene showed that the outbreak strain harboured the classical cholera toxin gene and therefore belonged to the newly assigned El Tor variant biotype. Clonal analysis by PFGE demonstrated that a single clone of a

V. cholerae strain was responsible for the outbreak. Importantly, this was the first molecular evidence that the toxigenic *V. cholerae* O1 El Tor variant had invaded Malaysia.

There was an outbreak of cholera in Miri, Sarawak, Malaysia between November 1997 and April 1998 (Radu et al. 2002). The data on antimicrobial susceptibility patterns of *V. cholerae* O1 from patients during the outbreak period were found to be high but with variable rates of multi-drug resistance. Thirty-two of 33 *V. cholerae* isolates harboured the *tcp*, *ctx*, *zot* and *ace* genes, suggesting their possible roles in the outbreak cases. The molecular diversity of the isolates was analysed by RAPD. The 30 typable isolates could be separated into four major clusters containing 5, 17, 2 and 6 isolates, respectively. However, no particular RAPD pattern was predictive of a particular pattern of antibiotic susceptibility. The findings of the study indicated that multiple clones seemed to be responsible for the cases in the outbreak.

Forty-three clinical strains of *V. cholerae* O1 biotype El Tor were isolated between 3 May and 10 June 1998 during an outbreak in the metropolitan area of Kuala Lumpur and its suburbs (Vadivelu et al. 2000). With the exception of three Inaba strains that were restricted to three members of a family, all the others belonged to the Ogawa serotype. The strains were analysed for clonality using ribotyping and PFGE. Two ribotypes, V/B21a and B27, were identified among 40 Ogawa isolates using BglI restriction endonuclease. Ribotype V/B21a has been described previously from Taiwan and Colombia and several Asian countries, while B27 has been reported among isolates from Senegal. The three Inaba strains belonged to one ribotype, designated type A, not previously reported. Pulsed-field gel electrophoresis analysis using NotI revealed that all isolates within a ribotype had identical profiles demonstrating clonality amongst the strains. Dice coefficient analysis of the two Ogawa genotypes revealed 89 % similarity on ribotype patterns and 91.3 % on PFGE profiles. Ribotype V/B21a isolates were associated with cases from dispersed areas of Kuala Lumpur and its suburbs while ribotype B27 was restricted to cases from one particular area suggesting a common-source outbreak.

4.8.2 Singapore

Singapore, officially the Republic of Singapore, is a South-East Asian island city-state off the southern tip of the Malay Peninsula. An island country made up of 63 islands, it is separated from Malaysia by the Straits of Johor to its north and from Indonesia's Riau Islands by the Singapore Strait to its south.

An epidemiological investigation of cholera was carried out in Singapore between 1992–2007 in order to elucidate its characteristics as well as the factors contributing to its occurrence (Wong et al. 2010). Epidemiological data of all notified cases of cholera maintained by the Communicable Diseases Division, Ministry of Health, for the period 1992–2007 were collated and analysed. Case–control studies were carried out in outbreaks to determine the source of infection and mode of transmission. Linear patterns in age and ethnic distribution of cholera cases were assessed using Chi Square test for trend. There were a total of 210 cholera cases reported between 1992 and 2007. About a quarter of the cases were imported from endemic countries in the region. Between 76 and 95 % of the reported cases were local residents. Four elderly patients with comorbidities and who sought medical treatment late died, giving a case-fatality rate of 1.9 %. *V. cholerae* O1, biotype El Tor, serotype Ogawa, accounted for 83.8 % of the cases. The vehicles of transmission identified in outbreaks included raw fish, undercooked seafood and iced drinks cross-contaminated with raw seafood.

An outbreak of cholera caused by *V. cholerae* O1, biotype El Tor, serotype Inaba, phage type 4, occurred in an institution for the aged in Singapore in August and September 1984 (Goh et al. 1987). Ninety-six inmates were infected (21 symptomatic and 75 asymptomatic) and five died. The index case was a 72-year-old male inmate who continued to assist in food preparation in the kitchen from the time on onset of diarrhoea until he was seriously ill and hospitalised 4 days later. Another kitchen helper was found to have asymptomatic *V. cholerae* O1 infection. The infection rate for males was significantly higher than that for females ($p < 0.025$), associated with the use of unsanitary toilets. The main mode of transmission was through food contaminated by the two kitchen helpers who probably accounted for most of the infections, while poor personal hygiene of the inmates helped to sustain person-to-person spread.

An outbreak of cholera broke out in a group of foreign construction workers in Singapore between 3 and 11 November 1982 (Goh et al. 1984). The outbreak pathogen was *V. cholerae* O1, biotype El Tor, serotype Ogawa, phage type 1. Epidemiological investigations revealed that a total of 22 workers were confirmed to have cholera and another 15 had asymptomatic *V. cholerae* O1 infection. The source of infection was traced to contaminated seafood prepared at the construction site canteen where two food handlers were found to be infected with *V. cholerae* O1. The incubation period of cholera in this outbreak ranged from 4 to 203 h with a median of 38 h. Luckily, only two workers had moderate to severe dehydration and required intravenous therapy.

4.8.3 Philippines

The Philippines, officially known as the Republic of the Philippines, is a sovereign island country in South-East Asia in the western Pacific Ocean. To its north across the Luzon Strait lies Taiwan. West across the South China Sea sits Vietnam. The Sulu Sea to the southwest lies between the country and the island of Borneo, and to the south the Celebes Sea separates it from other islands of Indonesia. It is bounded on the east by the Philippine Sea. Its location on the Pacific Ring of Fire and its tropical climate make the Philippines prone to earthquakes and typhoons but have also endowed the country with natural resources and made it a mega-diverse country. Its capital city is Manila.

A cholera outbreak occurred in Pohnpei Island (Micronesia) in which vaccination was used as a control measure (Calain et al. 2004). Mass vaccination with the single-dose live-attenuated oral cholera vaccine CVD 103-HgR was carried out as a potential adjunct measure. Importantly, the outbreak provided a unique opportunity to evaluate the practicality of use and effectiveness of the vaccine. Under field conditions encountered in Pohnpei, crude vaccine efficacy was estimated at 79.2 % (95 % CI: 71.9–84.6 %) in the target population. Retrospective analysis suggests that mass vaccination with oral cholera vaccines can be a useful adjunct tool for controlling outbreaks, particularly if implemented early in association with other standard control measures.

During surveillance for cholera in the community of Can-Itom (Negros Occidental, Philippines) in which the disease is endemic, a limited outbreak of cholera occurred (WHO 1970). Although it was not possible to determine how the infection arose, the index case was detected and the spread of infection traced. The infection was found to be transmitted initially from person-to-person until the water of a dug well became contaminated, as a result of which a waterborne outbreak of a rather explosive nature occurred. Although 25 out of 288 individuals living in the community were infected with the El Tor biotype of *V. cholerae*, there was no manifest case of cholera; 13 persons had mild diarrhoea and 12 were asymptomatic. The outbreak subsided without any control measures having been adopted.

The introduction of cholera into many of the islands of the Philippines in 1961 often occurred in an explosive manner. The disease was introduced into Bacolod City and Talisay in Negros Occidental Province in such a manner in November 1961 (WHO 1965). The hospital and health department records in Bacolod City and Talisay and the results of interviews conducted with adult patients 10 months after the explosive outbreak were carefully analysed. The results suggest that infection during the initial explosive wave of cases in Bacolod City and Talisay in November 1961 was transmitted principally by consumption of raw shrimp.

4.8.4 Vietnam

Vietnam, officially the Socialist Republic of Vietnam, is the easternmost country on the Indochina Peninsula in South-east Asia. The country is bordered by China to the north, Laos to the north-west, Cambodia to the southwest and South China Sea to the east. Its capital city has been Hanoi since the reunification of North and South Vietnam in 1976.

Since 2007, there has been a re-emergence of cholera outbreaks in northern Vietnam. To understand the molecular epidemiological relatedness and determine the antibiotic susceptibility profiles of responsible *V. cholerae* O1 outbreak strains, a representative collection of 100 *V. cholerae* O1 strains was characterised (Tran et al. 2012). *V. cholerae* O1 strains isolated from diarrhoeal patients in northern Vietnam between 2007 and 2010 were investigated for antibiotic susceptibility and characterised by using phenotypic and genotypic tests, including PFGE analysis.

The results revealed that all isolates were resistant to cotrimoxazole and nalidixic acid, 29 % were resistant to tetracycline and 1 % were resistant to azithromycin. All strains were susceptible to ampicillin-sulbactam, doxycycline, chloramphenicol and ciprofloxacin and 95 % were susceptible to azithromycin. MIC values did show reduced susceptibility to fluoroquinolones and 63 % of the strains were intermediately resistant to tetracycline. The isolates expressed phenotypic traits of both serogroup O1 Ogawa and El Tor and harboured an *rstR* El Tor and *ctxB* classical biotype. Among the outbreak isolates, only a single PFGE pattern was observed throughout the study period. This study showed that multi-drug resistant *V. cholerae* altered El Tor producing classical CT strains had become predominant in northern Vietnam.

Vietnam is a place where the killed oral cholera vaccine (OCV) has been evaluated in an outbreak situation. In 2007–2008, unprecedented cholera outbreaks occurred in the capital, Hanoi, prompting immunisation in two districts (Anh et al. 2011). From 16 to 28 January 2008, vaccination campaigns with the Vietnamese killed OCV were held in two districts of Hanoi. No cholera cases were detected from 5 February to 4 March 2008, after which cases were again identified. Beginning 8 April 2008, residents of four districts of Hanoi admitted to one of five hospitals for acute diarrhoea with onset after 5 March 2008 were recruited for a matched, hospital-based, case–control outbreak investigation. Cases were matched by hospital, admission date, district, gender and age to controls admitted for non-diarrhoeal conditions. Subjects from the two vaccinated districts were evaluated to determine vaccine effectiveness. Fifty-four case–control pairs from the vaccinated districts were included in the analysis. There were 8 (15 %) and 16 (30 %) vaccine recipients among cases and controls, respectively. The vaccine was 76 % protective against cholera in this setting (95 % CI: 5–94 %; $p = 0.042$). Importantly, this was the first study to explore the effectiveness of the reactive use of killed OCVs during a cholera outbreak.

It has been reported from Vietnam that cholera outbreaks can be caused by an altered *V. cholerae* O1 El Tor biotype strain producing classical cholera toxin B (Nguyen et al. 2009). It was found that *V. cholerae* O1 isolates collected during cholera outbreaks occurring from late 2007 to early 2008 in northern Vietnam were revealed to represent an altered strain containing the RS1 element followed by a CTX prophage harbouring El Tor type *rstR* and classical *ctxB* on the large chromosome.

4.8.5 Laos

Laos, officially the Lao People's Democratic Republic, is a landlocked country in South-East Asia, bordered by Myanmar and China to the north-west, Vietnam to the east, Cambodia to the south and Thailand to the west. The capital city is Vientiane.

A cholera outbreak in Laos in July 2010 involved 237 cases, including four deaths (Sithivong et al. 2011). Molecular sub-typing indicated relatedness between the *V. cholerae* isolates in this and in a 2007 outbreak, uncovering a clonal group of *V. cholerae* circulating in the Mekong basin. The study suggested that the subtyping methods would affect this relatedness.

Large-scale cholera outbreaks were reported in Laos in 1993 and 1994 and from 2000 to 2002 (Lenglet et al. 2010). On 23 December 2007, a drastic increase in acute watery diarrhoea patients at a health center in Sekong Province was reported to the provincial health office. An outbreak investigation was initiated to understand the magnitude of the outbreak, identify new cases, identify the suspected causal agent, implement control measures and prevent new cases. Through active village based surveillance, 370 cases and three deaths were reported from 31 villages between 15 December 2007 and 29 January 2008. Of these reported cases, 29 % were under the age of 5. From 28 fresh stool samples taken, 17 (58.6 %) were positive for *V. cholerae* O1 Ogawa strain. Two water sources close to affected villages were found to be contaminated with the same strain of *V. cholerae*. Control measures implemented included health education for safe household water consumption and early identification and treatment of suspected cholera patients at village level. The cause of the outbreak was suspected to be a combination of contaminated drinking water and person-to-person transmission.

5 Conclusion

The South-East Asia region has always been a hotbed for cholera outbreaks and continues to be so. Importantly, the region has been the source of all the seven pandemics. The ongoing review has been a revelation in the sense that many of the outbreaks have occurred both within as well as outside the purview of the WHO SEARO classification system for the member countries. An important reason could be the following. Those countries that fall within the WHO SEARO classification system could be hesitant in reporting cholera cases. In this regard, it should be noted that Bangladesh reports zero cholera and even in case of India, cholera is grossly under-reported. Various reasons have been cited in this regard, including political connotations, trade embargoes, etc. On the other hand, some countries outside the WHO SEARO system of classification have reported cholera outbreaks, indicating that there is little or no inhibition or hindrance in reporting cholera cases, being outside the purview of the WHO system. Currently, the *modus operandi* for monitoring outbreaks is by carrying out outbreak investigations. In the future, there is a need for good surveillance systems in the region in order to closely monitor the cholera outbreak situation. A robust surveillance system will ensure that outbreaks can be picked up at the very outset and nipped in the bud, so to speak, thereby bringing down both morbidity as well as mortality.

References

Albert MJ, Siddique AK, Islam MS et al (1993) Large outbreak of clinical cholera due to *Vibrio cholerae* non-O1 in Bangladesh. Lancet 341(8846):704

Ang GY, Yu CY, Balqis K et al (2010) Molecular evidence of cholera outbreak caused by a toxigenic *Vibrio cholerae* O1 El Tor variant strain in Kelantan, Malaysia. J Clin Microbiol 48(11):3963–3969

Anh DD, Lopez AL, Thiem VD et al (2011) Use of oral cholera vaccines in an outbreak in Vietnam: a case control study. PLoS Negl Trop Dis 5(1):e1006

Bagchi K, Echeverria P, Arthur JD, Sethabutr O, Serichantalergs O, Hoge CW (1993) Epidemic of diarrhea caused by *Vibrio cholerae* non-O1 that produced heat-stable toxin among Khmers in a camp in Thailand. J Clin Microbiol 31(5):1315–1317

Bhandari GP, Bhusal CL (2013) Cholera outbreak in far-western region of Nepal. J Nepal Health Res Counc 11(23):6–8

Bhunia R, Ramakrishnan R, Hutin Y, Gupte MD (2009) Cholera outbreak secondary to contaminated pipe water in an urban area, West Bengal, India, 2006. Indian J Gastroenterol 28(2):62–64

Bhunia R, Ghosh S (2011) Water-borne cholera outbreak following cyclone Aila in Sunderban area of West Bengal, India, 2009. Trans R Soc Trop Med Hyg 105(4):214–219

Boyce TG, Mintz ED, Greene KD et al (1995) *Vibrio cholerae* O139 Bengal infections among tourists to Southeast Asia: an intercontinental foodborne outbreak. J Infect Dis 172(5):1401–1404

Calain P, Chaine JP, Johnson E et al (2004) Can oral cholera vaccination play a role in controlling a cholera outbreak? Vaccine 22(19):2444–2451

Das A, Manickam P, Hutin Y et al (2009a) Two sequential outbreaks in two villages illustrate the various modes of transmission of cholera. Epidemiol Infect 137(6):906–912

Das A, Manickam P, Hutin Y et al (2009b) An outbreak of cholera associated with an unprotected well in Parbatia, Orissa Eastern India. J Health Popul Nutr 27(5):646–651

Datta SS, Ramakrishnan R, Murhekar MV (2012) A rapidly-progressing outbreak of cholera in a shelter-home for mentally-retarded females, Amta-II block, Howrah, West Bengal, India. J Health Popul Nutr 30(1):109–112

Deepthi R, Sandeep SR, Rajini M, Rajeshwari H, Shetty A (2013) Cholera outbreak in a village in south India—timely action saved lives. J Infect Public Health 6(1):35–40

Dixit S, Bhandari GP, Karmacharya DB, Shrestha S, Manandhar S, Maskey MK (2011) Molecular screening of major bacterial enteropathogens in human stool samples from diarrhoeal outbreak sites. J Nepal Health Res Counc 9:181–185

Goel AK, Jiang SC (2011) Association of heavy rainfall on genotypic diversity in *V. cholerae* isolates from an outbreak in India. Int J Microbiol 2011:230597

Goel AK, Jain M, Kumar P et al (2011) Molecular characterization reveals involvement of altered El Tor biotype *Vibrio cholerae* O1 strains in cholera outbreak at Hyderabad, India. J Microbiol 49(2):280–284

Goh KT, Lam S, Kumarapathy S, Tan JL (1984) A common source of foodborne outbreak of cholera in Singapore. Int J Epidemiol 13(2):210–215

Goh KT, Lam S, Ling MK (1987) Epidemiological characteristics of an institutional outbreak of cholera. Trans R Soc Trop Med Hyg 81(2):230–232

Ise T, Pokharel BM, Rawal S, Shrestha RS, Dhakhwa JR (1996) Outbreaks of cholera in Kathmandu valley in Nepal. J Trop Pediatr 42(5):305–307

Jain M, Goel AK, Bhattacharya P, Ghatole M, Kamboj DV (2011) Multidrug resistant *Vibrio cholerae* O1 El Tor carrying ctxB allele involved in a cholera outbreak in South Western India. Acta Trop 117(2):152–156

Jiraphongsa C, Jinwong T, Sangwonloy O et al (1994) A second outbreak of cholera in the home for mentally handicapped. J Med Assoc Thai 77(5):249–252

Kanungo S, Sah BK, Lopez AL et al (2010) Cholera in India: an analysis of reports, 1997–2006. Bull World Health Organ 88:185–191

Kondo S, Kongmuang U, Kalnauwakul S, Matsumoto C, Chen CH, Nishibuchi M (2001) Molecular epidemiologic analysis of *Vibrio cholerae* O1 isolated during the 1997–1998 cholera epidemic in southern Thailand. Epidemiol Infect 127(1):7–16

Korthuis PT, Jones TR, Lesmana M et al (1998) An outbreak of El Tor cholera associated with a tribal funeral in Irian Jaya, Indonesia. Southeast Asian J Trop Med Public Health 29(3):550–554

Kumar P, Jain M, Goel AK et al (2009) A large cholera outbreak due to a new cholera toxin variant of the *Vibrio cholerae* O1 El Tor biotype in Orissa, Eastern India. J Med Microbiol 58(Pt 2):234–238

Lenglet A, Khamphaphongphane B, Thebvongsa P et al (2010) A cholera epidemic in Sekong Province, Lao People's Democratic Republic, December 2007–January 2008. Jpn J Infect Dis 63(3):204–207

Mendis NM, Ratnasabapathy P, Maheswaran K, Wijayarajah C (1975) Outbreak of cholera El Tor in Sri Lanka, 1973. Ceylon Med J 20(2):82–93

Mendis NM, De La Motte PU, De Silva AV, Maheswaran K, Sivayoham S (1977) The spread of cholera El Tor in Sri Lanka in 1974. Ceylon Med J 22(1):24–40

Ministry of Health and Family Welfare, Government of India (2013) States Profile, New Delhi. http://www.mohfw.nic.in/NRHM/State_Profile.htm. Accessed 17 Sept 2013

Mridha P, Biswas AK, Ramakrishnan R, Murhekar MV (2011) The 2010 outbreak of cholera among workers of a jute mill in Kolkata, West Bengal, India. J Health Popul Nutr 29(1):9–13

Mukherjee R, Halder D, Saha S et al (2011) Five pond-centered outbreaks of cholera in villages of West Bengal, India: evidence for focused interventions. J Health Popul Nutr 29(5):421–428

Mutreja A, Kim DW, Thomson NR et al (2011) Evidence for several waves of global transmission in the seventh cholera pandemic. Nature 477(7365):462–465

Nguyen BM, Lee JH, Cuong NT et al (2009) Cholera outbreaks caused by an altered *Vibrio cholerae* O1 El Tor biotype strain producing classical cholera toxin B in Vietnam in 2007 to 2008. J Clin Microbiol 47(5):1568–1571

Okada K, Chantaroj S, Roobthaisong A, Hamada S, Sawanpanyalert P (2010) A cholera outbreak of the Vibrio cholerae O1 El Tor variant carrying classical CtxB in northeastern Thailand in 2007. Am J Trop Med Hyg 82(5):875–878

Okada K, Roobthaisong A, Nakagawa I, Hamada S, Chantaroj S (2012) Genotypic and PFGE/MLV analyses of *Vibrio cholerae* O1: geographical spread and temporal changes during the 2007-2010 cholera outbreaks in Thailand. PLoS ONE 7(1):e30863

Pal BB, Khuntia HK, Samal SK, Kar SK, Patnaik B (2010) Epidemics of severe cholera caused by El Tor *Vibrio cholerae* O1 Ogawa possessing the ctxb gene of the classical biotype in Orissa, India. Int J Infect Dis 14(5):e384–e389

Pal BB, Khuntia HK, Samal SK et al (2013) Large outbreak of cholera caused by El Tor variant of *Vibrio cholerae* O1 in the eastern coast of Odisha, India during 2009. Epidemiol Infect 6:1–8 [Epub ahead of print]

Palit A, Batabyal P (2010) Toxigenic Vibrio cholerae from environmental sources associated with the cholera outbreak after "Aila" cyclone in West Bengal, India. Lett Appl Microbiol 51(2):241–243

Panda S, Pati KK, Bhattacharya MK, Koley H, Pahari S, Nair GB (2011) Rapid situation and response assessment of diarrhoea outbreak in a coastal district following tropical cyclone Aila in India. Indian J Med Res 133:395–400

Pokhrel BM, Kubo T (1996) Outbreaks of cholera in Nepal. Southeast Asian J Trop Med Public Health 27(3):574–579

Radu S, Vincent M, Apun K et al (2002) Molecular characterization of *Vibrio cholerae* O1 outbreak strains in Miri, Sarawak (Malaysia). Acta Trop 83(2):169–176

Rajeshwari K, Gupta A, Dubey AP, Uppal B, Singh MM (2008) Diarrhoeal outbreak of *Vibrio cholerae* O1 Inaba in Delhi. Trop Doct 38(2):105–107

Ramamurthy T, Garg S, Sharma R et al (1993) Emergence of novel strain of Vibrio cholerae with epidemic potential in southern and eastern India. Lancet 341(8846):703–704
Sack RB, Siddique AK, Longini IM et al (2003) A 4-year study of the epidemiology of *Vibrio cholerae* in four rural areas of Bangladesh. J Infect Dis 187(1):96–101
Sekar R, Amudhan M, Sivashankar M, Mythily N, Mythreyee M (2012) An outbreak of cholera among a rural population in south India: Is it time to vaccinate the children in endemic areas? Indian J Med Res 135(5):678–679
Shah HD, Shah VP, Desai AN (2012) An epidemic outbreak of *Vibrio cholerae* El Tor O1 serotype ogawa biotype in a Lalpur town, Jamnagar, India. J Postgrad Med 58(1):14–18
Sharma SP (2006) Hepatitis E and cholera outbreak in Kathmandu. Canad Med Assoc J 175(8):860
Siddique AK, Zaman K, Baqui AH et al (1992) Cholera epidemics in Bangladesh: 1985–1991. J Diarrhoeal Dis Res 10(2):79–86
Simanjuntak CH, Larasati W, Arjoso S et al (2001) Cholera in Indonesia in 1993–1999. Am J Trop Med Hyg 65(6):788–797
Sithivong N, Morita-Ishihara T, Vongdouangchanh A et al (2011) Molecular sub-typing in cholera outbreak, Laos, 2010. Emerg Infect Dis 17(11):2060–2062
Sivagnanasundram C, Rajasingham P, Nagarajah K, Xavier RL (1975) Cholera El Tor carriers in the Kondavil North focus, 1973. Ceylon Med J 20(1):35–39
Swaddiwudhipong W, Kunasol P (1989) An outbreak of nosocomial cholera in a 755-bed hospital. Trans R Soc Trop Med Hyg 83(2):279–281
Swaddiwudhipong W, Limpakarnjanarat K (1991) An outbreak of El Tor cholera in an institution for the mentally retarded in Nonthaburi, June–July 1987. J Med Assoc Thai 74(6):306–310
Swaddiwudhipong W, Peanumlom P (2010) A case of nosocomial cholera during a community outbreak in a Thai-Myanmar border area. J Med Assoc Thai 93(9):1112–1114
Swaddiwudhipong W, Akarasewi P, Chayaniyayodhin T, Kunasol P, Foy HM (1989) Several sporadic outbreaks of El Tor cholera in Sunpathong, Chiang Mai, September–October, 1987. J Med Assoc Thai 72(10):583–588
Swaddiwudhipong W, Akarasewi P, Chayaniyayodhin T, Kunasol P, Foy HM (1990) A cholera outbreak associated with eating uncooked pork in Thailand. J Diarrhoeal Dis Res 8(3):94–96
Swaddiwudhipong W, Jirakanvisun R, Rodklai A (1992) A common source foodborne outbreak of El Tor cholera following the consumption of uncooked beef. J Med Assoc Thai 75(7):413–417
Swaddiwudhipong W, Ngamsaithong C, Peanumlom P, Hannarong S (2008) An outbreak of cholera among migrants living in a Thai-Myanmar border area. J Med Assoc Thai 91(9):1433–1440
Swaddiwudhipong W, Hannarong S, Peanumlom P, Pittayawonganon C, Sitthi W (2012) Two consecutive outbreaks of food-borne cholera associated with consumption of chicken rice in northwestern Thailand. Southeast Asian J Trop Med Public Health 43(4):927–932
Tamang MD, Sharma N, Makaju RK et al (2005) An outbreak of El Tor cholera in Kavre district, Nepal. Kathmandu Univ Med J 3(2):138–142
Taneja N, Mishra A, Sangar G, Singh G, Sharma M (2009) Outbreaks caused by new variants of *Vibrio cholerae* O1 El Tor, India. Emerg Infect Dis 15(2):352–354
Teh CS, Suhaili Z, Lim KT et al (2012) Outbreak-associated *Vibrio cholerae* genotypes with identical pulsotypes, Malaysia, 2009. Emerg Infect Dis 18(7):1177–1179
Tran HD, Alam M, Trung NV et al (2012) Multi-drug resistant *Vibrio cholerae* O1 variant El Tor isolated in northern Vietnam between 2007 and 2010. J Med Microbiol 61(Pt 3):431–437
United Nations (2008) UN Statistics Division, Millennium development goal indicators. http://mdgs.un.org/unsd/mdg/data.aspx. Accessed 17 Aug 2013
Vadivelu J, Iyer L, Kshatriya BM, Puthucheary SD (2000) Molecular evidence of clonality amongst *Vibrio cholerae* O1 biotype EL Tor during an outbreak in Malaysia. Epidemiol Infect 124(1):25–30
Waldor MK, Hotez PJ, Clemens JD (2010) A national cholera vaccine stockpile—a new humanitarian and diplomatic resource. N Engl J Med 363:2279–2282

Waturangi DE, Pradita N, Linarta J, Banerjee S (2012) Prevalence and molecular characterization of *Vibrio cholerae* from ice and beverages sold in Jakarta, Indonesia, using most probable number and multiplex PCR. J Food Prot 75(4):651–659

Waturangi DE, Wennars M, Suhartono MX, Wijaya YF (2013) Edible ice in Jakarta, Indonesia, is contaminated with multidrug-resistant *Vibrio cholerae* with virulence potential. J Med Microbiol 62(Pt 3):352–359

Wong CS, Ang LW, James L, Goh KT (2010) Epidemiological characteristics of cholera in Singapore, 1992–2007. Ann Acad Med Singapore 39(7):507–516

World Bank (2011) Press release No. 2009/343/SAR. http://go.worldbank.org/N2N84RDV00. Accessed 17 Aug 2013

World Bank (2013) World development indicators. http://data.worldbank.org/data_catalog/world_development_indicators. Accessed 17 Aug 2013

World Health Organization (1965) Studies of cholera El Tor in the Philippines, 2, A retrospective investigation of an explosive outbreak in Bacolod City and Talisay, November 1961. Bull World Health Organ 33(5):637–643

World Health Organization (1970) Study on the transmission of El Tor cholera during an outbreak in Can-Itom community in the Philippines. Bull World Health Organ 43(3):413–419

World Health Organization (1992) Diarrhoeal diseases, gastroenteritis and cholera epidemic, 1991. Wkly Epidemiol Rec 67(37):273–276

World Health Organization (2005) National health system profile, 2005. http://www.searo.who.int/en/Section313/Section1515_6038.htm. Accessed 17 Aug 2013

World Health Organization (2010) Cholera vaccines: WHO position paper. Wkly Epidemiol Rec 85(13):117–128

World Health Organization (2011) Cholera, 2010. Wkly Epidemiol Rec 86(31):325–339

World Health Organization (2012) Cholera fact sheet. http://www.who.int/mediacentre/factsheets/fs107/en/. Accessed 15 Aug 2013

Cholera Outbreaks in Africa

Martin A. Mengel, Isabelle Delrieu, Leonard Heyerdahl and Bradford D. Gessner

Abstract During the current seventh cholera pandemic, Africa bore the major brunt of global disease burden. More than 40 years after its resurgence in Africa in 1970, cholera remains a grave public health problem, characterized by large disease burden, frequent outbreaks, persistent endemicity, and high CFRs, particularly in the region of the central African Great Lakes which might act as reservoirs for cholera. There, cases occur year round with a rise in incidence during the rainy season. Elsewhere in sub-Saharan Africa, cholera occurs mostly in outbreaks of varying size with a constant threat of widespread epidemics. Between 1970 and 2011, African countries reported 3,221,050 suspected cholera cases to the World Health Organization, representing 46 % of all cases reported globally. Excluding the Haitian epidemic, sub-Saharan Africa accounted for 86 % of reported cases and 99 % of deaths worldwide in 2011. The number of cholera cases is possibly much higher than what is reported to the WHO due to the variation in modalities, completeness, and case definition of national cholera data. One source on country specific incidence rates for Africa, adjusting for underreporting, estimates 1,341,080 cases and 160,930 deaths (52.6 % of 2,548,227 estimated cases and 79.6 % of 209,216 estimated deaths worldwide). Another estimates 1,411,453 cases and 53,632 deaths per year, respectively (50 % of 2,836,669 estimated cases and 58.6 % of 91,490 estimated deaths worldwide). Within Africa, half of all cases between 1970 and 2011 were notified from only seven countries: Angola, Democratic Republic of the Congo, Mozambique, Nigeria, Somalia, Tanzania, and South Africa. In contrast to a global trend of decreasing case fatality ratios (CFRs), CFRs have remained stable in Africa at approximately 2 %. Early propagation of cholera outbreaks depends largely on the extent of individual bacterial shedding, host and organism characteristics, the likelihood of people coming into contact with an infectious dose of *Vibrio cholerae* and on the virulence of the implicated strain. Cholera transmission can then be amplified by several factors including

M. A. Mengel (✉) · I. Delrieu · L. Heyerdahl · B. D. Gessner
Agence de Médecine Préventive, 164 rue de Vaugirard, 75015 Paris, France
e-mail: mmengel@aamp.org

Current Topics in Microbiology and Immunology (2014) 379: 117–144
DOI: 10.1007/82_2014_369

Published Online: 16 May 2014

contamination of human water- or food sources; climate and extreme weather events; political and economic crises; high population density combined with poor quality informal housing and poor hygiene practices; spread beyond a local community through human travel and animals, e.g., water birds. At an individual level, cholera risk may increase with decreasing immunity and hypochlorhydria, such as that induced by *Helicobacter pylori* infection, which is endemic in much of Africa, and may increase individual susceptibility and cholera incidence. Since contaminated water is the main vehicle for the spread of cholera, the obvious long-term solution to eradicate the disease is the provision of safe water to all African populations. This requires considerable human and financial resources and time. In the short and medium term, vaccination may help to prevent and control the spread of cholera outbreaks. Regardless of the intervention, further understanding of cholera biology and epidemiology is essential to identify populations and areas at increased risk and thus ensure the most efficient use of scarce resources for the prevention and control of cholera.

Contents

1 Introduction

Since 1817, the world has faced seven cholera pandemics. During the current seventh pandemic, Africa bore the major brunt of global disease burden. Within barely half a century, cholera has changed from an imported to an endemic disease in most African countries. Cholera was first reported in Africa in 1836 when outbreaks occurred on the Indian Ocean coast, killing as many as 20,000 people in Zanzibar (Olago et al. 2007) and nearly depopulating the towns of Lamu, Malindi, and Kilwa. The next reports came from Egypt in 1848 with 30,000 deaths (Eichenberg 2011), fromWest Africa in 1868 (Macnamara 1876) and from the Senegambia region in 1893–1894 (Kolle et al. 1903). Cholera was declared a notifiable disease by the British Colonial government in East Africa (Bwire et al. 2013). No further outbreaks were reported in Africa until the seventh pandemic reached the continent in 1970, with the first case being reported in Guinea-Conakry (Fig. 1). Cholera subsequently spread along the coast and into the interior of the Sahel by waterways and was further disseminated by land travel of nomadic tribes (Goodgame and Greenough 1975). The impact of this seventh pandemic was particularly devastating, given that populations that had not experienced *Vibrio cholerae* before had low immunity and were served by health systems ill-equipped to effectively deal with the disease (Gangarosa 1971).

Between 1970 and 2011, African countries reported 3,221,050 suspected cholera cases to the World Health Organization (Fig. 2), representing 46 % of all cases reported globally (WHO, Global Health Observatory 2012). The number of African countries with indigenous cholera cases reported to the WHO rose from 24 in 1971 to 30 in 1998 and a record of 36 in 2008 (Fig. 3). In 2011, the number fell to 27. Excluding the Haitian epidemic, Africa accounted for 86 % of reported cases and 99 % of deaths worldwide in 2011 (WHO, Global Health Observatory).

The number of cholera cases in Africa could possibly be much higher than what is reported to the WHO. Reasons include underreporting and inadequate surveillance systems. One source on country-specific incidence rates for Africa, adjusting for underreporting, estimates 1,341,080 cases and 160,930 deaths (52.6 % of 2,548,227 estimated cases and 79.6 % of 209,216 estimated deaths worldwide)) (Sack 2013), another estimates 1,411,453 cases and 53,632 deaths per year, respectively (50 % of 2,836,669 estimated cases and 58.6 % of 91,490 estimated deaths worldwide) (Ali et al. 2012).

Cholera is not distributed equally throughout Africa. From 1970 to 2011, half of all cases were notified by only seven countries (Table 1): Angola (183,076), Democratic Republic of the Congo (DRC) (391,524), Mozambique (315,295), Nigeria (260,966), Somalia (255,788), Tanzania (204,569), and South Africa (186,462). Countries north of the Sahara were far less affected by cholera and only reported a total of 19,233 cases of which 12,729 came from Algeria alone. The last cases there were reported in 1991.

Throughout most of sub-Saharan Africa, cholera occurs in outbreaks of varying size with a constant threat of widespread epidemics. For example, in 2000, South

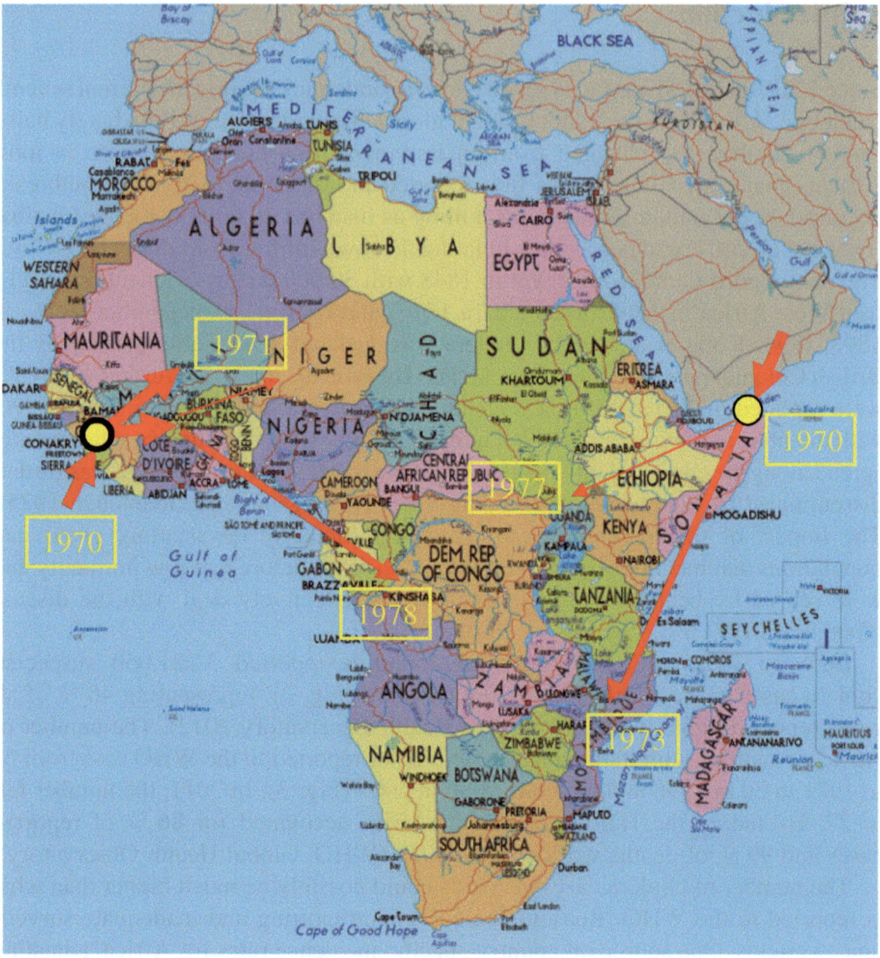

Fig. 1 Early expansion of cholera during the seventh pandemic in Africa 1970–1978

Africa reported 103,320 cases and 232 deaths, and from 2008 to 2009, its neighboring country Zimbabwe reported 128,208 cases and 5,634 deaths. Cholera can spread rapidly. In an analysis of 78 cholera outbreaks in Mozambique from 2009 to 2011, 68 % of all cases and 89 % of deaths occurred within the first 6 weeks of an outbreak (Gujral et al. 2013).

In the Rift Valley region of Central Africa, cholera occurs in an endemic pattern, which is defined by the WHO as culture-confirmed cases in populations for at least three of the past five years. For instance, in the DRC cases occur year-round with a rise in incidence during the rainy season (Ministry of Health, DRC 2012). While case fatality ratios (CFRs) have declined globally, they have remained stable in Africa at approximately 2 % (WHO 2012). This is double the

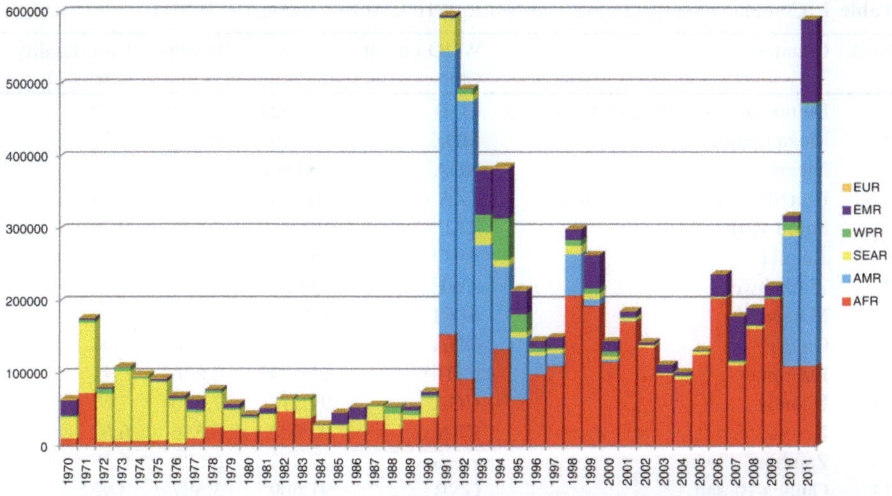

Fig. 2 Suspect cholera cases notified to the WHO by WHO-region, 1970–2011

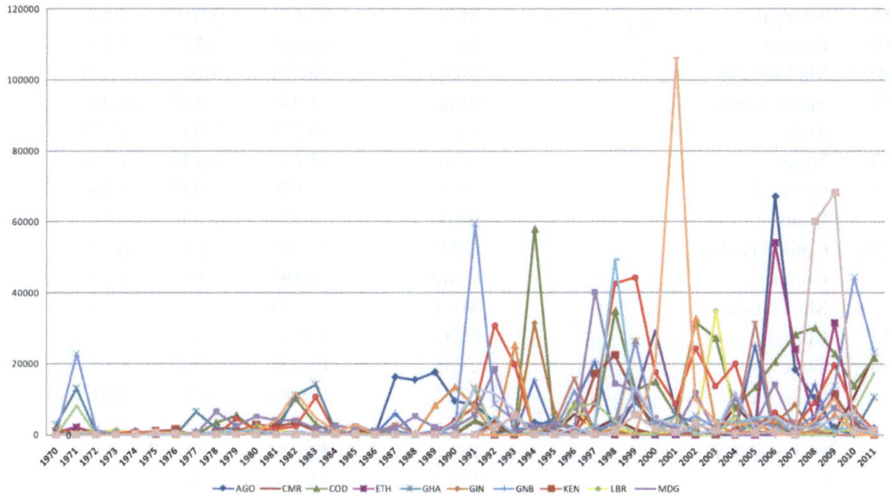

Fig. 3 Suspect cholera cases notified to the WHO from AFRO region by country, 1971–2011, 20 most notifying countries

threshold set by the WHO as an indicator of an appropriate case management system. Cholera is, therefore, a major public health problem in sub-Saharan Africa, as characterized by large disease burden, frequent outbreaks, persistent endemicity, and high CFRs. This chapter explores many of the underlying factors contributing to cholera outbreaks in Africa, addressing specifically the factors influencing cholera epidemics, cholera immunity and its role in Africa, cholera surveillance and anthropological issues related to cholera.

Table 1 Cumulative suspect cases notified to WHO, AFRO region 1970–2011

Rank	Country	WHO country code	Cases	Deaths	Case fatality ratio (%)
1	Democratic Republic of the Congo	COD	391,524	30,539	7.80
2	Mozambique	MOZ	315,295	11,752	3.73
3	Nigeria	NGA	260,966	259,92	9.96
4	United Republic of Tanzania	TZA	204,569	172,93	8.45
5	South Africa	ZAF	186,462	1,426	0.76
6	Angola	AGO	182,875	13,326	7.29
7	Zimbabwe	ZWE	153,335	13,783	8.99
8	Malawi	MWI	140,263	5,428	3.87
9	Ghana	GHA	128,525	6,400	4.98
10	Ethiopia	ETH	118,297	2,846	2.41
11	Uganda	UGA	99,517	7,630	7.67
12	Kenya	KEN	9,9022	6,556	6.62
13	Zambia	ZMB	97,408	6,698	6.88
14	Guinea-Bissau	GNB	91,609	3,587	3.92
15	Liberia	LBR	84,999	964	1.13
16	Chad	TCD	80,846	7,540	9.33
17	Cameroon	CMR	7,2551	5,876	8.10
18	Senegal	SEN	67,622	3,019	4.46
19	Guinea	GIN	60,635	3,237	5.34
20	Madagascar	MDG	46,531	5,268	11.32
21	Sierra Leone	SLE	38,343	2,432	6.34
22	Mali	MLI	33,378	5,087	15.24
23	Niger	NER	32,607	4,498	13.79
24	Burundi	BDI	31,990	1,042	3.26
25	Benin	BEN	28,835	1,257	4.36
26	Côte d'Ivoire	CIV	23,389	1,562	6,.68
27	Comoros	COM	17,866	799	4.47
28	Mauritania	MRT	17,765	734	4.13
29	Congo	COG	16,584	516	3.11
30	Togo	TGO	15,820	1,287	8.14
31	Cape Verde	CPV	1,4144	285	2.01
32	Algeria	DZA	12,729	650	5.11
33	Burkina Faso	BFA	12,564	1,513	12.04
34	Rwanda	RWA	11,449	585	5.11
35	Swaziland	SWZ	10,107	368	3.64
36	Sao Tome and Principe	STP	7,861	166	2.11
37	Equatorial Guinea	GNQ	6,962	100	1.44
38	Namibia	NAM	3,854	92	2.39
39	Central African Republic	CAF	902	267	29.60
40	Gabon	GAB	649	2	0.31
41	Gambia	GMB	252	28	11.11
42	Seychelles	SYC	178	2	1.12
43	Eritrea	ERI	120	18	15.00

(continued)

Table 1 (continued)

Rank	Country	WHO country code	Cases	Deaths	Case fatality ratio (%)
44	Botswana	BWA	8	6	75.00
45	Lesotho	LSO	0	0	
46	Mauritius	MUS	0	0	
	Grand total		3,221,207	202,456	Average: 8.15

Source WHO (2013)

2 Factors Influencing Cholera Epidemics in Africa

Several factors influence the occurrence and development of epidemics in sub-Saharan Africa (Fig. 4). These are listed below

- Exposures leading to infection of the index case.
- Transmission factors leading to initial spread.
- Outbreak amplification factors.
- Factors driving the spread of *V. cholerae* and the propagation of an epidemic.
- Risk or protective factors for individual infection or outbreak expansion.

2.1 Onset of an Outbreak: The Index Case and Initial Transmission

In sub-Saharan Africa, cholera frequently causes large outbreaks and epidemics presumably due to poor lack of safe water and sanitation and inadequate case management. The onset of an outbreak in a new location can result from person-to-person transmission when a symptomatic or asymptomatic carrier enters a susceptible population or when an individual comes in contact with contaminated environmental sources (Nelson et al. 2009). Once cholera has infected individuals in a new area, initial propagation depends on the extent of individual bacterial shedding, host and organism characteristics, and the likelihood of additional persons coming into contact with an infectious dose. Shedding may occur before and up to 7 months after symptom onset (Utsalo et al. 1999). Symptomatic persons shed substantially more (10^7–10^9 *V. cholerae* per ml of stool) than asymptomatic persons (10^3 *V. cholerae*/ml). The infectious dose for a susceptible individual is 10^4–10^{11} (Nelson et al. 2009; Kaper et al. 1995; Zuckerman et al. 2007). After excretion by the patient, *V. cholerae* acquires a hyper-infectious state that lasts for at least 5 h in an aquatic environment (Merrell et al. 2002; Nelson et al. 2009; Morris 2011). More virulent strains, or the introduction of equally virulent strains into an immunologically naïve population, can increase the risk of outbreaks and

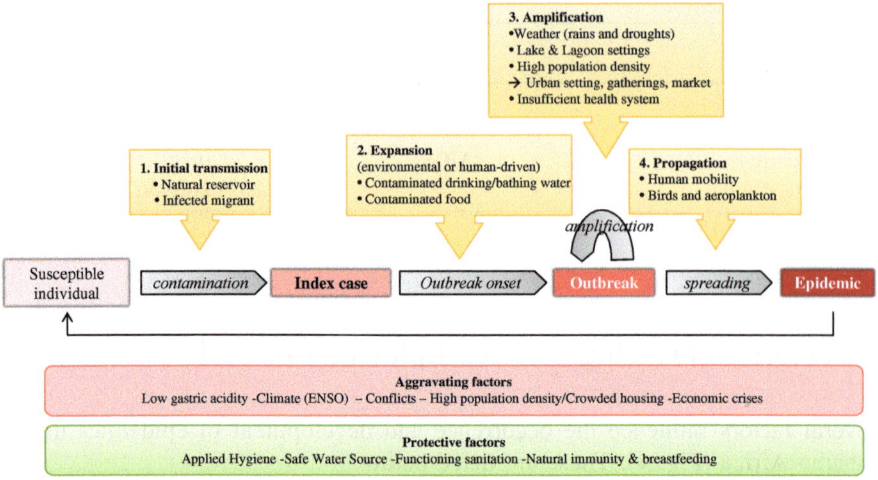

Fig. 4 Influence of various driving factors for cholera outbreaks in Africa. Once a susceptible individual is contaminated via a natural reservoir or a human carrier and thus becomes an index case, a series of factors can lead to the onset of an outbreak: The clonal expansion of vibrios, and the movement of cholera cases increasing human to human transmission and provoking an epidemic situation. A number of aggravating or protective factors may influence the dynamics of cholera outbreaks at each step

may have contributed to ongoing epidemics in Africa (Kaper et al. 1995; Keddy et al. 2007; Quilici et al. 2010; Piarroux and Faucher 2012).

The complex biological systems constituting the aquatic environmental reservoir are critical to long-term survival of epidemic *V. cholerae*. Pathogenic vibrios are commensal with numerous organisms such as algae, crustaceans, floating aquatic plants like water-hyacinth (Feikin et al. 2010), phytoplankton, and zooplankton such as copepods (Reyburn et al. 2011; Acosta et al. 2001; Colwell et al. 2003). In response to nutrient deprivation, vibrios can enter a dormant state and persist in an aquatic environment; subsequent changes in water temperature, salinity, pH, and nutrients can resuscitate vibrios and lead to their multiplication, causing epidemics (Reyburn et al. 2011). In Africa, water likely plays a major role in triggering cholera outbreaks, with lagoons and estuaries contributing to coastal disease, and lakes and rivers contributing to inland disease (Rebaudet 2013).

Contamination of human water or food sources can greatly accelerate cholera spread (Morris 2011). Water source contamination remains the most common risk factor for cholera outbreaks both in Africa and worldwide, incriminated in 29 % of 306 risk factor reports during the 1995–2005 period (Griffith et al. 2006). Transmission may occur by drinking from contaminated water sources, such as lakes, rivers, estuaries, irrigation canals, or ponds (Küstner et al. 1981; Birmingham et al. 1997; Swerdlow et al. 1997; Shapiro et al. 1999; Lawoyin et al. 1999; Bompangue et al. 2008; Bateman 2009a, b). Studies in Africa have associated cholera transmission with river bathing and use of water for domestic purposes (Acosta et al. 2001;

Birmingham et al. 1997; Küstner et al. 1981). Otherwise clean water may be contaminated within households when stored in open containers (Bateman 2009a, b; Swerdlow et al. 1997), or during transportation (Küstner et al. 1981). Vendors also may contaminate drinking water during extraction from wells or transfer to purchase containers (Umoh et al. 1983; Lipp et al. 2002; Hutin et al. 2003). Shallow, uncovered hand-dug wells—which constitute the main source of drinking water for many people in Africa—have been repeatedly incriminated in cholera outbreaks in sub-Saharan Africa (Barua 1972; Rodriguez et al. 1997; Sasaki et al. 2008; Ako et al. 2009; Adagbada et al. 2012). For example, in a slum area of Douala, Cameroon, over 70,000 wells are less than 1.5 m deep and frequently become contaminated by shallow groundwater, which itself is polluted through sewage and latrine discharge drains (Guévart et al. 2006).

Food may become contaminated with *V. cholerae* in the natural environment, during preparation of food or storage of leftovers (Kaper et al. 1995; Estrada-García and Mintz 1996; Albert et al. 1997). Because vibrios concentrate in the gastrointestinal tracts of mollusks, crustaceans, and fish that ingest copepods (Estrada-García and Mintz 1996), the consumption these seafoods has been incriminated in cholera outbreaks (Rabbani et al. 1999). Transmission of *V. cholerae* O1 has been associated with eating of unwashed raw vegetables or fruits (Albert et al. 1997; CDC MMWR 2004; Dubois et al. 2006), and with poor hygiene practices during meal preparation, as observed in fish gutting processes (Schürmann et al. 2002; Scheelbeek et al. 2009). Inadequately stored and reheated food has been shown to transmit cholera. In Africa, this has been observed, for example, with cooked rice in Guinea (St Louis et al. 1990), millet gruel in Mali (Tauxe et al. 1988) and cooked pigeon peas in Malawi (Swerdlow et al. 1991).

2.2 *Outbreak Amplification*

Once cholera has broken out in a community, several factors may amplify the outbreak (Fig. 4). Weather and climate play a critical role in cholera dynamics due to a variety of reasons (De Magny et al. 2012). An analysis of worldwide cholera data from 1974 to 2005 showed that countries closer to the equator experience greater and more frequent cholera outbreaks (Emch et al. 2008). In Africa, the climate influences cholera outbreaks in specific ways (Bompangue et al. 2011), with an increase in the frequency and size of outbreaks during the hot and rainy seasons, as has been documented in Zanzibar (Schaetti et al. 2009), the South Kivu district bordering Lake Tanganyika in DRC (Bompangue et al. 2009), Angola (Colombo et al. 1993), and five countries in West Africa (De Magny et al. 2007).

Climate may influence cholera dynamics by affecting water supplies. Heavy rainfall may increase contamination through overflow and disruption of water networks (Griffith et al. 2006; Guévart et al. 2006; Sasaki et al. 2009), as observed with rainfall in Dakar, Senegal, that exacerbated a cholera epidemic (De Magny et al. 2012). Flooding can cause draining of sewage into rivers and lakes

(Torres Codeço et al. 2001) and increase runoff from latrines or pit toilets, which then contaminates shallow and uncovered wells as noted in Senegal, Zambia, Cameroon, and Zimbabwe (Adagbada et al. 2012; Guévart et al. 2006; Sasaki et al. 2008, 2009; Ako et al. 2009; De Magny et al. 2012; Luque Fernandez et al. 2012). Spatial distribution studies have found a higher number of cases in areas bordering lakes (Birmingham et al. 1997; Bompangue et al. 2008; Shapiro et al. 1999; Piarroux and Faucher 2012), which may result from recurrent sewage seepage into these water sources that are used simultaneously for bathing and drinking. Lack of water also may amplify outbreaks, as drought and dry seasons can reduce the availability of potable water, leading people to drink contaminated water from streams and ponds (Lawoyin et al. 1999).

Certain weather conditions may lead to the proliferation of aquatic vibrios, subsequent contamination of fish food, and greater human transmission (Bompangue et al. 2011). Increased rain and ambient temperature can facilitate proliferation of free-living and zooplankton-attached *V. cholerae* populations (Colwell 1996; Mendelsohn and Dawson 2008; Reyburn et al. 2011; Lobitz et al. 2000). Nonseasonal increases in air and sea surface temperatures (SST) have been associated with elevated cholera incidence in Southeastern Africa (Paz 2009). In Tanzania, the relative risk of cholera outbreaks occurring increased by 15–29 % for each 1 °C increase in air temperature (Trærup et al. 2011).

High population density combined with poor quality informal housing may influence cholera incidence and outbreak amplification (Griffith et al. 2006; Penrose et al. 2010) by facilitating person-to-person transmission and increasing the burden on inadequate sanitation facilities. In Harare, 2008–2009, cholera attack rates ranged from 1.2 cases per 1,000 people in low-density residential suburbs to 90.3 per 1,000 in an overcrowded suburb (Luque-Fernandez et al. 2011), with similar trends observed in Ghana (Osei and Duker 2008) and Uganda (Legros et al. 2000).

A strong association exists between increased cholera incidence and the absence of sanitation facilities (Rodrigues et al. 1997; Sasaki et al. 2008; Griffith et al. 2006; Mahamud et al. 2012) or proximity to waste dumps (Osei and Duker 2008). In Africa, only 34 % of the population has access to improved sanitation facilities, ranging from 9 % in Niger, to 74 % in South Africa (WHO 2010). Poor hygiene practices, for example the absence of soap in the household, also increase cholera risk (Dubois et al. 2006; Guévart et al. 2006). Severe outbreaks can occur where a lack of functional hygiene and sanitation services coincides with high population density, such as in refugee camps (Boelaert et al. 1995; Swerdlow et al. 1997; Shultz et al. 2009; Goma Epidemiology Group 1995; Griffith et al. 2006), during gatherings (Manga et al. 2008) and in prisons (Griffith et al. 2006).

Markets, fairs, and other cultural and social events have been shown early on to provide a forum for increased food-borne cholera transmission (Barua 1972). *V. cholerae* can survive on produce for two to five days (Felsenfeld 1965) and easily spread because of crowding, and the absence of latrines and running water. In Lusaka, Zambia, 2004, raw vegetable consumption from the Soweto market was strongly associated with cholera, whereas water source contamination or treatment practices were not (Dubois et al. 2006); a similar situation has been observed in Guinea-Bissau (Luquero et al. 2011). Fecal-oral cholera spread is facilitated by sharing glasses and plates, as often occurs in traditional African settings (Kürtsner et al. 1981). Funerals may propagate cholera spread through local rites such as washing the deceased's body followed by preparing and serving a large community meal (Barua 1972; St Louis et al. 1990; Germani et al. 1998; Gunnlaugsson et al. 1998; Shapiro et al. 1999; Griffith et al. 2006).

Finally, health system deficiencies contribute to outbreak magnitude. For example, poor surveillance can delay diagnosis and reporting and lead to delays in the implementation of control measures (Gunnlaugsson et al. 2000; Einarsdottir et al. 2001; Ahmed et al. 2011, Nguyen et al. 2014). Inadequate treatment facilities may lead to an increase in the risk of nosocomial transmission (Daniels et al. 1999; Kyelem et al. 2011).

2.3 Factors Favoring Epidemics

Human travel via land, sea, rivers, and air drives the wide geographic spread of cholera (Barua 1972; Mari et al. 2012; Manga et al. 2008; Piarroux and Faucher 2012; Duval et al. 1999; Mugoya et al. 2008). Susceptible people may become infected while traveling and introduce the disease in their home communities (Manga et al. 2008); inversely, through fecal shedding, asymptomatic or recovered cholera patients may be responsible for long-range dissemination of vibrios to a foreign environment (Mari et al. 2012). For example, fishermen on the Rift Valley lakes travel long distances and may return to their lakeside cities and trigger cholera outbreaks (Piarroux et al. 2009).

In addition to humans, animals may propagate cholera. Vibrios can survive in a bird's gut and have been isolated from apparently healthy water birds, suggesting those might spread cholera (Halpern et al. 2008). By connecting wind direction with cholera dissemination patterns (Paz and Broza 2007) and considering that midges can carry *V. cholerae* on their surface for up to 2 weeks (Broza et al. 2005), it has been hypothesized that aeroplankton act as a vector for continental and intercontinental cholera spread (Paz and Broza 2007).

2.4 Factors Aggravating Cholera Outbreaks

Aggravating factors for cholera outbreaks may work at the individual or population level. Higher gastric acidity reduces the likelihood of symptomatic cholera (Van Loon et al. 1990) and increases the inoculum required for disease (Zuckerman et al. 2007). In many African settings, hypochlorhydria induced by *Helicobacter pylori* infections is endemic, which may increase individual susceptibility and cholera incidence (Adagbada et al. 2012). Similarly, vitamin A deficiency, more so than protein-calorie malnutrition, may increase cholera risk (Harris et al. 2008).

At the population level, global climatic events may influence local climatic risk factors described previously, particularly the El Niño/Southern Oscillation (ENSO) (Lobitz et al. 2000; Reyburn et al. 2011; Olago et al. 2007; Pascual et al. 2000). ENSO can increase the occurrence of rain and floods, or temperature and thus exacerbate outbreaks in cholera prone regions (Alajo et al. 2006; De Magny et al. 2012; Luque-Fernandez et al. 2009; Olago et al. 2007).

Political violence can increase the risk of cholera outbreaks due to the subsequent collapses in health and sanitation infrastructure (Kalipeni and Oppong 1998; Griffith et al. 2006; Gayer et al. 2007; Kelly-Hope 2008), including disruption of food supplies and subsequent malnutrition, destruction of water supplies and road networks, decreased availability of medical personnel, and destruction of sanitation and waste facilities in homes and communities (Kalipeni and Oppong 1998). In Liberia, civil war sparked a massive cholera epidemic, exacerbated by crowded refugee camps and the destruction of public health and clinical services (Wendo 2003), a situation seen also during Sierra Leone's 10-year long civil war (WHO 2009). Cholera associated with civil wars may impact neighboring countries, where refugee camps may harbor hundreds of thousands of people without adequate sanitation and hygiene facilities (Gayer et al. 2007; Kelly-Hope 2008). Following armed conflict in Mozambique in 1986, Malawi accepted political refugees and by October 1990, Mozambican refugees accounted for 10 % of the population; from 1988 to 1990, at least nine cholera outbreaks were reported in these refugee camps (Swerdlow et al. 1997). Similar events have occurred with internally displaced persons in Kenya following post-election violence (Shikanga et al. 2009), in Rwanda following an exodus of refugees from the DRC (Boelaert et al. 1995; Bhattacharya et al. 2009) and in a refugee camp in Sudan (Mulholland 1985).

Economic crises not related to war have contributed to cholera in several African countries. In Zimbabwe, since the start of the economic crisis in 1998, cholera has been reported every year (Mukandavire et al. 2011) with the massive 2008–2009 epidemic attributed in part to the dire economic situation and the resulting collapse of public health and clinical service systems (Mason 2009; Truscott 2008; Bateman 2009a, b). Fuel shortages may affect cholera case management, for example if health staff are unable to access their clinics or health centers (Muula 2009).

2.5 Protective Factors

Basic hygiene measures such as hand washing with soap have shown protection against cholera in Nigeria (Hutin et al. 2003), Zambia (Dubois et al. 2006; Sasaki et al. 2008), Kenya (Mahamud et al. 2012) and Guinea-Bissau (Rodrigues et al. 1997).

Having access to a clean latrine in or outside the household also may decrease cholera risk (Mahamud et al. 2012).

Growth of *V. cholerae* is inhibited in acidic foods. In an epidemic in Guinea, eating tomato sauce (pH 5.0) was shown to protect against symptomatic cholera (St Louis et al. 1990). For similar reasons, lime juice, which has been used as prophylaxis in northern Indian regions during the cholera season (Anand 1995), had a strong protective effect when added to sauce, as exemplified in Guinea-Bissau, 1996 (Rodrigues et al. 2000). *Vibrio* survival is reduced in food with lower water content and higher osmolarity such as dried, salt-preserved, and sugar-preserved foods (Estrada-Garcia and Mintz 1996). Consumption of dried fish has been shown to have a protective effect (Lucas et al. 2005; Dubois et al. 2006).

In sub-Saharan Africa, risk factors for cholera infection, transmission and propagation are very specific to the local socioeconomic context and might vary among sub-regions and geographical areas. In more developed regions, natural contamination through infected seafood or vegetables are more likely to account for cholera cases, while in poor settings, risk factors will rather be a lack of potable water and proper sanitation (Griffith et al. 2006), mostly resulting from human crises and possibly exacerbated by natural disasters such as flooding. Political instability and civil wars have been shown to increase the risk of cholera outbreaks especially in vulnerable populations such as refugees that have even less access to adequate water and sanitation facilities. Climatic factors periodically aggravate these difficult conditions and can lead to more frequent and more deadly cholera outbreaks. In Africa, cholera can be considered primarily as a disease of poverty (Bateman 2009a).

3 Cholera Immunity and its Role in African Cholera

While there is significant literature on cholera immunity globally, with a regional focus on the Indian subcontinent, literature specifically on sub-Saharan Africa is limited. Studies have found that infection with *V. cholerae* provides immunity of variable duration, although the exact mechanism of adaptive immunity remains unknown (Pasetti and Levine 2012; Kaper et al. 1995). In a summary of studies in which volunteers were exposed to cholera, it was reported that 90–100 % of persons given an inoculum of El Tor Ogawa or Inaba serotypes were protected from disease for up to 3 years, and that cross-protection between serotypes existed. Epidemiological studies support the concept of immunity following natural exposure to cholera but with some differences (Cash et al. 1974). In Bangladesh, persons with a first episode of cholera experienced a 90 % reduction in the expected number of hospitalizations with a subsequent episode of cholera (Glass et al. 1982). Another study in Bangladesh within the context of a vaccine trial documented that classical cholera was completely protective against subsequent classical cholera; unlike volunteer studies, El Tor infections led to negligible future protection (Clemens et al. 1991). Overall, this study found a 61 % reduction in the risk of any cholera recidivism. More recently, a study in Bangladesh identified a 65 % reduction of El Tor cholera following an initial El Tor infection over 3 years of follow-up; interestingly, El Tor serotype Inaba infections led to lower risk of both subsequent Inaba and Ogawa infections, but Ogawa serotype infections were associated only with a lower risk of re-infection with serotype Ogawa (Ali et al. 2011). Lastly, data from a study of anti-vibriocidal antibody titers over the year subsequent to an episode of severe cholera suggested that previous exposure at a minimum is protective against recurrent severe disease (Weil et al. 2012).

Another feature of cholera immunity is that asymptomatic or mildly symptomatic infections are common (McCormack et al. 1969), and that asymptomatic infections may precede the occurrence of clinically recognizable cases during an outbreak or epidemic (Bart et al. 1970). A recent study found that the model that best explains 50 years of mortality data in Bengal included a high asymptomatic to symptomatic case ratio, rapidly waning immunity particularly among asymptomatic cases, and transmission from both human and environmental sources (King et al. 2008).

Although few data from Africa exist, natural immunity likely plays a critical role in the dynamics of cholera epidemiology in this region as well. For example, a study in Mozambique has demonstrated that at the district level, cholera epidemics are of short duration and rarely affected the same district, at least over the 3 years of observation (Gujral et al. 2013). This suggests a strong role for waxing and waning population immunity. Indeed, a modeling exercise in Bangladesh emphasizes the primacy of population immunity over climate variations in determining the duration of refractory periods for cholera risk (Koelle et al. 2005). In contrast, the interplay of population immunity, and yearly cultural and climatic changes, in combination with a local environmental reservoir, could lead to endemic transmission punctuated by larger epidemics, such as is seen in the Great Lakes Region of the DRC (Bompangue et al. 2008). Additionally, natural immunity will influence age distribution of cases where disease is sporadic rather than epidemic, all age groupsage groups may be affected equally while endemic areas may experience a weighting among nonimmune younger children such as has been reported from Kenya (Mutonga et al. 2013). Breast milk may provide protection against cholera for infants living in endemic or epidemic cholera settings. A study in Guinea-Bissau demonstrated that heavily exposed mothers exhibit vibriocidal IgA antibody in breast milk, which may protect their children from cholera during the breastfeeding period (Qureshi et al. 2006).

4 Cholera Surveillance in Sub-Saharan Africa

In most African countries, publicly available data on cholera stem largely from national surveillance systems. Since 1950, the WHO has used these data to develop reports. It is important to understand the processes and limitations of these national surveillance systems to understand how to appropriately interpret reported data.

Cholera was included as one of three notifiable diseases in the International Health Regulations 1969 (WHO 2005). Currently, cholera cases and deaths are reported to WHO through the national Integrated Diseases and Response Systems (IDSR) (WHO 2010) and published in the Weekly Epidemiological Record (WER). The WHO produces a dedicated report on the cholera situation in each country and a summary of the globally notified cases is published each year in August.

The 2005 revised International Health Regulations (IHR) explicitly states that no travel—or economic—restrictions are to be established if a country notifies cholera. Yet, ministries of health may delay declaring the presence of cholera and initiating a response due to fears of the impact on the tourism and export sectors (Harris et al. 2012).

The IDSR guidelines define the modalities of reporting from the local to the national level and state in detail and which competences should be available at each level (WHO 2010). The IDSR guideline for community health workers asks them to report cases "with plenty of watery diarrhea" to the district health officers who enter this information into the IDSR system. When a country changes from its own generic case definition to the WHO standard case definition, this can lead to a considerable increase in reported cases as was seen in Cameroon (Djomassi et al. 2013). Countries are supposed to report cases to WHO when "they are unusual or unexpected or when they pose a significant risk of international spread" (WHO 2012). The numbers reported to WHO are thought to be misleading due, in part, to underreporting and limitations in surveillance systems. The modalities, completeness, and case definition of national cholera surveillance have substantial limitations and may vary from country to country.

4.1 Underestimation of Disease Burden in Children Under 5 Years of Age

The WHO uses the following case definition for reporting suspect cases of cholera:

- "in an area where the disease is not known to be present, a patient aged 5 years or more who develops severe dehydration or dies from acute watery diarrhea;
- In an area where there is a cholera epidemic, a patient aged 5 years or more who develops acute watery diarrhea, with or without vomiting".

The WHO case definition excludes cases in children under 5 years of age despite several studies that have shown considerable disease and death burden in that age group (Deen et al. 2011; Lanata et al. 2002). While the reason for this is to avoid wasting resources on investigation of routine infant diarrhea (mainly that due to rotavirus), this case definition has the obvious disadvantage that it will underestimate case counts among young children. A recent global multicenter study in children under five found that *V. cholerae* was the second most frequent pathogens causing moderate to severe diarrhea in Beira, Mozambique (Kotloff et al. 2013).

4.2 Limited Health Care Access and Diminished Sensitivity

To be counted in surveillance system data, a person with cholera must present itself to a health care structure. However, health system access is limited in many African settings due to lack of transportation means and infrastructure, financial barriers, cultural barriers, and lack of education. Programs such as the "Diseases of the Most Impoverished" have tried to compensate for these shortcomings by using data from reporting sources outside national surveillance systems and then using modeling for more precise estimations (IVI 2013).

4.3 Limited Laboratory Confirmation and Diminished Sensitivity and Specificity

Outside endemic settings, WHO guidelines specify that identification of a cholera epidemic requires laboratory confirmation through standard methods (Bopp et al. 1999). Remote areas may have nonexistent or poorly developed laboratory facilities, stockouts, or lack of appropriately trained personnel, all of which may contribute to a delay or failure in identifying cholera outbreaks, thereby reducing the sensitivity of the surveillance system. To overcome this challenge, new tools have been developed, such as rapid diagnostic tests (Qadri et al. 1995), biosensors (Retzky 2012), and mobile microbiological laboratories (Ouedraogo et al. 2009).

Additionally, WHO recommends laboratory confirmation only at the beginning of the outbreak and sporadically thereafter to monitor antibiotic resistance and confirm the end of the outbreak. However, the conditions that contribute to cholera outbreaks may also contribute to the spread of many other enteric diseases. Without confirmatory testing, it is likely that a substantial percentage of cases reported as cholera actually are due to other organisms, thereby reducing surveillance system specificity.

4.4 Reporting Limitations

Data at the local level are collected at cholera treatment centers, government clinics and hospitals, and private health care facilities. In most countries in sub-Saharan Africa, the district health office compiles these data and reports them as weekly summaries to the regional or national level. These summaries contain limited data including district name and outcome (death or not). Detailed demographic data, risk factors, environmental variables, and other information are not collected. Additionally, laboratory data are usually not included, so that national surveillance systems must independently access laboratory structures to determine case confirmation. Third, data reports to the central level may be incomplete, and few countries have attempted to audit district level reporting. Even when data are reported, substantial delays may occur so that reports for any particular week or month may not document accurate numbers until months later. Fourth, no system exists in most countries to exclude duplicate case counts. For example, patients may present to one health structure 1 day, and to a different structure the following day and would be counted twice.

Lastly, a relatively common reporting limitation is the occurrence of cholera outbreaks at national borders. Cross-border flow and lack of cooperation between countries means that cholera cases may not be accounted for in national systems. Moreover, many national borders are along natural waterways (rivers and lakes), which facilitate cholera epidemics, as mentioned above.

New tools for notification have been employed to decrease the delay in notification of outbreaks to national authorities. One example is Kenya's strategy to use coded short-text messages sent via mobile phones (Zurovac et al. 2012). Such tools have also been developed for the transmission of laboratory results (Breslauer et al. 2009).

4.5 Limitations in Analysis

African ministries of health may have limited capacity to enter, store, and analyze data. For example, many African epidemiology systems lack databases designed specifically to input data from weekly case report forms. Even where the database exists, these forms usually are handwritten and thus require substantial data entry time or expensive scanners to enter into a database. Consequently, weekly case reports may be analyzed by hand, or not analyzed at all.

4.6 Limited Spatial Resolution of Aggregate Data

As indicated above, data reported to the national level usually do not report spatial resolution finer than district level. This may give an inaccurate assessment of cholera dynamics. For example, one district may have an endemic focus in one localized area, while another could have epidemics moving from one village to the next, yet the data at national level may appear similar (Gujral et al. 2013).

4.7 Surveillance in Humanitarian Emergencies and Natural Disasters

Surveillance is even more complicated when it has to be implemented in already overburdened health systems that are additionally faced with a humanitarian emergency caused by a natural or man-made disaster. Additionally, humanitarian crises may result in large refugee camps just inside national boundaries. Monitoring of cholera cases under these circumstances—with frequent in- and out-migration for work, social reasons, or medical care—poses particular challenges.

4.8 Possible Improvement in Cholera Surveillance in Africa

The above limitations influence the sensitivity, specificity, and timeliness of the surveillance system, and thereby affect the ability to accurately interpret data. The introduction of additional variables beyond reports of suspect cases and deaths in persons below and above 5 years of age would greatly improve existing data. Ideally, this would include individual case reports with case-specific demographic data and risk factors. Even summary data, though, could include more specific location (such as village), age group, and sex. An additional improvement would include systematic reporting from laboratory facilities. However, collection of robust data should come with strengthening of analytic capacity (including systems and number and skill of human resources) and monitoring the completeness of reporting.

5 Anthropological Considerations

5.1 Perceptions of Cholera Causes and Prevention

Perceptions of disease causation can vary greatly between groups of people and even within the same group according to a person's educational or professional background and experience with disease. Perceptions may also change over time based on personal experience and government initiatives like public health education.

In the DRC, lack of hygiene, nonrespect of ancestral laws, malnutrition, rubella, and adultery are believed to be causes of cholera (Schubert and Diwete 2008; Guillermet et al. 2012). In Burkina Faso, disease perception has been shown to vary depending on the respondent's age (Poda et al. 2003). In Zanzibar, a study comparing rural and urban areas showed that people with a higher level of education and socioeconomic status tend to perceive disease causes using a modern science paradigm (e.g., identifying the role of bacteria, an unclean environment, and unsafe water in disease spread) (Schaetti et al. 2010). Even so, traditional knowledge and perceptions of causation are not necessarily contradictory to, or exclusive of modern science-based practices. For example, handwashing has been traditionally practiced in KwaZulu-Natal, South Africa (O'Donoghue 2005). In Gabon, shellfish are always eaten cooked, never raw (Sabinot 2009). Throughout sub-Saharan Africa, smoking and salting of fish is generally practiced (Essuman 1992).

5.2 Stigmatization

At the individual and community level, stigma against cholera may exist. In Guinea-Bissau, stigmatization delays or prevents care seeking at modern medical facilities (Nzirorera 2008; Perry and Donini-Lenhoff 2010), which in turn can increase mortality and impede timely outbreak identification and response. Although data are lacking, marginalized communities such as refugees or migrants might be particularly susceptible to stigmatization if perceived as the source of a cholera outbreak.

5.3 Care-Seeking Behavior

Clinical case management at adequately equipped facilities (such as cholera treatment centers) plays a vital role in decreasing cholera mortality if they are accessible and clinical care is sought timely. Cultural beliefs may greatly influence care-seeking behavior, including whether patients present to modern or traditional health care providers (Staro 2011; Guillermet et al. 2012). In parts of Katanga, Kasai Oriental, and Kinshasa in the DRC, and regardless of proximity to modern health centers, studies have found that mothers prefer to seek traditional care for diarrheal diseases, especially in rural areas (Harris et al. 2012); stated reasons include cost, distance, and perceived efficacy (Schubert and Diwete 2008). Traditional and modern medical treatments are not necessarily mutually exclusive. For example, a study in rural areas of Zanzibar revealed that herbal treatment, oral rehydration solution, and prayers were used by 83.1, 72.9, and 47.5 % of interviewees, respectively (Schaetti 2010). Another phenomenon that affects care-seeking behavior is the increase in street pharmacies, which do not require access to a health care provider. In Burkina Faso, for example, 7 % of the population regularly uses street medicine (Soura et al. 2008).

5.4 Demographic Changes and Urbanization

Fishermen, seasonal agricultural workers, truck drivers, and merchants all travel from urban hubs to more remote areas via roads, air, and water. The average number of kilometers traveled per habitant per year in sub-Saharan Africa almost doubled between 1960 and 1990, from 900 to 1,600 km (Orfeuil 2002). This has two direct effects on cholera: (i) more rapid disease spread to distant locations (Matzger 2012; IRIN 2012) and (ii) reduced contact with safe water, sanitation, and treatment facilities (IOM 2010).

Moreover, African societies have experienced rapid urbanization. In West Africa, 1 in 3 inhabitants lived in a city in 2010, versus 1 in 13 in 1950 (CEPED 2009). This massive growth has not been accompanied by a commiserate growth in clean water and sanitation infrastructure (Assako et al. 2004) or adequate housing. Consequently, many new residents live in shantytowns that provide fertile ground for cholera outbreak initiation and amplification (Guévart et al. 2006).

In this context, it is important to distinguish attitudes toward individual versus communal responsibility for sanitation. In Burkina Faso for instance, it is thought that individual responsibility stops at the entrance to one's home, with the space beyond being the responsibility of the state or municipality. This naturally leads to conflicts between local communities and governments when clean water and sanitation are lacking (Bouju et al. 2009).

6 Conclusion

More than 40 years after its resurgence in Africa, cholera remains a grave public health problem. While the disease occurs throughout most of sub-Saharan Africa, it is particularly widespread in the Great Lakes region. This may be explained by the presence of large bodies of water, which can act as reservoirs for cholera when contaminated. Additional climatic, environmental, social, and biological factors contribute to endemic and epidemic disease patterns.

Since contaminated water is the main vehicle for the spread of cholera, the obvious long-term solution to eradicate the disease is the provision of safe water to all African populations. Yet, this requires considerable human and financial resources as well as time. In the short and medium term, vaccination may help to control the spread of cholera outbreaks. Encouraging results from a recent trial on a bivalent killed whole-cell oral cholera vaccine in Kolkata, India showed that immunity conveyed by this vaccine lasted up to 5 years (Bhattacharya et al. 2013).

Ultimately, it will take an integrated approach using all available means (i.e., improved water/hygiene, vaccine use, improved clinical care) to tackle cholera on all fronts. This approach marks a shift from current reactive strategies to cholera control, where national and international aid workers rush into the affected areas after the onset of epidemics and countries often exhaust their national resources trying to contain the outbreak and keep CFRs as low as possible. The international community has advanced significantly towards promoting such an integrated approach. The foundation was laid by the declaration of the 64th World Health Assembly in 2010 which was taken up by a number of international groups and led to numerous studies and guidelines for cholera prevention and control, a large number of which are contained in a compilation issued by Unicef very recently (see Unicef 2013).

Further understanding of the biology and epidemiology of *V. cholerae* is essential to identify populations and areas at increased risk. This knowledge will enable countries to implement prevention and control measures accordingly, and thus ensure the most efficient use of scarce resources. Moreover, to promote the adoption of such measures, it is necessary to understand community perceptions, knowledge, attitudes, and practices regarding cholera. This will help countries to develop appropriate public health messages that aim to change behavior, without inadvertently deterring currently used traditional prevention practices or creating confusion (Schaetti et al. 2010; v. Seidlein 2013).

Acknowledgments The authors would like to thank Lan Ngo and Sabrina Gaber for their enormous help in completing this chapter. Lan Ngo for the many hours of ceaseless search of cholera literature and news and Sabrina Gaber for her valuable work editing the text.

References

Acosta CJ, Galindo CM, Kimario J, Senkoro K, Urassa H, Casals C, Corachán M, Eseko N, Tanner M, Mshinda H, Lwilla F, Vila J, Alonso PL (2001) Cholera outbreak in southern Tanzania: risk factors and patterns of transmission. Emerg Infect Dis 7(3):583–587

Adagbada AO, Adesida SA, Nwaokorie FO, Niemogha MT, Coker AO (2012) Cholera epidemiology in Nigeria: an overview. Pan Afr Med J 12:59

Ahmed S, Bardhan PK, Iqbal A, Mazumder RN, Khan AI, Islam MS, Siddique AK, Cravioto A (2011) The 2008 cholera epidemic in Zimbabwe: experience of the icddr, b team in the field. J Health Popul Nutr 29(5):541–546

Ako AA, Nkeng GE, Takem GE (2009) Water quality and occurrence of water-borne diseases in the Douala 4th District, Cameroon Water SciT echnol 59(12):2321–2329

Alajo SO, Nakavuma J, Erume J (2006) Cholera in endemic districts in Uganda during El Niño rains: 2002–2003. Afr Health Sci 6(2):93–97

Albert MJ, Neira M, Motarjemi Y (1997) The role of food in the epidemiology of cholera. World Health Stat Q 50(1–2):111–118

Ali M, Emch M, Park JK, Yunus M, Clemens J (2011) Natural cholera infection-derived immunity in an endemic setting. J Infect Dis 204:912–918

Ali M, Lopez AL, You YA, Kim YE, Sah B, Maskery B, Clemens J (2012) The global burden of cholera. Bull WHO 90:209–218A

Anand JK (1995) Cholera treatment in Goma. Lancet 345(8964):1568

Assako RJ, Abomo DM, Tchuikoua LB (2004) Etude géographique de l'épidémie de choléra à Douala ou la qualité de vie à l'épreuve des pratiques urbaines

Bart KJ, Huq Z, Moslemuddin K, Mosley WH (1970) Seroepidemiologic studies during a simultaneous epidemic of infection with El Tor Ogawa and Classical Inaba Vibrio cholerae. J Infect Dis 121:17–24

Barua D (1972) The global epidemiology of cholera in recent years. Proc R Soc Med 65(5):423–428

Bateman C (2009a) Cholera—getting the basics right. S Afr Med J 99(3):138–140

Bateman C (2009b) SA medical schools to rescue Zimbabwe's aspirant doctors. S Afr Med J 99(4):214, 216, 218

Bhattacharya S, Black R, Bourgeois L, Clemens J, Cravioto A, Deen JL, Dougan G, Glass R, Grais RF, Greco M, Gust I, Holmgren J, Kariuki S, Lambert PH, Liu MA, Longini I, Nair GB, Norrby R, Nossal GJ, Ogra P, Sansonetti P, von Seidlein L, Songane F, Svennerholm AM, Steele D, Walker R (2009) Public health. The cholera crisis in Africa. Science 324(5929):885

Birmingham ME, Lee LA, Ndayimirije N, Nkurikiye S, Hersh BS, Wells JG, Deming MS (1997) Epidemic cholera in Burundi: patterns of transmission in the great rift valley lake region. Lancet 349(9057):981–985

Boelaert M, Suetens C, van Soest M, Henkens M, Rigal J, de Graaf P (1995) Cholera treatment in Goma. Lancet 345(8964):1567

Bompangue D, Giraudoux P, Handschumacher P, Piarroux M, Sudre B, Ekwanzala M, Kebela I, Piarroux R (2008) Lakes as source of cholera outbreaks, Democratic Republic of Congo. Emerg Infect Dis 14(5):798–800

Bompangue D, Giraudoux P, Piarroux M, Mutombo G, Shamavu R, Sudre B, Mutombo A, Mondonge V, Piarroux R (2009) Cholera epidemics, war and disasters around Goma and Lake Kivu: an eight-year survey. PLoS Negl Trop Dis 3(5):436

Bompangue Nkoko D, Giraudoux P, Plisnier PD, Tinda AM, Piarroux M, Sudre B, Horion S, Tamfum JJ, Ilunga BK, Piarroux R (2011) Dynamics of cholera outbreaks in great lakes region of Africa, 1978–2008. Emerg Infect Dis 17(11):2026–2034

Bopp CA, Ries AA, Wells JG (1999) Laboratory methods for the diagnosis of epidemic dysentery and cholera. Centers for Disease Control and Prevention

Bouju J, Bocoum H, Ouattara F, Touré L (2009) Les incivilités de la société civile Espace public urbain, société civile et gouvernance communale à Bobo-Dioulasso et Bamako (Communes 1 et 2)

Breslauer DN, Maamari RN, Switz NA et al (2009) Mobile phone based clinical microscopy for global health applications. PLoS One 4:6320

Broza M, Gancz H, Halpern M, Kashi Y (2005) Adult non-biting midges: possible windborne carriers of Vibrio cholerae non-O1 non-O139. Environ Microbiol 7(4):576–585

Bhattacharya S, Sur D, Ali M, Kanungo S, Ae You Y, Manna B, Sah B, Niyogi SK, Park JK, Sarkar B, Puri MK, Kim DR, Deen JL, Holmgren J, Carbis R, Singh Dhingra M, Donner A, Nair GB, Lopez AL, Wierzba TF, Clemens JD (2013) 5 year efficacy of a bivalent killed whole-cell oral cholera vaccine in Kolkata, India: a cluster-randomized. double-blind, placebo-controlled trial. Lancet Infect Dis. 2013 Dec 13(12):1050–1056

Bwire G, Malimbo M, Makumbi I, Kagirita A, Wamala JF, Kalyebi P, Bingi A, Gitta S, Mukanga D, Dahlke M (2013) Cholera surveillance—Uganda, 2007–2011. J Infect Dis. 208(1):S78–S85

Cash RA, Music SI, Libonati JP, Craig JP, Pierce NF, Hornick RB (1974) Response of man to infection with Vibrio cholerae. II. Protection from illness afforded by previous disease and vaccine. J Infect Dis 130:325–333

CEPED (2009) Estimated urbanization levels in West African Societies between 1950 and 2020. July 2009—Issue 57—GB

Clemens JD, van Loon F, Sack DA, Rao MR, Ahmed F, ChakrabortY J, Kay BA, Khan MR, Yunus MD, Harris JR et al (1991) Biotype as determinant of natural immunizing effect of cholera. Lancet 337:883–884

Codeço, Cláudia T (2001) Endemic and Epidemic Dynamics of Cholera: the Role of the Aquatic Reservoir. BMC Infect Dis 1(1) doi: 10.1186/1471-2334-1-1. Accessed 2 Feb 2001

Colombo MM, Francisco M, Ferreira BD, Rubino S, Cappuccinelli P (1993) The early stage of the recurrent cholera epidemic in Luanda. Angola Eur J Epidemiol 9(5):563–565

Colwell RR (1996) Global climate and infectious disease: the cholera paradigm. Science 274:2025–2031

Colwell RR, Huq A, Islam MS, Aziz KM, Yunus M, Khan NH, Mahmud A, Sack RB, Nair GB, Chakraborty J, Sack DA, Russek-Cohen E (2003) Reduction of cholera in Bangladeshi villages by simple filtration. Proc Natl Acad Sci USA 100:1051–1055

Daniels NA, Simons SL, Rodrigues A, Gunnlaugsson G, Forster TS, Wells JG, Hutwagner L, Tauxe RV, Mintz ED (1999) First do no harm: making oral rehydration solution safer in a cholera epidemic. Am J Trop Med Hyg 60(6):1051–1055

deMagny GC, Guégan JF, Petit M, Cazelles B (2007) Regional-scale climate-variability synchrony of cholera epidemics in West Africa. BMC Infect Dis 19(7):20
deMagny GC, Thiaw W, Kumar V, Manga NM, Diop BM, Gueye L, Kamara M, Roche B, Murtugudde R, Colwell RR (2012) Cholera outbreak in senegal in 2005: was climate a factor? PLoS One 7(8):e44577
Deen JL, Von Seidlein L, Clemens JD (2011) Multidisciplinary studies of disease burden in the Diseases of the Most Impoverished Program. J Health Popul Nutr 22:232–239
Djomassi LD, Gessner BD, Andze GO, Mballa GA (2013) Cholera epidemiology in Cameroon based on national surveillance data. J Infect Dis 208(1):S92–S97
Dubois AE, Sinkala M, Kalluri P, Makasa-Chikoya M, Quick RE (2006) Epidemic cholera in urban Zambia: hand soap and dried fish as protective factors. Epidemiol Infect 134(6):1226–1230
Duval P, Champetier de Ribes G, Ranjalahy J, Quilici ML, Fournier JM (1999) Cholera in Madagascar. Lancet 353(9169):2068
Eichenberg M (2011) Africa in the time of cholera: a history of pandemics from 1817 to the present. Cambridge University Press, Cambridge
Einarsdóttir J, Passa A, Gunnlaugsson G (2001) Health education and cholera in rural Guinea-Bissau. Int J Infect Dis 5(3):133–138
Emch M, Feldacker C, Islam MS, Ali M (2008) Seasonality of cholera from 1974 to 2005: a review of global patterns. Int J Health Geogr 20(7):31
Essuman KM (1992) Fermented fish in Africa: a study on processing marketing and consumption
Estrada-García T, Mintz ED (1996) Cholera: foodborne transmission and its prevention. Eur J Epidemiol 12(5):461–469
Feikin DR, Tabu CW, Gichuki J (2010) Does water hyacinth on East African lakes promote cholera outbreaks? Am J Trop Med Hyg 83(2):370–373
Felsenfeld O (1965) Notes on food, beverages, and fomites contaminated with Vibrio cholerae. Bull WHO 33:725–734
Gangarosa EJ (1971) The epidemiology of cholera: past and present. Bull N Y Acad Med 47:1140
Gayer M, Legros D, Formenty P, Connolly MA (2007) Conflict and emerging infectious diseases. Emerg Infect Dis 13(11):1625–1631
Germani Y, Quilici ML, Glaziou P, Mattera D, Morvan J, Fournier JM (1998) Emergence of cholera in the Central African Republic. Eur J Clin Microbiol Infect Dis 17(12):888–890
Glass RI, Becker S, Huq MI, Stoll BJ, Khan MU, Merson MH, Lee JV, Black RE (1982) Endemic cholera in rural Bangladesh, 1966–1980. Am J Epidmiol 116:959–970
Goodgame RW, Greenough WB (1975) Cholera in Africa: a message for the West. Ann Intern Med 82:101–106
Goma Epidemiology Group (1995) Public health impact of Rwandan refugee crisis: what happened in Goma, Zaire, in July, 1994? Lancet 345:339–344
Griffith DC, Kelly-Hope LA, Miller MA (2006) Review of reported cholera outbreaks worldwide, 1995–2005. Am J Trop Med Hyg 75(5):973–977
Guévart E, Noeske J, Solle J, Essomba JM, Edjenguele M, Bita A, Mouangue A, Manga B (2006) Factors contributing to endemic cholera in Douala, Cameroon. Med Trop 66(3):283–291. French: Déterminants du choléra à douala. Med Trop 66:283–291
Gujral L, Sema C, Rebaudet S, Taibo CLA, Manjate AA, Piarroux R, Gessner BD (2013) Jani IV cholera epidemiology in Mozambique using national surveillance data. J Infect Dis 208(1):107–114
Guillermet E, Colombini A, Gessner BD and Breugelmans G (2012) Literature review of anthropological studies on diarrhea in the DRC, in anticipation of a potential rotavirus vaccine introduction
Gunnlaugsson G, Angulo FJ, Einarsdóttir J, Passa A, Tauxe RV (2000) Epidemic cholera in Guinea-Bissau: the challenge of preventing deaths in rural West Africa. Int J Infect Dis 4(1):8–13
Gunnlaugsson G, Einarsdóttir J, Angulo FJ, Mentambanar SA, Passa A, Tauxe RV (1998) Funerals during the 1994 cholera epidemic in Guinea-Bissau, West Africa: the need for disinfection of bodies of persons dying of cholera. Epidemiol Infect 120(1):7–15

Halpern M, Senderovich Y, Izhaki I (2008) Waterfowl: the missing link in epidemic and pandemic cholera dissemination? PLoS Pathog 4(10):e1000173

Harris JB, LaRocque RC, Qadri F, Ryan ET, Calderwood SB (2012) Seminar Cholera. Lancet 379:2466–2476

Harris JB, LaRocque RC, Chowdhury F, Khan AI, Logvinenko T, Faruque AS, Ryan ET, Qadri F, Calderwood SB (2008) Susceptibility to Vibrio cholerae infection in a cohort of household contacts of patients with cholera in Bangladesh. PLoS Negl Trop Dis 2(4):e221

Hutin Y, Luby S, Paquet C (2003) A large cholera outbreak in Kano City, Nigeria: the importance of hand washing with soap and the danger of street-vended water. J Water Health 1:45–52

International Organization for Migration (IOM) (2010) Eye on migration news bulletin, (3)

IRIN AFRIQUE DE L'OUEST: Choléra, quelles sont les solutions ? 2012

IVI international vaccine institute: program activities and progress (2013) http://www.ivi.int/publication/brochure/program.html. Accessed 19 Mar 2013

Kalipeni E, Oppong J (1998) The refugee crisis in Africa and implications for health and disease: a political ecology approach. Soc Sci Med 46(12):1637–1653

Kaper JB, Morris JG Jr, Levine MM (1995) Cholera. Clin Microbiol Rev 8(1):48–86

Keddy KH, Nadan S, Govind C, Sturm AW (2007) Group for enteric, respiratory and meningeal disease surveillance in South Africa. Evidence for a clonally different origin of the two cholera epidemics of 2001–2002 and 1980–1987 in South Africa. J Med Microbiol 56(12):1644–1650

Kelly-Hope LA (2008) Conflict and emerging infectious diseases. Emerg Infect Dis 14(6):1004–1005

King AA, Ionides EL, Pascual M, Bouma MJ (2008) Inapparent infections and cholera dynamics. Nature 2008(454):877–880

Koelle K, Rodo X, Pascual M, Yunus M, Mostafa G (2005) Refractory periods and climate forcing in cholera dynamics. Nature 436:696–700

Kolle W, Wassermann A, Kossel H, Neisser A (1903) Handbook of pathogenic microorganisms. Am J Med Sci 125:706

Kotloff K, Nataro J, Blackwelder W, Nasrin D, Farag H, Panchalingam S, Wu Y, Sow S, Sur D, Breiman R, Faruque A, Zaidi A, Saha D, Alonso P, Tamboura B, Sanogo D, Onwuchekwa U, Manna B, Ramamurthy T, Kanungo S, Ochieng J, Omore R, Oundo J, Hossain A, Das S, Ahmed S, Qureshi S, Quadri F, Adegbola R, Antonio M, Hossain J, Akinsola A, Mandomando I, Nhampossa T, Acácio S, Biswas K, O'Reilly C, Mintz E, Berkeley L, Muhsen K, Sommerfelt H, Robins-Browne R, Levine M (2013) Burden and etiology of diarrheal disease in infants and young children in developing countries (the Global Enteric Multicenter Study, GEMS): a prospective, case-control study. Lancet 382(9888):209–222. doi: 10.1016/S0140-6736(13)60844-2)

Küstner HG, Gibson IH, Carmichael TR, Van Zyl L, Chouler CA, Hyde JP, du Plessis JN (1981) The spread of cholera in South Africa. S Afr Med J 60(3):87–90

Kyelem CG, Bougouma A, Thiombiano RS, Salou-Kagoné IA, Sangaré L, Ouédraogo R. (2011) Cholera epidemic in Burkina Faso in 2005: epidemiologic and diagnostic aspects. Pan Afr Med J 8:1

Lanata CF, Mendoza W, Black RE (2002) Improving diarrhea estimates. World Health Organization, Geneva

Lawoyin TO, Ogunbodede NA, Olumide EA, Onadeko MO (1999) Outbreak of cholera in Ibadan, Nigeria. Eur J Epidemiol 15(4):365–370

Legros D, McCormick M, Mugero C, Skinnider M, Bek'Obita DD, Okware SI (2000) Epidemiology of cholera outbreak in Kampala, Uganda. East Afr Med J 77(7):347–349

Lipp EK, Huq A, Colwell RR (2002) Effects of global climate on infectious disease: the cholera model. Clin Microbiol Rev 15(4):757–770

Lobitz B, Beck L, Huq A, Wood B, Fuchs G, Faruque AS, Colwell R (2000) Climate and infectious disease: use of remote sensing for detection of Vibrio cholerae by indirect measurement. Proc Natl Acad Sci USA 97:1438–1443

Lucas ME, Deen JL, von Seidlein L, Wang XY, Ampuero J, Puri M, Ali M, Ansaruzzaman M, Amos J, Macuamule A, Cavailler P, Guerin PJ, Mahoudeau C, Kahozi-Sangwa P, Chaignat CL, Barreto A, Songane FF, Clemens JD (2005) Effectiveness of mass oral cholera vaccination in Beira, Mozambique. N Engl J Med 352:757–767

Luque Fernández MA, Bauernfeind A, Jiménez JD, Gil CL, El Omeiri N, Guibert DH (2009) Influence of temperature and rainfall on the evolution of cholera epidemics in Lusaka, Zambia, 2003–2006: analysis of a time series. Trans R Soc Trop Med Hyg 103(2):137–143

Luque Fernandez MA, Schomaker M, Mason PR, Fesselet JF, Baudot Y, Boulle A, Maes P (2012) Elevation and cholera: an epidemiological spatial analysis of the cholera epidemic in Harare, Zimbabwe, 2008–2009. BMC Public Health 12(1):442

Luquero FJ, Banga CN, Remartínez D, Palma PP, Baron E, Grais RF (2011) Cholera epidemic in Guinea-Bissau (2008): the importance of "place". PLoS One 6(5):e19005

Macnamara NC (1876) A history of Asiatic cholera. MacMillan, London

Mahamud AS, Ahmed JA, Nyoka R, Auko E, Kahi V, Ndirangu J, Nguhi M, Burton JW, Muhindo BZ, Breiman RF, Eidex RB (2012) Epidemic cholera in Kakuma refugee camp, Kenya, 2009: the importance of sanitation and soap. J Infect Dev Ctries 6(3):234–241

Manga NM, Ndour CT, Diop SA, Dia NM, Ka-Sall R, Diop BM, Sow AI, Sow PS (2008) Cholera in Senegal from 2004 to 2006: lessons learned from successive outbreaks. Med Trop 68(6):589–592

Mari L, Bertuzzo E, Righetto L, Casagrandi R, Gatto M, Rodriguez-Iturbe I, Rinaldo A. (2012) Modelling cholera epidemics: the role of waterways, human mobility and sanitation. J R Soc Interface 9(67):376–388

Mason PR (2009) Zimbabwe experiences the worst epidemic of cholera in Africa. J Infect 3(2):148–151

Matzger H, BMGF, Why Fishermen & Data are Key for Combating Cholera . 2012

McCormack WM, Islam MS, Fahimuddin M, Mosley WH (1969) A community study of inapparent cholera infections. Am J Epidemiol 89:658–664

Mendelsohn J, Dawson T (2008) Climate and cholera in KwaZulu-Natal, South Africa: the role of environmental factors and implications for epidemic preparedness. Int J Hyg Environ Health 211(1–2):156–162

Merrell DS, Butler SM, Qadri F, Dolganov NA, Alam A, Cohen MB, Calderwood SB, Schoolnik GK, Camilli A (2002) Host-induced epidemic spread of the cholera bacterium. Nature 417(6889):642–645

Ministry of Health DRC (2012) Situation épidémiologique du choléra en République Démocratique du Congo en 2011. Cholera Division of the Ministry of Health, Democratic Republic of the Congo (DRC)

MMWR (Morbidity and Mortality Weekly Report) September 3, 2004 Centers for disease control and prevention (CDC). Cholera epidemic associated with raw vegetables—Lusaka, Zambia, 2003–2004. 53(34):783–786

Morris JG Jr (2011) Cholera—modern pandemic disease of ancient lineage. Emerg Infect Dis 17(11):2099–2104

Mugoya I, Kariuki S, Algal T, Njuguna C, Omolon J, Jorge J, Kalan R, Niota C, Teethe C, Bedno S, Breiman RF (2005) Feikin DR (2008) Rapid spread of Vibrio cholerae O1 throughout Kenya. Am J Trop Med Hyg 78(3):527–533

Mukandavire Z, Liao S, Wang J, Gaff H, Smith DL (2011) Morris JG Jr (2011) Estimating the reproductive numbers for the 2008–2009 cholera outbreaks in Zimbabwe. Proc Natl Acad Sci USA 108(21):8767–8772

Mulholland K (1985) Cholera in Sudan: An account of an epidemic in a refugee camp in eastern Sudan, May–June 1985. Disasters 9(4):247–258

Mutonga D, Langat D, Mwangi D, Tonui J, Njeru M, Abade A et al (2013) Cholera epidemiology in Kenya based on national surveillance data from 1997–2010. J Infect Dis 208(1):S55–S61

Muula AS (2009) My Africa. Poverty, health, disease, and medical journalism. Croat Med J 50(6):598–599

Nelson EJ, Harris JB, Morris JG Jr, Calderwood SB, Camilli A (2009) Cholera transmission: the host, pathogen and bacteriophage dynamic. Nat Rev Microbiol 7(10):693–702

Nguyen VD, Sreenivasan N, Lam E, Ayers T, Kargbo D, Dafae F, Jambai A, Alemu W, Kamara A, Islam MS, Stroika S, Bopp C, Quick R, Mintz ED, Brunkard JM (2014) Cholera epidemic associated with consumption of unsafe drinking water and street-vended water–eastern freetown, Sierra Leone, 2012. Am J Trop Med Hyg 90(3):518–523. doi: 10.4269/ajtmh.13-0567. Epub 2014 Jan 27

Nzirorera S (2008) Prevention and hygiene-awareness efforts aim to stave off cholera in Guinea-Bissau

O'Donoghue R (2005) Rhodes university, South Africa. cholera in KwaZulu-Natal: probing institutional governmentality and indigenous hand-washing practices

Olago D, Marshall M, Wandiga SO, Opondo M, Yanda PZ, Kanalawe R, Githeko AK, Downs T, Opere A, Kavumvuli R, Kirumira E, Ogallo L, Mugambi P, Apindi E, Githui F, Kathuri J, Olaka L, Sigalla R, Nanyunja R, Baguma T, Achola P (2007) Climatic, socio-economic, and health factors affecting human vulnerability to cholera in the Lake Victoria basin, East Africa. Ambio 36(4):350–358

Orfeuil JP (2002) La mobilité dans le monde

Osei FB, Duker AA (2008) Spatial and demographic patterns of cholera in Ashanti region - Ghana. Int J Health Geogr 7:44

Ouedraogo RT, Njanpop-Lafourcade B-M, Jaillard P et al (2009) Mobile laboratory to improve response to meningitis epidemics, Burkina Faso epidemic season 2004. Field actions science reports. J Field Actions 1

Pascual M, Rodó X, Ellner SP, Colwell R, Bouma MJ (2000) Cholera dynamics and El Niño-Southern Oscillation. Science 289:1766–1769

Pasetti MF, Levine MM (2012) Insights from natural infection-derived immunity to cholera instruct vaccine efforts. Clin Vaccine Immunol 19:1707–1711

Paz S (2009) Impact of temperature variability on cholera incidence in Southeastern Africa, 1971–2006. Ecohealth 6(3):340–345

Paz S, Broza M (2007) Wind direction and its linkage with Vibrio cholerae dissemination. Environ Health Perspect 115(2):195–200

Penrose K, de Castro MC, Werema J, Ryan ET (2010) Informal urban settlements and cholera risk in Dar-as-Salaam, Tanzania. PLoS Negl Trop Dis 4(3):e631

Perry Phil MSJ, Donini-Lenhoff F (2010) Stigmatization complicates infectious disease management

Piarroux R, Bompangue D, Oger PY, Haaser F, Boinet A, Vandevelde T (2009) From research to field action: example of the fight against cholera in the democratic Republic of Congo. Field Actions Sci Rep 2:69–77

Piarroux R, Faucher B (2012) Cholera epidemics in 2010: respective roles of environment, strain changes, and human-driven dissemination. Clin Microbiol Infect 18(3):231–238

Poda JN, Gagliardi R, Kam FO, Niameogo AT (2003) La perception des populations des maladies diarrhéiques au Burkina Faso: une piste pour l'éducation aux problèmes de santé,VertigO–la revue électronique en sciences de l'environnement

Qadri F, Hasan JA, Hossain J et al (1995) Evaluation of the monoclonal antibody-based kit Bengal SMART for rapid detection of Vibrio cholerae O139 synonym Bengal in stool samples. J Clin Microbiol 33:732–734

Quilici ML, Massenet D, Gake B, Bwalki B, Olson DM (2010) Vibrio cholerae O1 variant with reduced susceptibility to ciprofloxacin, Western Africa. Emerg Infect Dis 16(11):1804–1805

Qureshi K, Mølbak K, Sandström A, Kofoed PE, Rodrigues A, Dias F, Aaby P, Svennerholm AM (2006) Breast milk reduces the risk of illness in children of mothers with cholera: observations from an epidemic of cholera in Guinea-Bissau. Pediatr Infect Dis J 25(12):1163–1166

Rabbani GH, Greenough WB (1999) Food as a vehicle of transmission of cholera. J Diarrheal Dis Res 17(1):1–9

Rebaudet S, Sudre B, Piarroux R (2013) A review of cholera in coastal Africa. J Infect Dis 208(1):S98–S106

Retzky A (2012) Professor Virginia cornish working to engineer yeast to detect cholera. In: Columbia University. http://news.columbia.edu/research/2806. Accessed 19 Mar 2013

Reyburn R, Kim DR, Emch M, Khatib A, von Seidlein L, Ali M (2011) Climate variability and the outbreaks of cholera in Zanzibar, East Africa: a time series analysis. Am J Trop Med Hyg 84(6):862–869. (Erratum in: Am J Trop Med Hyg 2011 Jul;85(1):191)

Rodrigues A, Brun H, Sandstrom A (1997) Risk factors for cholera infection in the initial phase of an epidemic in Guinea-Bissau: protection by lime juice. Am J Trop Med Hyg 57(5):601–604

Rodrigues A, Sandström A, Cá T, Steinsland H, Jensen H, Aaby P (2000) Protection from cholera by adding lime juice to food - results from community and laboratory studies in Guinea-Bissau, West Africa. Trop Med Int Health 5(6):418–422

Sabinot C (2009) Dynamique des savoirs et des Savoir-faire dans un contexte pluriculturel, étude comparative des activités littorales au Gabon

Sack DA (2013) Global cholera burden estimates. In: Johns hopkins bloomberg school of public health. http://www.jhsph.edu/departments/international-health/research/cholera/index.html. Accessed 15 Nov 2013

Sasaki S, Suzuki H, Fujino Y, Kimura Y, Cheelo M (2009) Impact of drainage networks on cholera outbreaks in Lusaka, Zambia. Am J Public Health 99(11):1982–1987

Sasaki S, Suzuki H, Igarashi K, Tambatamba B, Mulenga P (2008) Spatial analysis of risk factor of cholera outbreak for 2003-2004 in a peri-urban area of Lusaka, Zambia. Am J Trop Med Hyg 79(3):414–421

Schaetti C, Hutubessy R, Ali SM, Pach A, Weiss MG, Chaignat CL, Khatib AM (2009) Oral cholera vaccine use in Zanzibar: socioeconomic and behavioral features affecting demand and acceptance. BMC Public Health 9:99

Schaetti C, Khatib IS, Hutubessy R, Chaignat CL, Weiss M-G (2010) Social and cultural features of cholera and shigellosis in peri-urban and rural communities of Zanzibar

Scheelbeek P, Treglown S, Reid T, Maes P (2009) Household fish preparation hygiene and cholera transmission in Monrovia, Liberia. J Infect Dev Ctries 3(9):727–731

Schubert J, Diwete J (2008) Étude qualitative sur la prise en charge de la diarrhée et l'introduction du zinc en RDC (Katanga, Kasaï oriental, Kinshasa)

Schürmann D, Ebert N, Kampf D, Baumann B, Frei U, Suttorp N (2002) Domestic cholera in Germany associated with fresh fish imported from Nigeria. Eur J Clin Microbiol Infect Dis 21(11):827–828

Shapiro RL, Otieno MR, Adcock PM, Phillips-Howard PA, Hawley WA, Kumar L, Waiyaki P, Nahlen BL, Slutsker L (1999) Transmission of epidemic Vibrio cholerae O1 in rural western Kenya associated with drinking water from Lake Victoria: an environmental reservoir for cholera? Am J Trop Med Hyg 60(2):271–276

Shikanga OT, Mutonga D, Abade M, Amwayi S, Ope M, Limo H, Mintz ED, Quick RE, Breiman RF, Feikin DR (2009) High mortality in a cholera outbreak in western Kenya after post-election violence in 2008. Am J Trop Med Hyg 81(6):1085–1090

Shultz A, Omolon JO, Burke H, Qassim M, Ochieng JB, Weinberg M, Feikin DR, Breiman RF (2009) Cholera outbreak in Kenyan refugee camp: risk factors for illness and importance of sanitation. Am J Trop Med Hyg 80(4):640–645

Soura B, Baya B, Rossier C (2008) Institut Superieur des Sciences de la Population Université de Ouagadougou. Utilisation des médicaments de la rue à Ouagadougou effet de niveau de vie ou effet de niveau d'éducation ?

St Louis ME, Porter JD, Helal A, Drame K, Hargrett-Bean N, Wells JG, Tauxe RV (1990) Epidemic cholera in West Africa: The role of food handling and high-risk foods. Am J Epidemiol 131:719–728

Staro F (2011) Entre savoirs experts et mauvais sort Pratiques d'utilisation de l'eau et perception de l'épidémie du

Swerdlow DL, Malanga G, Begokyan G et al (1991) Epidemic of antimicrobial resistant Vibrio cholera O1 infections in a refugee camp, Malawi. In: Program and abstracts of the 31st interscience conference on antimicrobial agents and chemotheraphy, vol. 529. p 187

Swerdlow DL, Malenga G, Begkoyian G, Nyangulu D, Toole M, Waldman RJ, Puhr DN, Tauxe RV (1997) Epidemic cholera among refugees in Malawi, Africa: treatment and transmission. Epidemiol Infect 118(3):207–214

Tauxe RV, Holmberg SD, Dodin A, Wells JV, Blake PA (1988) Epidemic cholera in Mali: high mortality and multiple routes of transmission in a famine area. Epidemiol Infect 100:279–289

Trærup SL, Ortiz RA, Markandya A (2011) The costs of climate change: a study of cholera in Tanzania. Int J Environ Res Public Health 8(12):4386–4405

Truscott R (2008) Zimbabwe faces a "major health disaster", as hospitals close. BMJ 337:a2710

Umoh JU, Adesiyun AA, Adekeye JO, Nadarajah M (1983) Epidemiological features of an outbreak of gastroenteritis/cholera in Katsina, Northern Nigeria. J Hyg (Lond) 91(1):101–111

UNICEF (2013) http://www.unicef.org/cholera/. Accessed 25 May 2013

Utsalo SJ, Eko FO, Umoh F, Asindi AA (1999) Faecal excretion of Vibrio cholerae during convalescence of cholera patients in Calabar, Nigeria. Eur J Epidemiol 15(4):379–381

Van Loon FP, Clemens JD, Shahrier M, Sack DA, Stephensen CB, Khan MR, Rabbani GH, Rao MR, Banik AK (1990) Low gastric acid as a risk factor for cholera transmission: application of a new non-invasive gastric acid field test. J Clin Epidemiol 43:1361–1367

Von Seidlein L (2013) J Infect Dis 208(1):S8-S14

Weil AG, Ragheb J, Niazi TN, Bhatia S (2012) Am J Trop Med Hyg 87(5):921–6. doi: 10.4269/ajtmh.2012.12-0323. Epub 2012 Sep 10

Wendo C (2003) Cholera spreads in Liberia. Lancet 362(9388):966

WHO (2005) International health regulations, 2nd edn. World Health Organization, Geneva

WHO (2009) Global task force on cholera control. Cholera country profile: Sierra Leone. http://www.who.int/cholera/countries/SierraLeoneCountryProfile2009.pdf. Accessed 7 Sept 2009

WHO (2010) Global health observatory, MDG-7 Environment sustainability, population using improved sanitation. http://apps.who.int/gho/data/?vid=640. Accessed 21 Dec 2012

WHO Global Health Observatory (GHO) (2012) http://www.who.int/gho/en/. Accessed 15 Jan 2013

WHO (2013) Global health observatory. http://www.who.int/gho/en. Accessed 15 Jan 2013

WHO (2013) Integrated disease surveillance. In: World Health Organization. http://www.who.int/csr/labepidemiology/projects/diseasesurv/en/index.html. Accessed 18 Mar 2013

WHO (2013) Technical guidelines for integrated disease surveillance and response in the African region. http://www.afro.who.int/en/clusters-a-programmes/dpc/integrated-disease-surveillance/features/2775-technical-guidelines-for-integrated-disease-surveillance-and-response-in-the-african-region.html. Accessed 1 Mar 2013

Zuckerman JN, Rombo L, Fisch A (2007) The true burden and risk of cholera: implications for prevention and control. Lancet Infect Dis 7(8):521–530

Zurovac D, Talisuna AO, Snow RW (2012) Mobile phone text messaging: tool for malaria control in Africa. PLoS Medicine 9:e1001176

The Cholera Outbreak in Haiti: Where and how did it begin?

Daniele Lantagne, G. Balakrish Nair, Claudio F. Lanata and Alejandro Cravioto

Abstract In October 2010, cholera appeared in Haiti for the first time in nearly a century. The Secretary-General of the United Nations formed an Independent Panel to "investigate and seek to determine the source of the 2010 cholera outbreak in Haiti". To fulfill this mandate, the Panel conducted concurrent epidemiological, water and sanitation, and molecular analysis investigations. Our May 2011 findings indicated that the 2010 Haiti cholera outbreak was caused by bacteria *introduced* into Haiti as a result of human activity; more specifically by the contamination of the Meye Tributary System of the Artibonite River with a pathogenic strain of the current South Asian type *Vibrio cholerae.* Recommendations were presented to assist in preventing the future introduction and spread of cholera in Haiti and worldwide. In this chapter, we discuss both the results of the Independent Panel's investigation and the context the report sat within; including background information, responses to the report's release, additional research subsequent to our report, and the public health implications of the Haiti cholera epidemic.

D. Lantagne (✉)
Department of Civil and Environmental Engineering, Tufts University, 200 College Avenue, Medford, MA 02155, USA
e-mail: daniele.lantagne@tufts.edu

G. Balakrish Nair
Translational Health Science and Technology Institute, Haryana, India

C. F. Lanata
Instituo de Investigación Nutricional, The US Navy Medical Research Unit 6, Lima, Peru

A. Cravioto
International Vaccine Institute, Seoul, Korea

Current Topics in Microbiology and Immunology (2014) 379: 145–164
DOI: 10.1007/82_2013_331

Published Online: 22 May 2013

Contents

1 Introduction

1.1 History of Haiti

In 1492, Columbus first landed in the new world at Cap-Haiten on the northern coast of the island of Hispaniola; now comprised of Haiti and the Dominican Republic (Prince 1985). The native Taíno population was exploited for gold mining and by 1548 (56 years after Columbus landed) the Taíno population dropped from an estimated 500,000 to less than 500. In 1519, sugar and cattle farming, worked by slaves, replaced worked-out gold mines as the economic foundation of the island. From 1519 to 1549, 864,000 slaves were brought to Haiti.

Over time, France began to wrest with Spain over Hispaniola, and took control of the western portion of the island (modern day Haiti) in 1697. In 1801, slave leaders led a revolt against the French, and Haiti declared independence on January 1, 1804. Haiti thus became the first black republic in the world and the second free state in the western hemisphere. France officially recognized Haiti in 1825, on the condition that compensation for lost income due to confiscation of property be paid. Haiti paid this debt until 1922.

A number of different political leaders led Haiti between 1804 and 1915, and a stable political system was never established. From 1915 to 1934, the United States occupied Haiti after seven different presidents were in power from 1910 to 1915.

A number of dictators led Haiti from 1934 to 1956. In 1956, Francois Duvalier, with support from the black middle class and isolated rural poor, won the presidency, and his son, Jean Claude, succeeded him after his death in 1971. The Duvalier regime was characterized by rule by private militia, violence, amendment of the constitution, personal wealth, and intermittent support from the United States.

In 1986, a combination of popular uprising and withdrawal of United States support led Jean Claude Duvalier to flee to exile in France (Macquire et al. 1996). In February 1991, after a period of civil unrest, a young priest named Jean-Bertrand Aristide was inaugurated into the presidency in what is widely regarded as the first democratic election in Haiti. His Lavalas ('cleansing flood') party survived only until a coup in September 1991. Aristide escaped to the United States, and the army regained power.

In October 1991, the United States established economic sanctions against the military regime and then occupied Haiti again in 1994. On October 15, 1994, Aristide was reestablished as the Haitian president, with one and a half years left in his constitutionally mandated 5-year term. Aristide was replaced by his successor, Rene Préval, in 1996, reelected President in November 2000, and forced into exile in 2004. The United Nations Stabilization Mission in Haiti (MINUSTAH) peacekeeping force was established in response to the political turmoil of 2004. Rene Préval was reelected president in 2006, with a constitutionally mandated 5 year maximum term ending in 2011.

1.2 Haiti Geography and Environment

Haiti encompasses 27,750 square kilometers of the western third of the island of Hispaniola in the Caribbean Sea (Library of Congress—Federal Research Division 2006). The majority of Haiti's land (63 %) is considered too steep for agricultural production; however, nearly 80 % of the country's area functions as agricultural land. Deforestation is extreme in Haiti, as forests covered nearly 60 % of the country in 1923, and only 2 % by 2006. Most Haitians still depend on charcoal as their primary fuel and cooking source. This deforestation has led to soil erosion, which has decreased agricultural yields and resulted in deadly landslides.

The 2010 population of Haiti was estimated at just under 10 million, with 3 million in the capital city of Port-au-Prince (UNICEF 2012). Haiti is the poorest country in the Western Hemisphere, with a per capita income of 650 USD/year and 55 % of the population living below the world poverty line of 1.25 dollars per day. The life expectancy in Haiti is 62 years and adult literacy is 49 %. In 2008, 63 % of the population had access to improved drinking water (71 % of urban residents and 55 % of rural residents) and 17 % of the population had access to improved sanitation.

The development of sustainable water and sanitation infrastructure in Haiti has been hindered by ongoing political instability and lack of investment. In 1964, the government agency CAMEP was established with responsibility for the drinking water supply in Port-au-Prince. In 1977, the government agency SNEP was established with responsibility for water supply in secondary cities. During this time, the rural water supply situation was managed by the government agency POCHEP in the Ministry of Public Health.

In January 2009, the Haitian Parliament approved a water and sanitation sector reform bill,which formalized sector reform. The law created a National Directorate of Water Supply and Sanitation (DINEPA) in the Ministry of Public Works, Transport, and Communications, as well as four Regional Offices of Drinking Water and Sanitation (OREPAs). The role of DINEPA is to execute the government guidelines in the water and sanitation sector by developing water and sanitation sector regulation and monitoring stakeholders in the sector.

1.3 January 12, 2010 Earthquake

On January 12, 2010, a 7.0 magnitude earthquake struck 17 km southwest of Port-au-Prince, Haiti. Nearly one-third of Haiti's population, almost three million people, were affected by 'extreme', 'violent', or 'severe' shaking (USGS 2010). An estimated 222,650 people died and 310,930 were injured (OCHA 2013a). This powerful quake in an area of poor quality construction materials caused extensive damage to shelters. The building damage assessment conducted from March 2010 to February 2011 indicated 403,176 buildings were damaged or destroyed (OCHA 2013a). Out-migration of an estimated 482,000 people from affected areas also strained resources in rural Haiti (CDEMA 2010). In addition, many schools and hospitals were destroyed (OCHA 2013a).

The immediate humanitarian response was complicated by the: (1) inability to import goods due to damage to the airport and port; (2) inability to transport goods due to rubble and temporary shelters blocking roadways; (3) loss of life and resources within humanitarian organizations; (4) communications difficulties; (5) lack of staff capacity to respond; and (6) the overwhelming scale of the disaster. The water, sanitation, and hygiene emergency response Cluster estimated 1.1 million people hosted in approximately 651 spontaneous settlements in Port-au-Prince, Jacmel, Gressier, Léogâne, Grand Goâve, and Petit Goâve were in immediate need of services (OCHA 2010).

Over time, as the response continued, the number of people housed in spontaneous settlements fell from a high of 1,536,447 in July 2010 to 420,513 in April 2012 (IASC 2012). However, as of April 2012, 70 % of water points in these settlements had no free chlorine residual, 95 % of residents did not have access to 10 l of water per day, and only 3 % had adequate handwashing facilities with soap and water.

In the Center for Disease Control and Prevention's (CDC) "Haiti Pre-decision Brief for Public Health Action Cholera", the CDC wrote "Cholera is extremely unlikely to occur" as "Epidemic cholera has not been reported from Haiti before" and "An outbreak of cholera is very unlikely at this time (CDC 2010). For a cholera outbreak to occur, two conditions must be met: (1) there must be significant breeches in the water, sanitation, and hygiene infrastructure used by groups of people, permitting large-scale exposure to food or water contaminated with *Vibrio cholera* [sic] organisms; and (2) cholera must be present in the population. While the current water, sanitation, and hygiene infrastructure in Haiti would certainly facilitate transmission of cholera (and many other illnesses), cholera is not circulating in Haiti, and the risk of cholera introduction to Haiti is low. Most current travelers to Haiti are relief workers from countries without endemic cholera, and they are likely to have access to adequate sanitation and hygiene facilities within Haiti, such that any cholera organisms they import would be safely contained."

1.4 Cholera

Cholera is a severe, acute, dehydrating diarrhea that can kill children and adults in less than 12 h, and is the result of infection with a pathogenic strain of the bacterium *Vibrio cholerae*. The organism is capable of producing a potent toxin known as cholera toxin (CT). Depending on the severity of the infection, cholera may be treated with oral rehydration salt (ORS) solutions, intravenous fluids, and/or antibiotics. *V. cholerae* infection displays a clinical spectrum that ranges from asymptomatic infection to severe cholera known as *cholera gravis*. The number of asymptomatic cases that play a role in the transmission of cholera varies according to age and the endemic nature of the disease. In countries such as Bangladesh, asymptomatic cases may represent roughly half of all cases (Nelson et al. 2009).

Although cholera has been a localized phenomenon in South Asia for centuries, the pathogen has repeatedly demonstrated the ability to spread both regionally and internationally. The seventh worldwide pandemic of cholera began in 1961 and is ongoing. The control of the disease requires a combination of interventions that range from water supply and sanitation improvements at the community level to the use of currently available oral cholera vaccines at the individual level.

1.5 Cholera in Haiti

In October 2010, cholera appeared in Haiti. At the beginning of the outbreak, the source of the 2010 outbreak was a topic of debate. Three credible hypotheses were proposed. The first hypothesis held that an environmental strain of *V. cholerae* that normally inhabits the Gulf of Mexico traveled to Haiti naturally via ocean currents as a consequence of the January 12th, 2010 earthquake and caused the present cholera epidemic. The second hypothesis held that a local, non-toxigenic *V. cholerae* strain endemic to the Haitian environment naturally mutated into a virulent pathogenic strain, which quickly spread throughout the human population of Haiti. The third hypothesis held that the source of the outbreak was an infected human who carried a pathogenic strain of *V. cholerae* into Haiti from a cholera endemic region outside the country.

1.6 MINUSTAH in Haiti

The United Nations Stabilization Mission in Haiti (MINUSTAH) was created in April 2004 by the United Nations Security Council. After the January 12th, 2010 earthquake, the United Nations (UN) Security Council passed additional resolutions increasing the number of MINUSTAH forces in order to support recovery, reconstruction, and stability efforts. A specific form of the third hypothesis for the source of the cholera outbreak, that soldiers at the Mirebalais MINUSTAH camp were the direct source for the cholera outbreak, was a commonly held belief in Haiti immediately after the introduction of cholera. Testimony cited to support this belief includes the following: (1) the Mirebalais MINUSTAH camp is located near the area where the first cholera cases were identified; (2) a new group of soldiers had recently arrived at the time of the first cases; and (3) witnesses reported sanitation practices at the camp that allowed soldiers' feces to enter the environment.

1.7 Convening of Independent Panel

In order to definitively determine the source of the outbreak, the Secretary-General of the UN convened the Independent Panel of Experts on the Cholera Outbreak in Haiti (the "Independent Panel"), with the mandate to "investigate and seek to determine the source of the 2010 cholera outbreak in Haiti", and to present the findings of this investigation in a written report submitted to the UN Secretary-General and to the Government of Haiti.

Before convening the Independent Panel, a definitive determination of the source of the 2010 cholera outbreak in Haiti had been lacking. Two previous investigations that commented on the source of the outbreak came to opposing conclusions: Sack (Hurtado 2010 and personal communication) concluded that the outbreak was caused by a local event; whereas Piarroux (2010 and personal communication) concluded that the outbreak was caused by cholera being imported to Haiti by an infected MINUSTAH soldier. Neither investigation presented sufficient evidence to support its conclusions with absolute certainty at the time of the Independent Panel's convening.

The four members of the Panel were selected for their various areas of expertise, including microbiological (Balakrish Nair), epidemiological (Claudio Lanata), cholera (Alejandro Cravioto), and water and sanitation (Daniele Lantagne). To conduct the investigation the Panel members: (1) conducted meetings in Asia and the United States with key informants; (2) convened for field investigations in Haiti from February 14–18, 2011; (3) conducted further meetings in the United States with key informants; (4) convened in March 2011 to draft the report; and (5) convened in May 2011 to finalize the report and present the results to the Secretary-General. A copy of the finalized report was presented to the UN Secretary-General's office the evening before the formal meeting with the Secretary-General (Cravioto et al. 2011), and later adopted for peer-reviewed publication (Lantagne et al. 2012). All informants and documentation received relevant to the investigation were kept confidential and not provided to the Secretary-General's office.

2 Results of the Report of the Independent Panel

To determine the source of the 2010 Haiti cholera outbreak, the Independent Panel undertook concurrent epidemiological, water and sanitation, and molecular analysis investigations. Epidemiological information was obtained from records of diarrheal illnesses among MINUSTAH personnel, as well as during visits to hospitals along the Artibonite River to determine the exact onset dates of the cholera outbreak throughout the watershed. Discussions were held with local experts to understand the hydrology of the Artibonite River and its tributaries, the water and sanitation situation in the Mirebalais MINUSTAH camp, and water use practices of the population along the river. Published and unpublished information was obtained from groups currently working on the evolution of *V. cholerae* in Haiti and worldwide. Information on the basic microbiology and data from advanced molecular typing techniques was used to compare the Haitian strains against other known worldwide strains of *V. cholerae*. Each of these three investigations will be described in the following sections.

2.1 Epidemiological Investigation

MINUSTAH uniformed personnel in Haiti originate from 22 countries, and are deployed in contingents based on their country-of-origin to specific geographical areas in Haiti. In Centre and Artibonite Departments, there were permanently deployed contingents from Nepal, Argentina, and Peru. Contingents from Nepal were stationed in three camps (Hinche, Mirebalais, and Terre Rouge).

MINUSTAH contingents are deployed in 6 month rotations. The replacement Nepal contingent arrived in Centre Department between October 8th and 24th, 2010 after 3 months of training in Kathmandu, Nepal. Once the training and a medical examination were completed, soldiers were given a 10 day free period to visit their families before traveling to Haiti. Within 1 day of arrival in Haiti, soldiers were transported to their posts in Centre Department.

The medical records of MINUSTAH personnel stationed in Haiti for the time period between September and October 2010 were obtained and reviewed. No cases of severe diarrhea and dehydration occurred among MINUSTAH personnel during this period.

In each hospital visited along the Artibonite River, a detailed review of medical records from October 2010 was carried out to identify cases, especially adults, that required hospitalization due to diarrhea and dehydration in order to establish an outbreak onset date. Since detailed medical records did not exist, which would have allowed an epidemiological definition of a cholera case to be created, hospitalizations due to severe diarrhea were used as a proxy for cholera cases.

At Mirebalais Government Hospital in Mirebalais, the first severe diarrhea case that required hospitalization and the first death from dehydration in patients older than 20 years of age occurred during the night of October 17th, 2010 and early morning of October 18th, 2010, respectively. No fish or shellfish products from the coast were found in the Mirebalais market by the Independent Panel. At Hospital Albert Schweitzer, two-thirds of the way between Mirebalais and St. Marc, the first cases of severe diarrhea requiring observation and hospitalization were seen on October 20th, 2010. At St. Nicolas Hospital in St. Marc in the Artibonite River Delta, a low background rate of diarrhea was abruptly interrupted by an explosive outbreak of cholera cases with dehydration and death on October 20th, 2010. On this date, medical staff recorded 404 hospitalizations (one every 3.6 min) and 44 deaths on individual pieces of paper. These 404 cases came from 50 identified communities throughout the Artibonite River Delta region, with only 9 (2.2 %) of the 404 patients originated from St. Marc. It is important to mention that cholera cots, designed to minimize fecal contamination in cholera wards and to measure fluid loss easily, were not seen in any of the three hospitals visited.

2.2 Water and Sanitation Investigation

The Artibonite River is the largest river in Haiti, flowing from the mountains of the Dominican Republic to the coast near the town of Grande Saline (Fig. 1). The river is controlled at two points: (1) the Peligre Hydroelectric Dam, which is located approximately 10 km upstream from Mirebalais and is operated by Électricité d'Haïti (EDH); and (2) at the Canneau Canal Sitew here the river is split into a series of canals for use by small farmers to irrigate their fields in the Artibonite Valley.

At the Peligre Dam, EDH engineering staff reported that it takes 1.5–2 days for water released from the dam to reach the Canneau Canal Site. At the Canneau Canal Site, operations and maintenance staff also reported that water flows from the Peligre Dam to Canneau in 2 days. In St. Marc, Artibonite Valley engineering staff reported that it takes about 1 day for water to flow from the Peligre Dam to the Canneau Canal Site, and another 1 day for water to flow from Canneau through the canal system to the sea in the Artibonite River Delta.

Two branches of the Meye Tributary of the Artibonite River flow northwards from the mountains that are located to the southwest and southeast of Mirebalais (Fig. 1). The branches join together to form the Meye Tributary just north of the Mirebalais MINUSTAH camp. There is significant human activity along this tributary, with women washing, people bathing, people collecting water for drinking, and children playing.

At the time of the Independent Panel's visit, there was one main area at the Mirebalais MINUSTAH camp that housed toilet and showering facilities for the

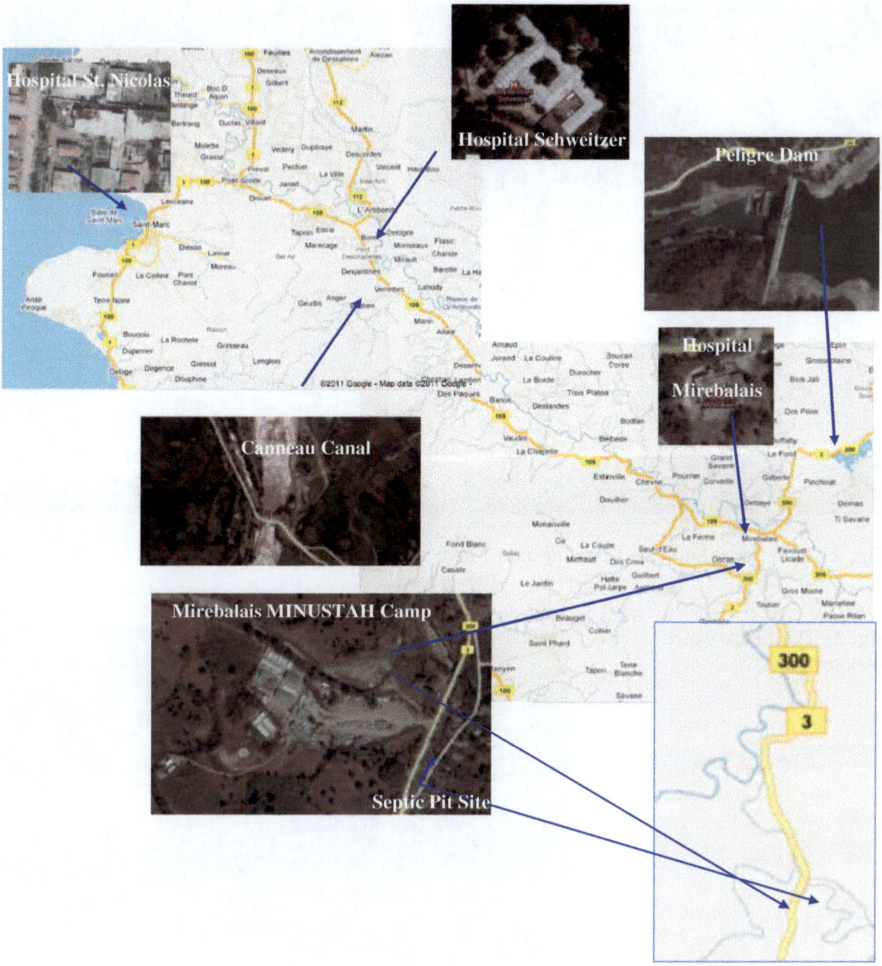

Fig. 1 Sites visited along Artibonite River

contingent. Gray water waste (cooking water, wash water, shower water) flowed into on-site soak pits and was allowed to drain into the soil. Black water waste (containing human feces) flowed into six 2,500 l fiberglass tanks. The construction of the water pipes in the main toilet/showering area was haphazard, with significant potential for cross-contamination through leakage from broken pipes and poor pipe connections, especially from pipes that ran over an open drainage ditch that runs throughout the camp and flows directly into the Meye Tributary System (Fig. 2). It was evident from inspection, as well as reported by local Haitians, that construction work in this area had been undertaken after October 2011.

The black water tanks were emptied on demand by a contracting company approved by MINUSTAH headquarters in Port-au-Prince. The contracting company dispatched a truck from Port-au-Prince to collect and transport the waste across the

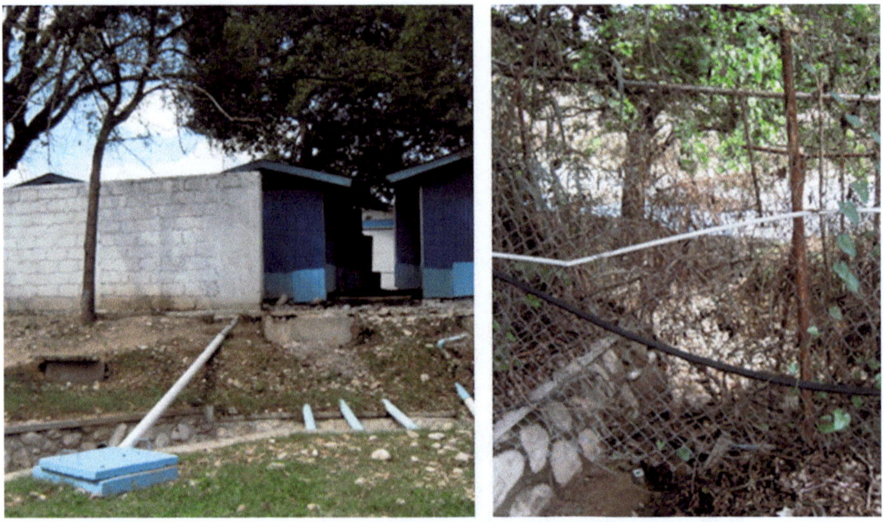

Fig. 2 Toilet area and canal flowing into Meye Tributary

Fig. 3 The black water disposal pit

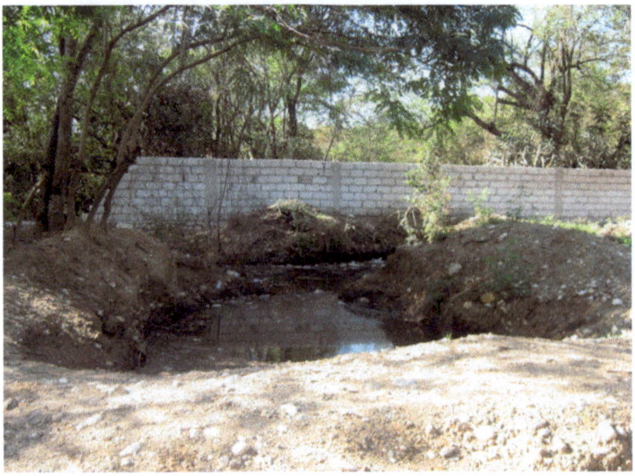

street and up a residential dirt road to a location at the top of the hill, where the waste was deposited in an open septic pit (Fig. 3). Black water waste for the two other MINUSTAH facilities—Hinche and Terre Rouge—was also disposed of in this pit. There was no fence around the site, and children were observed playing and animals roaming in the area around the pit. The southeast branch of Meye Tributary System is located a short walk down the hill from the pit, and local residents reported the area is susceptible to flooding and overflow into the Tributary during rainfall. Calculations indicate that it would take 2–8 h for water to flow from near the septic disposal pit to the junction with the Artibonite River.

2.3 Molecular Analysis Investigation

At the time of the Independent Panel's investigation, the current Nepal strain of cholera was not available for molecular analysis. Thus, the Independent Panel was able to review information on the Haitian strain itself, and on comparing the Haitian strain to other known strains. The available molecular data from whole genome sequence and smaller comparisons of specific parts of the genomes of the *V. cholerae* strains responsible for the outbreak of cholera in Haiti showed a remarkable consistency. They all indicated that the Haitian strains were: (1) clonal (genetically identical) indicating a point-source for the outbreak; and (2) very similar but not identical to the South Asian strains of *V. cholerae* O1. It was emphasized, however, that the Haitian strains has certain minor traits not found in collections from across the world, which is consistent with the micro-evolution that takes place continuously within the El Tor biotype as it moves throughout the world.

Our analysis of available data at the time of our investigation refuted the argument that the Haitian strains arose indigenously from the Haitian environment. The Haitian strains did not originate from the native environs of Haiti but as a result of human activity in an area that promoted the dissemination of the organism. The presence of riverine settings that merges into an estuarine environment, which is an optimal setting for rapid growth of *V. cholerae* O1, is likely to have contributed to the rapid spread of the pathogen. This has happened before in many parts of the world. The precise country from where the Haiti isolate of *V. cholerae* O1 arrived is debatable. Such a conclusion, if warranted, can only be made if representative strains from other countries in South Asia were available for global DNA sequence comparisons. Since none of these stains from Nepal were available for comparison at the time of the preparation of our report it was not possible to established a direct comparison between strains of *V. cholerae* O1 circulating in Nepal strains and those circulating in Haiti.

2.4 Results

The epidemiological data indicated the cholera epidemic began in the upstream region of the Artibonite River on October 17th, 2010. As this region has little to no consumption of fish or shellfish products, the most likely cause of the outbreak was the consumption of contaminated water from the river. Two to three days later, an explosive cholera outbreak began on October 20th, 2010 in the Artibonite River Delta.

The sanitation conditions at the Mirebalais MINUSTAH camp were not sufficient to prevent contamination of the Meye Tributary System with human fecal waste. Contamination in the Meye could have reached Canneau within 1–2 days, and would have been fully distributed in the canal system in the Artibonite River Delta within a maximum of 2–3 days, consistent with the epidemiological timeline.

The available molecular data from whole genome sequence and comparisons of smaller specific parts of the genomes of the *V. cholerae* strains responsible for the outbreak of cholera in Haiti all indicate that the Haitian strains are: (1) clonal (genetically identical) indicating a point-source for the outbreak; and, (2) very similar but not identical to the South Asian strains of *V. cholerae* O1. The precise country from where the Haiti isolate of *V. cholerae* O1 arrived is unknown.

2.5 Conclusions

At the time of the report, the evidence did not support the hypotheses suggesting that the current outbreak is of a natural environmental source. In particular, the outbreak was not due to the Gulf of Mexico strain of *V. cholerae,* nor was it due to a pathogenic mutation of a strain indigenously originating from the Haitian environment. Instead, the evidence overwhelmingly supported the conclusion that the source of the Haiti cholera outbreak was due to contamination of the Meye Tributary of the Artibonite River with a pathogenic strain of current South Asian type *V. cholerae* as a result of human activity.

This contamination initiated an explosive cholera outbreak downstream in the Artibonite River Delta, and eventually, throughout Haiti. The explosive spread was due to several factors:

- Tens of thousands of Haitians use the Meye Tributary System and Artibonite River waters for washing, bathing, drinking, and recreation, and were thus exposed to cholera;
- Thousands of Haitian agriculture workers are regularly exposed to the Artibonite River water, particularly in the rice paddy fields;
- The canal system and delta of the Artibonite River provided optimal environmental conditions for rapid proliferation of *V. cholerae*;
- The Haitian population lacked immunity to cholera;
- Many areas of Haiti suffer from poor water and sanitation conditions;
- Infected individuals fled to their home communities from the initial outbreak locations, and in the process dispersed the disease;
- Infected individuals rapidly concentrated where treatment was available;
- The South Asian type *V. cholerae* strain that caused the outbreak causes a more severe diarrhea due to an increase in the production of a classical type of CT and has the propensity of protracting outbreaks of cholera; and
- The conditions in which cholera patients were initially treated in medical facilities did not help in the prevention of the spread of the disease to other patients or to the health workers.

The introduction of this cholera strain as a result of environmental contamination with feces could not have been the source of such an outbreak without simultaneous water and sanitation and health care system deficiencies. These deficiencies, coupled with conducive environmental and epidemiological conditions, allowed the spread of the *V. cholerae* organism in the environment, from which a large number of people became infected. The Independent Panel concluded that the Haiti cholera outbreak was caused by the confluence of circumstances as described above, and was not the fault of, or deliberate action of, a group or individual.

The source of cholera in Haiti is no longer relevant to controlling the outbreak. What are needed at this time are measures to prevent the disease from becoming endemic.

2.6 Recommendations

The Independent Panel of Experts on the Cholera Outbreak in Haiti made the following recommendations to the UN, the Government of Haiti, and the international community:

- The Haiti cholera outbreak highlights the risk of transmitting cholera during mobilization of population for emergency response. To prevent introduction of cholera into non-endemic countries, United Nations personnel and emergency responders traveling from cholera endemic areas should either receive a prophylactic dose of appropriate antibiotics before departure or be screened with a sensitive method to confirm absence of asymptomatic carriage of *V. cholerae*, or both.
- UN missions commonly operate in emergencies with concurrent cholera epidemics. All UN personnel and emergency responders traveling to emergencies should receive prophylactic antibiotics, be immunized against cholera with currently available oral vaccines, or both, in order to protect their own health and to protect the health of others.
- To prevent introduction of contamination into the local environment, UN installations worldwide should treat fecal waste using on-site systems that inactivate pathogens before disposal. These systems should be operated and maintained by trained, qualified UN staff or by local providers with adequate UN oversight.
- To improve case management and decrease the cholera case fatality rate, UN agencies should take stewardship in:
  - Training health workers, especially at the treatment center level;
  - Scaling-up the availability and use of oral rehydration salts at the household and community level in order to prevent deaths before arrival at treatment centers; and
  - Implementing appropriate measures (including the use of cholera cots) to reduce the risk of intra-facility transmission of cholera to health staff, relatives, and other patients.

- To prevent the spread of cholera, the UN and the Government of Haiti should prioritize investment in piped, treated drinking water supplies, and improved sanitation throughout Haiti. Until such time as water supply and sanitation infrastructure is established:
  - Programs to treat water at the household or community level with chlorine or other effective systems, handwashing with soap, and safe disposal of fecal waste should be developed and/or expanded; and
  - Safe drinking water supplies should continue to be delivered and fecal waste should be collected and safely disposed of in areas of high population density, such as the spontaneous settlement camps.
- The international community should investigate the potential for using vaccines reactively after the onset of an outbreak to reduce cholera caseload and spread of the disease.
- Recent advances in molecular microbial techniques contributed significantly to the investigative capabilities of this report. Through its agencies, the UN should promote the use of molecular microbial techniques to improve surveillance, detection, and tracking of *V. cholerae*, as well as other disease-causing organisms that have the potential to spread internationally.

3 Responses to Report

The immediate response to the report of the UN was to establish a Task Force to evaluate the recommendations and state that the report "does not present any conclusive scientific evidence linking the outbreak to the MINUSTAH peacekeepers or the Mirebalais camp" and "anyone carrying the relevant strain of the disease in the area could have introduced the bacteria into the river" (Reuters 2011; UN News Centre 2011). The Task Force did submit one request for additional information from the Independent Panel, which was answered. To date, no further contact has been initiated, and no results from the Task Force released.

The immediate press response to the Independent Panel's report was a fascinating perspective on how science is translated to the public through media. As members of the Independent Panel we knew we were writing an important, political report that would be scrutinized closely. We made a group decision we would write the report in scientific language, speaking as experts in the field, reporting what we could with scientific certainty. All text was reviewed and approved by all members of the Independent Panel, and key text—including the Executive Summary, Conclusions, and Recommendations—were written as a consensus-based verbal process, with a recorder writing the language, which was then reviewed by all.

The immediate media response focused around the key theme of blame, and whether, and to whom, the panel apportioned blame to, including some representative samples below:

- But the four scientific experts refrained from blaming UN peacekeepers … Instead their report said the outbreak was a result of a "confluence of circumstances" (Leopold 2011).
- But—perhaps so as not to fan the flames—it stops short of blaming the Nepalese or MINUSTAH. Instead, the report stresses that the disease became a major disaster as a result of a series of circumstances, including Haiti's poor drinking water and sanitation infrastructure and lack of medical services. The outbreak "was not the fault of, or deliberate action of, a group or individual," it says (Enserink 2011).
- The 32-page report … clearly states that the source of the epidemic was most likely a camp for UN peacekeepers in Haiti, whose human waste was dumped by independent contractors into an unsecured pit that was susceptible to flooding in heavy rainfall. But the report buries that central finding under a welter of circumstances that caused investigators to conclude that the outbreak, which is ongoing, "was not the fault of, or deliberate action of, a group or individual" (Russell 2011).
- Fortunately, most news articles have looked beyond the conclusion of the report, and accurately noted that while the panel members refused to lay blame on MINUSTAH, the evidence in the report clearly does. As Joe Lauria of the Wall Street Journal wrote: The report plays down as a "hypothesis that soldiers deployed from a cholera-endemic country to the Mirebalais Minustah camp were the source of the cholera" which it said was "a commonly held belief in Haiti." But the report then describes in detail how the outbreak occurred because of contamination of the Artibonite River from the peacekeeping camp (CEPR 2011).
- But the panel refused to single out the troops for blame, stating that Haitians—who had recently suffered a devastating earthquake—should not have been using the river for drinking or washing (Lynn 2011).
- It is also a masterpiece of diplomatic writing that never once directly names the Nepali peacekeepers as the carriers of the South Asian strain of *V. cholera* that has killed almost 5,000 persons and sickened a quarter of a million. In fact, the report blames the victims much more directly (Crof 2011).

The comments above can be summarized into questions on: 1) Why did we not blame the Nepali MINUSTAH soldiers? 2) Why did we not blame the United Nations? and 3) Why did we blame the Haitians?

There are two answers to the first question. First, the majority of the evidence presented in the report was circumstantial. As we did not have microbiological evidence to support a direct link between the Nepal and Haiti strain at the time of writing, we did not feel we could present with scientific certainty that someone associated with the MINUSTAH facility was responsible for the introduction of cholera into Haiti. As the United Nations stated, it could, theoretically, have been someone else infected with that strain in the same area, however unlikely that might be. Second, we strongly felt that the introduction of cholera into Haiti was an accidental, as opposed to a deliberate, act. Thus, whomever—whether it be a peacekeeper or another individual—introduced the strain should not be held personally responsible.

To answer the second questions, we felt the transmission of cholera in this manner was so unprecedented and unlikely, as evidenced by the CDC statement, that we did not feel that this was a predictable event. While we know now that cholera can be introduced in this manner, and thus should strive to prevent this happening in the future, at the time of the report, this was a novel thought.

For the third question, we do not feel we blamed the Haitians for the outbreak. To cause an outbreak you need a source, a means of dissemination, and a susceptible population. Haiti, sadly, had all three, and the confluence of all three is what led to the outbreak.

Some journalists, in our opinion, translated the scientific language into popular media accurately, such as the Independent: "An official report into the ongoing epidemic, which began last October, has concluded that it was almost certainly caused by a poorly constructed sanitation system installed at a rural camp used by several hundred UN troops from Nepal" (Adams 2011).

On the whole, the media response caused us to reflect on the role of writing for scientific certainty in situations with imperfect information.

4 Additional Evidence and Response

Since the completion of the Independent Panel's report, there has been a plethora of research on the Haitian cholera outbreak. In total, the weight of this additional evidence supports the conclusions of the Independent Panel. Three articles in particular expand upon our conclusions. On August 23, 2011, results from whole-genome sequence typing to compare Nepal 2010 cholera strains to the Haiti cholera strain were reported; the authors found that "three Nepalese isolates and three Haitian isolates that were almost identical, with only 1- or 2-bp [base-pair] differences. Results in this study are consistent with Nepal as the origin of the Haitian outbreak." (Hendriksen et al. 2011). In July 2011, results from an epidemiological investigation conducted by a French and Haitian team in December 2010 were published, with their epidemiological model "strongly suggest[ing] that contamination of the Artibonite and one of its tributaries downstream from a military camp triggered the epidemic" (Piarroux et al. 2011). Finally, staff of the non-governmental organization Partners in Health used qualitative methods including community focus groups, discussions with key local leaders, and their extensive local community health worker network to identify the "first" case of cholera in Haiti—a mentally ill man who lived downstream of the MINUSTAH facility, often drank and bathed in the Meye tributary waters, developed cholera on October 12, 2010, and subsequently died in his home (Ivers and Walton 2012).

The weight of this additional evidence has led to significant pressure on the UN. The BBC, the New York Times, and al Jazerra have all run high profile stories on the topic of the introduction of cholera in Haiti (Doyle 2012; Saloomey 2012; Sontag 2012). In November 2011, the BAI [Bureau des Avocats Internationaux] and IJDH [Institute for Justice and Democracy in Haiti] filed a case against the UN on behalf of 5,000 Haitian cholera victims demanding that the UN: (1) install a national water and sanitation system; (2) compensate individual victims of cholera for their losses; and (3) issue a public apology from the UN (IJDH 2013). In December 2011, the UN Office of Legal Affairs acknowledged receipt and said they would reply "in due course". On February 21, 2013, the UN did reply, stating the claim was "not receivable" because of the diplomatic immunity of the UN (Ivers 2013).

The response of the UN to date has been not to focus on the legal issues of the introduction of cholera, but instead to state "my focus is on today, as it has been since the outbreak, and is on making sure that Haitians stay alive" (Olson 2012). On December 11, 2010, the U.N. Secretary-General Ban Ki-moon announced a $2.27 billion initiative to eradicate cholera in Haiti and the Dominican Republic, and vowed to work aggressively to secure donations for the ambitious but largely unfunded 10-year plan that focuses on water and sanitation infrastructure development and vaccine distribution (UN News Centre 2013).

It is not clear at this point in time how successful water and infrastructure development and vaccination campaigns in Haiti can be in preventing the transmission of cholera, even if the mandate is funded. Political will and capacity building will be required to support the development of sustainable water and sanitation infrastructure. On March 16, 2010, the World Health Organization (WHO) revised an April 2001 position paper on the use of vaccines in response to cholera (WHO 2010). In the new Position Paper, the WHO reiterates the need for the "mainstay of control measures"—cholera case control, water and sanitation interventions, and community mobilization; but also states: "Given the availability of two oral cholera vaccines and data on their efficacy, field effectiveness, feasibility and acceptance in cholera-affected populations, immunization with these vaccines should be used in conjunction with other prevention and control strategies in areas where the disease is endemic and should be considered in areas at risk for outbreaks. Vaccination should not disrupt the provision of other high-priority health interventions to control or prevent cholera outbreaks. Vaccines provide a short-term effect that can be implemented to bring about an immediate response while the longer term interventions of improving water and sanitation, which involve large investments, are put into place." In Haiti, Partners in Health distributed 45,000 vaccines in cholera-endemic high-risk rice farming villages near the Artibonite Delta (PIH 2013). A positive public health outcome was that 90 % of those vaccinated received both required doses, however as of this writing, there has been no impact evaluation conducted on the program.

Overcoming the weight of history to establish programs to reduce the burden of cholera to the population of Haiti will be both a challenging and necessary endeavor.

5 Current Statement on the Source of Cholera in Haiti

The exact source of introduction of cholera into Haiti will never be known with scientific certainty, as it is not possible to travel back in time to conduct the necessary investigations, and those on the ground at the time focused on outbreak response not source introduction. However, the preponderance of the evidence and the weight of the circumstantial evidence does lead to the conclusion that personnel associated with the Mirebalais MINUSTAH facility were the most likely source of introduction of cholera into Haiti. We would like to highlight here that we do not feel that this was a deliberate introduction of cholera into Haiti; based on the evidence we feel that the introduction of cholera was an accidental and unfortunate confluence of events. Action should be taken in the future to prevent such introduction of cholera into non-endemic countries in the future.

6 Public Health Implication

As of December 2012, the cholera outbreak in Haiti continues. The partners involved in cholera response have reduced the mortality rates by treating the symptoms and launching an awareness campaign. However, as of March 13, 2013, there still have been 650,218 cases of cholera reported, and 8,048 deaths (MSPP 2013). In 2011, Haiti accounted for 340,311 of 589,534 (57.7 %) of reported cholera cases worldwide (WHO 2012). Although the case number has declined in 2012, the capacity to respond to the epidemic has also decreased, as in December 2010, 61 cholera treatment centers were operational, compared to only 20 in December 2012 (OCHA 2013b). At this point in time, Haiti continues to work to recover from the January 2010 earthquake, the October 2010 introduction of cholera, new natural disasters such as Hurricane Thomas and Hurricane Sandy, and ongoing political instability. It is a challenging road ahead.

Lastly, the use of concurrent epidemiological, water and sanitation, and molecular analyses was a powerful combination in our investigation to identify and verify the source of the outbreak almost 6 months after outbreak initiation. While it was not possible to identify the exact individual(s) who transported the bacteria into Haiti, the use of the concurrent investigations allowed us to: (1) pinpoint and verify the outbreaks' geographical origin and transmission route; (2) determine the most likely source of introduction; and (3) make recommendations to prevent such introduction in the future. Concurrent analyses are recommended to public health professionals for future cholera investigations.

Disclaimer The views expressed in this article are those of the authors and do not necessarily reflect the official policy or position of the Department of the Navy, Department of Defense, nor the U.S. Government.

References

Adams G (2011) Haiti's cholera misery: 5,000 dead—and UN peacekeepers to blame. The Independent. Independent Print Limited, London

CDC (2010) Acute watery diarrhea and cholera: Haiti pre-decision brief for public health action. Centers for Disease Control and Prevention, Atlanta

CDEMA (2010) Haiti earthquake sit rep #12. Caribbean Disaster Emergency Management Agency, St. Michael

CEPR (2011) UN panel links cholera to MINUSTAH base; MINUSTAH continues to shift blame. Center for Economic Policy and Research, Washington DC

Cravioto A, Lanata C, Lantagne D, Nair G (2011) Final report of the independent panel of experts on the cholera outbreak in Haiti. Presented to the Secretary-General of the United Nations, New York City

Crof (2011) The UN's report on origins of cholera in Haiti. H5N1 Blog, Canada

Doyle M (2012) Haiti cholera epidemic 'most likely' started at UN camp—top scientist. British Broadcasting Corporation, London

Enserink M (2011) U.N. forces introduced cholera to Haiti, panel concludes. Science Insider. American Association for the Advancement of Science, Washington

Hendriksen RS, Price LB, Schupp JM, Gillece JD, Kaas RS, Engelthaler DM, Bortolaia V, Pearson T, Waters AE, Upadhyay BP, Shrestha SD, Adhikari S, Shakya G, Keim PS, Aarestrup FM (2011) Population genetics of *Vibrio cholerae* from Nepal in 2010: evidence on the origin of the Haitian outbreak. MBio 2:e00157-11

Hurtado M (2010) Haiti's cholera epidemic caused by weather, says scientists. The Guardian. Guardian News and Media, London

IASC (2012) FACT SHEET—Cuseter E-shelter and CCCM—May 2012. Inter-Agency Standing Committee, Haiti E-shelter/CCCM Cluster, Geneva

IJDH (2013) Cholera litigation. Institute for Justice and Democracy in Haiti, Boston

Ivers L (2013) A chance to right a wrong in Haiti. New York Times, Arthur Ochs Sulzberger Jr

Ivers LC, Walton DA (2012) The "first" case of cholera in Haiti: lessons for global health. Am J Trop Med Hyg 86:36–38

Lantagne D, Nair G, Lanata C, Cravioto A (2012) The origin of cholera in Haiti. J Disaster Res 7:759–767

Leopold E (2011) Did UN peacekeepers bring cholera to Haiti? Expert panel hedges bets. Huffington Post AOL, New York

Library of Congress—Federal Research Division (2006) Country profile: Haiti. Library of Congress, Washington

Lynn J (2011) http://www.democraticunderground.com/discuss/duboard.php?az=view_all&address=102x4839762. Democratic Underground, Kensington

Macquire R, Balutansky E, Fomerand J, Minear L, O'Neill W, Weiss T, Zaidi S (1996) Haiti held hostage: international responses to the quest for nationhood 1986–1996. Occasional paper #23. Thomas J. Watson Jr. Institute for International Studies, Providence

MSPP (2013) Rapport de cas: 13 mars 2013. Ministére de la Santé Publique et de la Population, Port-au-Prince, Haiti

Nelson EJ, Harris JB, Morris JG Jr, Calderwood SB, Camilli A (2009) Cholera transmission: the host, pathogen and bacteriophage dynamic. Nat Rev Microbiol 7:693–702

OCHA (2010) Haiti earthquake situation report #29–15 March 2010. United Nations Office for the Coordination of Humanitarian Affairs, New York

OCHA (2013a) Haiti humanitarian response. United Nations Office for the Coordination of Humanitarian Affairs, Geneva

OCHA (2013b) Haiti: cholera snapshot. United Nations Office for the Coordination of Humanitarian Affairs, New York

Olson A (2012) UN launches $2.27 billion cholera plan for Haiti, Dominican Republic but needs funds. Huffington Post AOL, New York

Pairroux R (2010) Rapport de mission sur l'épidémie de choléra en Haïti. Le Monde, Paris

Piarroux R, Barrais R, Faucher B, Haus R, Piarroux M, Gaudart J, Magloire R, Raoult D (2011) Understanding the cholera epidemic, Haiti. Emerg Infect Dis 17:1161–1168

PIH (2013) Cholera. Partners in Health, Boston

Prince R (1985) Haiti: family business. Latin America Bureau, London

Reuters (2011) U.N. Haiti cholera panel avoids blaming peacekeepers. Reuters. Thomas Reuters, London

Russell G (2011) U.N.—Sponsored report on Haiti's cholera outbreak points to U.N. Itself as culprit. Fox News. News Corporation, New York

Saloomey K (2012) UN likely to blame for Haiti cholera outbreak. Al Jazeera. Sheikh Hamad bin Thamer Al Thani, Al Jazeera Media Network, Doha

Sontag D (2012) In Haiti, global failures on a cholera epidemic. New York Times, Arthur Ochs Sulzberger Jr

UN News Centre (2011) UN to set up taskforce in wake of report into source of Haitian cholera outbreak. UN News Centre, United Nations New Service, New York

UN News Centre (2013) UN launches new initiative to eliminate cholera in Haiti and Dominican Republic. UN News Centre, United Nations New Service, New York

UNICEF (2012) At a glance: Haiti. UNICEF, New York

USGS (2010) Haiti estimated population exposed to earthquake shaking. United States Geological Survey, Reston

WHO (2010) Cholera vaccines: WHO position paper. Weekly epidemiological record. World Health Organization, Geneva

WHO (2012) Cholera, 2011. Weekly epidemiological record. World Health Organization, Geneva

Role of Phages in the Epidemiology of Cholera

Shah M. Faruque

Abstract Understanding the genetic and ecological factors which support the periodic emergence of toxigenic *Vibrio cholerae* causing outbreaks of cholera in regions where the disease is endemic, is vital to develop preventive measures. Besides environmental factors which are not precisely defined, bacteriophages, and horizontally transmissible genetic elements are known to have a significant role in the epidemiology and evolution of the pathogen. Cholera epidemics are also known to be self-limiting, and hence identifying natural factors which contribute to the collapse of epidemics may have important implications in controlling the disease. Phages have been shown to play a crucial role in modulating cholera epidemics, and enhance *V. cholerae* evolution through a bactericidal selection process which favors the emergence of new clones.

Contents

S. M. Faruque (✉)
Centre for Food and Water Borne Diseases, International Centre for Diarrhoeal Disease Research, Bangladesh,
68, Shaheed Tajuddin Ahmed Sharani,
Mohakhali, 1212 Dhaka, Bangladesh
e-mail: faruque@icddrb.org

Current Topics in Microbiology and Immunology (2014) 379: 165–180
DOI: 10.1007/82_2013_358

Published Online: 9 November 2013

1 Introduction

V. cholerae represents a group of bacteria which is autochthonous to coastal, river, and estuarine ecosystems, but at the same time, pathogenic for humans (Faruque et al. 1998; Kaper et al. 1995). Toxigenic strains of *V. cholerae*, cause the devastating diarrheal disease cholera, which frequently occurs in an epidemic form, particularly associated with poverty and lack of adequate clean water and sanitation. In recent times, remarkable progress has been made in identifying the major genetic determinants that account for virulence of this organism and understanding how virulent strains emerge in nature. Bacteriophages which act on *V. cholerae* (vibriophages) contribute to the evolution of this pathogen by mediating horizontal transfer of clusters of genes, genomic rearrangements, as well as by bactericidal selection (Brussow et al. 2004; Waldor and Mekalanos 1996; Faruque et al. 2005a). In this latter process, phage susceptible strains are selectively eliminated, whereas bacterial strains that are able to resist phage predation have a survival advantage. *V. cholerae* interacts with diverse phages, and the interaction can promote genetic diversity and/or cause selective enrichment of particular bacterial clones (Faruque et al. 2005a; Zahid et al. 2008, 2011).

Cholera is an ancient disease, and the occurrence of seven distinct pandemics has been recorded since the first pandemic began in 1817 (Faruque et al. 1998; Kaper et al. 1995). The 7th pandemic of cholera which originated in Indonesia in 1961 is the most extensive in geographic spread and duration, and the disease continues to affect an estimated 3–5 million people worldwide, and causes between 100,000 and 130,000 deaths, each year (World Health Organization 2010). Whereas the causative agent of the current 7th pandemic of cholera is *V. cholerae* O1 of the El Tor biotype, the 6th pandemic and presumably the earlier pandemics were caused by the classical biotype, which is now extinct (Siddique et al. 2009). The two biotypes of *V. cholerae* O1 differ in certain phenotypic and genetic characteristics (Kaper et al. 1995). The factors associated with the replacement of the classical biotype as the predominant epidemic strain by the El Tor biotype, and eventual disappearance of the classical strains have not been adequately explained. Possible contribution of particular groups of phages which selectively eliminated the classical biotype strains, while enriching the El Tor biotype (Zahid et al. 2011) has been proposed. However, the displacement of the classical strains by the El Tor might have also been driven by other environmental forces to which the El Tor strains adapted more efficiently.

Cholera epidemics occur most efficiently in regions of the world where transmission between humans occurs frequently due to inadequate sanitation and lack of access to clean water. Epidemics are often associated with the introduction of a fully virulent strain into a susceptible population. Rarely, strains of low pathogenicity acquire virulence genes and thus emerge as a unique new pathogenic clone. Perhaps the emergence of the El Tor biotype of *V. cholerae* to cause disease in Indonesia in 1961, was due to such an event (Faruque et al. 1998). Once endemicity is established in a region, cholera outbreaks appear to occur in a seasonal pattern. For example, in the Ganges Delta region of Bangladesh and India, two cholera epidemics occur every year with almost predictable seasonal regularity. Factors associated with the maintenance of the periodicity of cholera epidemics are not clear, but a multitude of environmental, genetic, ecological, and socioeconomic factors may be involved.

The role of the human host in selective amplification of *V. cholerae* from the majority of environmental non-pathogenic *V. cholerae* prior to an epidemic has been proposed to be an important factor in cholera epidemiology. Asymptomatic infections of humans supposedly account for the pre-epidemic build up of pathogenic strains which then initiate the index case of cholera. This model of cholera epidemiology (Faruque and Mekalanos 2008) takes into account both environmental and host factors in the initiation of seasonal epidemics and also explains the limited clonality apparent in the strains causing these epidemics. Cholera epidemics are also known to be self-limiting in nature, since the epidemics subside after reaching a peak, even without any active intervention. Among other factors, bacteriophages that can kill *V. cholerae* (cholera phages) have been shown to play a significant role in modulating the course of epidemics (Faruque et al. 2005a, b; Faruque and Mekalanos 2008). In this chapter, we discuss the role of phages in modulating the prevalence of *V. cholerae*, as well as infectivity and transmission of the pathogen, and thus the effect of phages on the occurrence and magnitude of seasonal cholera epidemics.

2 Bacteriophages of *V. cholerae* (Vibriophages)

V. cholerae is the host for a variety of bacteriophages, which are generally referred to as "vibriophages". These phages include temperate phages represented by kappa-type phage produced by most El Tor biotype strains, and virulent phages, e.g., Mukherjee's cholera phages (Basu and Mukerjee 1968) which were popularly used for phage typing of *V. cholerae* O1. The use of phage susceptibility as a method of strain differentiation has contributed greatly to the understanding of the epidemiology of cholera. A phage typing scheme for *V. cholerae* O1 biotype E1 Tor (Basu and Mukerjee 1968) was efficiently used to study the initial spread of the E1 Tor biotype of *V. cholerae* O1. Later, new phage typing schemes were developed for *V. cholerae* O1 (Chattopadhyay et al. 1993), and O139 (Chakrabarti et al. 2000), in which new lytic phages were used. The lytic phages have a typical head and tailed structure, and usually kill the host *V. cholerae* strain in the process of phage multiplication. Another group of phages known as filamentous phages play important roles in the evolutionary biology of *V. cholerae*, and they usually do not kill the host bacterial cells. Whereas the lytic phages have a double stranded genome, the filamentous phages carry a single stranded genome and have been shown to be involved in horizontal transfer of genes among *V. choleare* strains (Faruque and Mekalanos 2003).

A remarkable discovery in recent times that cholera toxin (CT), the major virulence factor of toxigenic *V. cholerae*, is encoded by a lysogenic filamentous phage (CTXϕ), led to the exploration of other filamentous phages as a means of lateral gene transfer among *V. cholerae*. Accordingly, several other filamentous phages or satellite phages that lack genes required for phage morphogenesis have been described in *V. cholerae* O1 and O139 serogroup strains (Faruque and Mekalanos 2012). Possible roles of these phages in *V. cholerae* evolution have been studied (Hassan et al. 2010; Faruque and Mekalanos 2012), and several of these have been shown to cooperate in horizontal gene transfer, leading to increased evolutionary fitness of *V. cholerae*.

In contrast to filamentous phages, the lytic phages often kill the host cells and thus contribute a strong selective force in nature, for the emergence of bacterial clones which are resistant to one or more of these phages. Historically, in the nineteenth century it was recognized that certain elements in the waters of the Ganges and Yamuna rivers in India had marked antibacterial activity against *V. cholerae*, and could protect against cholera (Hankin 1896; Sulakvelidze et al. 2001; Boyd 2008). It was suggested that an unknown heat labile substance which passed through fine porcelain filters was responsible for this antibacterial activity, and for limiting the spread of cholera epidemics. Frederick Twort (1915) reported a similar phenomenon and hypothesized that it may have been due to, among other possibilities, a virus. However, bacteriophages were "officially" discovered 2 years later by Felix D'Herelle, at the Institut Pasteur in Paris (D'Herelle 1917). The discovery or rediscovery of phages by D'Herelle is often linked with an outbreak of hemorrhagic dysentery among French troops stationed on the outskirts of Paris in July–August 1915 (D'Herelle 1930). Phages were used to treat dysentery by D'Herelle, as the first attempt of a therapeutic application of phages. However, the role of phages in combating bacterial infections including cholera was eventually ignored mainly due to the discovery and availability of antibiotics.

The revived interest in cholera phages stems from observations that phage blooms coincide with the decline of *V. cholerae* in water in cholera-endemic areas (Faruque et al. 2005a, b; Jensen et al. 2006). These findings have provided an impetus to examine the potential application of lytic phages in developing control measures against cholera epidemics. A considerable number of lytic and temperate vibriophages have now been found, of which the JSF series of phages isolated from the environment or cholera patients in Bangladesh are of particular interest because of their role in the epidemiology and ecology of *V. cholerae*. At least 27 distinct phages (JSF1 through JSF 27) have been isolated in Bangladesh (Table 1) and efforts are under way to isolate and characterize more cholera phages (Faruque and Mekalanos 2012).

Table 1 Lytic vibriophages isolated from surface water or cholera patients in Bangladesh

Phage designation	Primary host strains	Alternative host strains	Plaque type	Isolation of lysogens
JSF-1	*V. cholerae* O1	Not found	Clear	–
JSF-2	*V. cholerae* O1[a]	Not found	Turbid	+
JSF-3	*V. cholerae* O139	Not found	Clear	+
JSF-4	*V. cholerae* O1	Not found	Clear	+
JSF-5, JSF-11, JSF-13, JSF-14, JSF-17, JSF-18	*V. cholerae* O1	Not found	Clear	–
JSF-6	*V. cholerae* O1	*V. cholerae* non-O1 non-O139	Clear	–
JSF-7	*V. cholerae* O1[a]	*V. cholerae* O141 strain V50; *V. cholerae* O139 strain AI1853	Clear on O1 strain; Clear/turbid on non-O1 strains	+
JSF-8	*V. cholerae* O1[a]	*V. cholerae* non-O1 non-O139 strains 3565, 3548; *V. mimicus* strains 957V1621, 778V1349, and 1016V1721	Clear on O1 strain; Clear/ turbid on non-O1 strains	+
JSF-9	*V. cholerae* O1 classical biotype	*V. cholerae* O141 strain V50; non-O1 strains 79, 3565, 3548; *V. mimicus* strains 957V1621, 778V1349, and 1016V1721	Clear	–
JSF10	*V. cholerae* O1	*V. cholerae* O139 strain Arg-3; *V. cholerae* O141 strains V46 and V47	Clear	–
JSF12	*V. cholerae* O1[a]	*V. cholerae* non-O1 strains 79; *V. mimicus* strains 957V1621, 1016V1721	Clear	–
JSF-15	*V. cholerae* O1[a]	*V. cholerae* O141 strain V50; non-O1 strain 79, *V. mimicus* strains 957V1621, and 778V1349	Clear	–
JSF-16	*V. cholerae* O1	*V. cholerae* O141 strain V50	Clear/turbid	+

(continued)

Table 1 (continued)

Phage designation	Primary host strains	Alternative host strains	Plaque type	Isolation of lysogens
JSF-19	*V. cholerae* O1, classical biotype	Not found	Clear	–
JSF-20	*V. cholerae* O1	*V. cholerae* O139 strains MD01 and 1771	Clear on O1 strain; turbid on O139 strains	+
JSF-21	*V. cholerae* O1 classical biotype	*V. cholerae* O139 strain Arg-3	Clear/turbid	–
JSF23 JSF-24, JSF-25, JSF-27	*V. cholerae* O1[a]	Not found	Clear/turbid	–

[a] Recently isolated variants of El Tor biotype strains were found to be resistant to the *V. cholerae* O1-specific phages designated as JSF-2, JSF-7, JSF-8, JSF-12,JSF-15, JSF-17, JSF-19, JSF-25, and JSF-27

3 Prevalence of Phage and *V. cholerae* During the Epidemic Cycle of Cholera

A distinctive epidemiological feature of cholera is its appearance with seasonal regularity in endemic areas, such as the Ganges Delta region of Bangladesh and India. In Bangladesh, outbreaks usually occur twice during a year, with the highest number of cases just after the monsoon and a somewhat smaller number of cholera cases during the spring. The timing of the epidemics correlates with increased concentration of the causative *V. cholerae* in water (Khan et. al. 1984). Cholera epidemics are known to be self-limiting in nature, and interestingly lytic phages that can eradicate the epidemic strain of *V. cholerae* have been suggested to play a significant role in modulating the course of cholera epidemics (Faruque et al. 2005a, b; Jenson et al. 2006; Nelson et al. 2008, 2009).

In one of these studies, changing prevalence of lytic vibriophages in surface water and the number of cholera cases reporting to a nearby cholera hospital was monitored in Dhaka, Bangladesh. Over a nearly 3-year period between January 2001 and November 2003, the number of cholera patients was found to increase whenever the number of lytic vibriophages in water decreased. Similarly, cholera epidemics tended to end concurrent with large increases in the concentration of these phages in the water (Fig. 1). The dynamics of phage and *V. cholerae* concentration and its effect on the occurrence of cholera were also studied during an epidemic in Dhaka City in 2004 (Faruque et al. 2005b). The changing prevalence in the environment of the *V. cholerae* O1 strain causing an epidemic and a particular lytic cholera phage named JSF4 to which it was sensitive, was measured every 48–72 h for a period of 17 weeks. The incidence of phage excretion in stools of 387 cholera patients during the course of the epidemic was also monitored. This study showed that the peak of the epidemic was preceded by high *V. cholerae* prevalence in the environment and was followed by high JSF4 phage levels as the epidemic ended. Interestingly, the build up to high phage concentration in the environment coincided with increasing excretion of the same phage in the stools of cholera patients (Faruque et al. 2005b).

As mentioned above, choleraphages in the environment, and their amplification in cholera patients have been shown to remarkably influence the epidemiology of cholera. It has been proposed that when the balance of phage and bacteria tips in favor of the phage, there is a dramatic decline of numbers of bacteria to a point, where they are no longer able to sustain the epidemic. This prediction has been supported by a mathematical model that attempted to explain the dynamics observed for parameters such as cholera case load, density of *V. cholerae* and phage in the environment, and number of patients shedding *V. cholerae* alone, or shedding both *V. cholerae* and a phage to which the bacteria were susceptible (Jensen et al. 2006). As described in the following sections, phages appear to influence cholera epidemiology by interrupting transmission and by raising the infectious dose of the pathogen required to establish a productive infection.

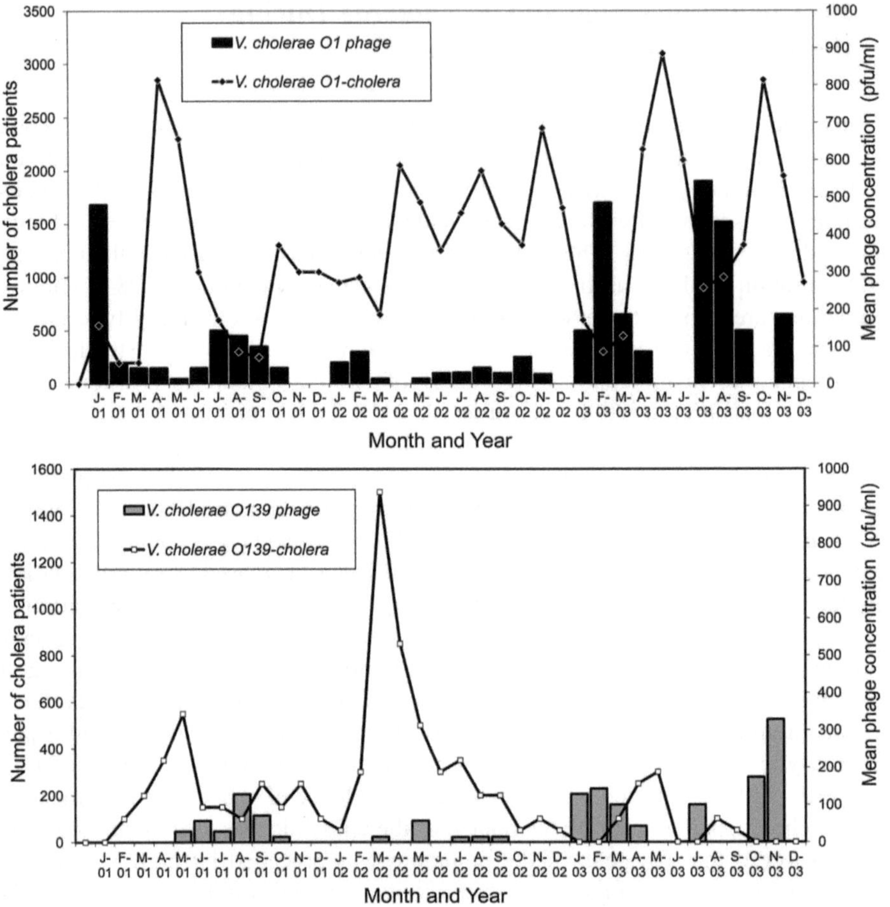

Fig. 1 Mean concentration of lytic vibriophages in the aquatic environment of Dhaka, Bangladesh, and the estimated number of cholera cases reporting to the Dhaka hospital of the International Centre for Diarrhoeal Disease Research, Bangladesh from 2001 to 2003. Number of cholera cases is extrapolated from a 2 % surveillance sample of all patients presenting for treatment

4 Effect of Phage on Transmissibility of Cholera

The factors which enhance water borne spread of cholera epidemics and sustain the epidemic strain in nature are somewhat unclear. It has been suggested that *V. cholerae* excreted in stools of cholera patients are hyperinfectious because the process of human colonization creates a hyperinfectious bacterial state (Merrel et al. 2002). It has been further proposed that the hyperinfectious state of *V. cholerae* in stools is maintained after dissemination into the aquatic environment and this phenomenon may contribute to the epidemic spread of cholera.

On the other hand, results of laboratory experiments have suggested that the rapid transmission of *V. cholerae* through water contaminated with stools of cholera victims to sustain an epidemic is quenched by lytic vibriophages (Nelson et al. 2008, 2009), which are often present in the same stools (Faruque et al. 2005b). In these studies, stools of cholera victims that naturally contained lytic phage or in vitro grown *V. cholerae* were incubated in a microcosm composed of pond water, and the culturability, infectious dose, and transcriptome were assayed over 24 h. The results showed that *V. cholerae* failed to colonize the small intestine after 24 h of incubation in pond water—the point when the phage titers were highest, suggesting that lytic phage block transmission (Nelson et al. 2008). This finding agreed with previous observations (Faruque et al. 2005b) suggesting that phages are most likely to antagonize the transmission of cholera during the late stage of an epidemic, when most patients excrete high titer of lytic phages together with the causative strain of *V. cholerae*.

It has been shown that stools from cholera patients contain a heterogenous mixture of biofilm-like aggregates and free swimming planktonic cells of *V. cholerae* (Faruque et al. 2006). Estimation of relative infectivity of these different forms of *V. cholerae* cells suggested that the enhanced infectivity of *V. cholerae* shed in human stools is largely due to presence of clumps of cells which disperse in vivo providing a high dose of the pathogen. It is widely accepted that cholera is rapidly transmitted through water contaminated with the pathogenic *V. cholerae* excreted in the feces of cholera patients. However, the pathogen has been found to exists in water mostly in a dormant state referred to as conditionally viable environmental cells (CVEC) alternatively known as the viable but non-culturable (VBNC) state. CVEC, the environmental survival form of pathogenic *V. cholerae* that resist cultivation by conventional techniques was found to exist in water as biofilm-like aggregates of partially dormant cells (Faruque et al. 2006). Such CVEC can be recovered as fully virulent bacteria by inoculation of water into rabbit intestines. More recently, it has been demonstrated that quorum sensing signal molecules called autoinducers can lead to resuscitation of the CVEC form of *V. cholerae* (Bari et al. 2013). Quorum sensing refers to regulatory responses in bacteria which are dependent on cell density.

V. cholerae shed in the stools of cholera patients, when inoculated in environmental water samples in the laboratory, exhibited characteristics similar to CVEC, suggesting that CVEC in nature may have been derived at least in part from human cholera stools. Thus these results support a model of cholera transmission in which in vivo formed biofilms contribute to enhanced infectivity and environmental persistence of pathogenic *V. cholerae* (Faruque et al. 2006). Further studies proposed that when the apparent concentration of *V. cholerae* in water is low by conventional enrichment and cultivation, certain human victims ingesting clumps of CVEC in the water might still get a fully infectious dose of the pathogen. In contrast to this scenario, when environmental phage concentration is high, even the clumped *V. cholerae* cells in water would fail to provide an infectious dose of the bacteria presumably due to predation by phages when the clumped bacterial cells are dispersed in vivo. These assumptions led to further experimental studies of the effect of phages on the infectious dose of *V. cholerae*, as described in the following section.

5 Effect of Phage on the Infectious Dose of *V. cholerae*

To better understand the mechanisms involved in reducing the transmissibility of cholera by phages and phage-mediated collapse of epidemics, studies were conducted to examine the effect of phage on the infectivity of *V. cholerae* shed in stools of cholera patients. These investigations were conducted by using assays that enabled to study the dose of *V. cholera*e required to colonize infant mice. It was found that the infectious dose (ID_{50}) of *V. cholerae* cells in stools of cholera patients as well as that of laboratory-grown cells was higher in the presence of a phage, and $\sim$10-fold more cells of *V. cholerae* would be required to cause a productive infection under the conditions in which cholera patients excrete *V. cholerae* together with phages in their stools (Zahid et al. 2008).

The sustainability of a cholera epidemic depends on amplification of the causative strain in each cholera victim, and waterborne spread of the pathogen to infect more individuals. The increase in the required infectious dose due to the deleterious effect of co-ingesting phage with *V. cholerae* therefore leads to a reduced number of new victims. Moreover, in the face of phage predation, the environment fails to support a heavy load of viable *V. cholerae*, and hence the epidemic ends. Thus these results provided a more clear understanding of the mechanisms involved in the conclusion of a seasonal epidemic of cholera.

6 Emergence of Phage Resistance in *V. cholerae*

The observed data and the theoretical model analysis strongly support a role for phage as a natural biological controller of epidemic cholera in Bangladesh. However, since epidemics reoccur in a seasonal pattern and often caused by the same or a similar strain, it's most likely that a proportion of the causative *V. cholerae* survive phage predation by various mechanisms, and these survivors seed the environment before the next epidemic season. Factors or genetic changes which enhance the ability of the bacteria to resist phage predation may also be a strong driving force in the evolution of *V. cholerae*. Therefore, studies were conducted to understand more about the interactions of *V. cholerae* with lytic phages and the emergence of phage-resistant derivatives.

Under laboratory conditions, co-culture of a phage with *V. cholerae* or culture of dilutions of phage-positive cholera stools were shown to cause emergence of phage-resistant derivatives of the concerned *V. cholerae* strains (Zahid et al. 2008). Frequently, these resistant derivatives were found to have lost their O1 antigen which often acts as the receptor for these phages. While a proportion of the phage-resistant colonies were rough and agglutinated in normal saline, there were also phage-resistant derivatives that formed smooth colonies similar to the parent strains, but did not agglutinate with the O1 antiserum suggesting that these derivatives had undergone possible serotype conversion. However, it was observed that subsequent epidemics were in fact caused by strains which remain sensitive to the predominant vibriophage detected during the epidemic, and hence further studies were conducted to understand this phenomenon. Subsequently, challenge studies in mice with a mixture of *V. cholerae* and phage, suggested that the intestinal environment did not favor the emergence of phage-resistant derivatives that lost the O1 antigen (Zahid et al. 2008).

The observed resistance to phage may also be manifested by the metabolic status of the *V. cholerae* cells both inside the human host and in vitro, and other mutations that affect the ability of phages to replicate in the bacterial host. It's also likely that in the human host or in the environment a proportion of *V. cholerae* cells may survive phage predation by forming biofilms or cellular organization that becomes transiently inaccessible to the predatory phage or become unsuitable for phage replication due to transient dormancy of the bacterial hosts. Thus, the outcome of phage bacterial interactions is more complex in nature and involves a multitude of factors including environmental parameters, intrinsic properties of relevant phage and bacterial strains, and presumably the role of the human host.

7 Phages with Multiple Bacterial Hosts

The environment in a cholera endemic area (such as Bangladesh) not only promotes the persistence of pathogenic *V. cholerae,* but also enhances dramatic shifts in the strains that emerge to cause disease. It has been suggested that this process might be driven by bacteriophages either specific for *V. cholerae* of the epidemic serogroup or phages that can infect other aquatic bacterial species which act as alternative hosts. Such phages were hypothesized to grow in other *Vibrio* species or in *V. cholerae* non-O1 strains particularly in the absence of *V. cholerae* O1 strains, but are able to modulate the prevalence of the O1 serogroup strains when these become abundant. Environmental and clinical surveillance in Bangladesh has indeed identified certain phages that can grow on both *V. cholerae* O1 and non-O1 non-O139 strains as alternative hosts (Table 1). Some of these phages appear to exist as lysogens in the *V. cholerae* non-O1 non-O139 strains. However, it remains to be demonstrated what effect a "bloom" of these aquatic, non-cholera *Vibrio* species might have on epidemic strains of *V. cholerae*, whether it is direct (via competition for a limited aquatic niche) or indirect (through promoting phage replication that has a deleterious effect on the survival of pathogenic *V. cholerae*). It seems possible that vibriophages can also replicate in other common environmental species. These "non-*Vibrio* species" may be common to the aquatic environments, e.g., *Aeromonas*, *Pleiseomonas*, *Pseudomonas*, etc. Search for alternative hosts for vibriophages which can act on epidemic *V. cholerae* strains is of particular importance, since identifying and characterizing such non-cholera *Vibrio* species may have predictive value in cholera epidemiology.

8 Co-evolution of Lytic Phages and *V. cholerae*

The ability of *V. cholerae* to evade phage predation constitutes important development in attaining evolutionary fitness. Conversely, phage resistance is often attained by altering expression of bacterial surface appendages such as flagella or pili or O antigens which may act as receptors for different lytic phages. Thus, there may also be a fitness cost associated with achieving phage resistance by *V. cholerae*, and the evolutionary success of the pathogen has presumably been dependent on a balance between these various factors.

The complete genomic sequences of a number of *V. cholerae* strains have been determined, and the crucial changes that define virulence altering traits are beginning to be revealed. Pathogenic strains typically differ from environmental strains in their virulence gene content and the lipopolysaccharide O1 or O139 antigens that are typically carried by the pathogens (Faruque et al. 1998; Kaper et al. 1995). Only strains belonging to these two serogroups (O1 and O139) are known to be associated with epidemic and endemic disease despite the fact that over 250 different serogroups of *V. cholerae* have so far been reported. Filamentous phages are known to be involved in some of the horizontal gene transfer events, that causes the emergence of strains carrying virulence genes. However, the role of lytic phages is also important because of the selection pressure they impart to different clones of *V. cholerae*. For example, the explanation for the evolutionary success of the 7th pandemic clone over the preexisting 6th pandemic strain remains largely a mystery since both classical and El Tor biotypes of *V. cholerae* O1 carry CTX and TCP. Notably, recent studies are beginning to suggest possible role of lytic phages in this process (Zahid et al. 2011). Phage resistance has also been associated with serotype conversion, suggesting that phages may provide a strong selective force for *V. cholerae* strains to undergo genetic or phenotypic alteration.

The ecological interactions of *V. cholerae* with chitin-rich zooplankton has been suggested to have an evolutionary significance and not just limited to deriving nutrients from this abundant carbon source. *V. cholerae* has been reported to become naturally competent to uptake exogenous DNA, while growing on a chitin substrate (Meibom et al. 2005). It has recently been suggested that free DNA released in the aquatic environment by phage-mediated lysis of *V. cholerae* can be harnessed and assimilated by surviving *V. choleare* strains (Udden et al. 2008). Thus, phages contribute to bacterial evolution in numerous ways and the full potential of these mechanisms in the evolution of *V. cholerae* as a pathogen is yet to be appreciated. As explained above, the role of phages in the evolution of *V. cholerae* involves not only a means of horizontal gene transfer among

Table 2 Predominant phages isolated from surface water and cholera patients in Bangladesh during 2002–2013

Year	Abundant Phages	Predominant Phage
2002–2004	JSF1 through JSF6	JSF4
2005	JSF1 through JSF9	JSF4
2006	JSF1, JSF4, JSF6 through JSF9	JSF4
2007	JSF1 through JSF11	JSF4/JSF11
2008	JSF1, JSF4 through JSF11	JSF11
2009	JSF1, JSF4 through JSF11	JSF11
2010	JSF1, JSF4 through JSF11	JSF11
2011	JSF1, JSF4 through JSF16	JSF11
2012	JSF11, JSF13	JSF13
2013	JSF11, JSF13	JSF13

V. choleare strains, but also provide a selection pressure for particular bacterial clones.

In keeping with changes in the host *V. cholerae* strains, temporal changes in the prevalence and properties of diverse lytic vibriophages have also been noticed. The environmental surveillance system to monitor phages and *V. cholerae* in the aquatic environment in Bangladesh yielded various phage isolates and data on phage prevalence. Different phage strains (JSF1 through JSF27) which interact with *V. cholerae* have been identified and partially characterized (Table 1). Fluctuation in the prevalence of the different predatory phages have been observed, with a temporal change in the most prevalent phage type (Table 2) which is a factor in the collapse of epidemics by phage predation (Faruque et al. 2005a; Faruque and Mekalanos 2012). Studies were also conducted to identify bacterial factors which mediate resistance to phage susceptibility, and thus provide a mechanism to survive predation by phages. As mentioned above, often phage-resistant strains were found to have lost their O antigen. The lipopolysaccharide O1 antigen is a major target of bacteriophages as well as the human immune system. Seed and colleagues (2012) showed that under the selective pressure of a lytic phage *V. cholerae* can modulate O antigen expression and exhibit intrastrain heterogeneity. Two phase variable genes *manA* and *wbeL* were found to be involved and these phase variants were found to be attenuated for virulence, providing functional evidence to support the critical role of the O1 antigen for infectivity. These authors suggested that the maintenance of the phase variable loci is an important means by which *V. cholerae* can generate diverse subpopulations of cells needed for infecting the host intestinal tract and for escaping predation by an O1-specific phage.

Incorporation of mutations in the *cyaA* or *crp* genes encoding adenylate cyclase or cyclic AMP receptor protein (CRP), respectively, into *V. cholerae* O1 strains was also found to cause alterations in their phage susceptibility patterns, and the susceptibility correlated with the ability of the bacteria to adsorb these phages. These results suggested that cAMP-CRP-mediated downregulation of phage adsorption may contribute to a mechanism for the *V. cholerae* strains to survive predation by phages in the environment (Zahid et al. 2010).

Although the significance of the observed change in prevalence of particular phage types is not fully understood, occasional change in the predominant phage appears to maintain susceptibility of the epidemic strain to the most prevalent phage responsible for ending epidemics in a self-limiting manner. A bacterial adaptive immune system against phage invasion is the CRISPR/Cas (clustered regularly interspaced short palindromic repeats/CRISPR-associated proteins) system, which provides sequence-specific protection from invading nucleic acids, including phage. Interestingly, a phage-encoded CRISPR/Cas system has also been documented, and this system is used to counteract a phage inhibitory chromosomal island of the bacterial host (Seed et al. 2013). Thus, *V. cholerae* and their phages co-evolve, and while a range of bacterial immunity mechanisms against phages has evolved, this in turn seems to have also resulted in the evolution of diverse phages with the immunity evasion strategies.

9 Conclusion

It has now been recognized that phage predation may not only play a role in the natural control of cholera epidemics, but that changes in pathogenic *V. cholerae* may have been driven to a large extent by phages. Although there are multiple other factors which can drive the evolution of *V. cholerae* and the epidemiological nature of the pathogen, phages have been shown to contribute extensively to the dynamics of cholera epidemics. Briefly, phage predation of *V. cholerae* influences the prevalence of the pathogen in the environment, and hence occurrence of cholera in Bangladesh, where a large proportion of the population use surface water due to inadequate access to safe water and sanitation facilities (Faruque et al. 2005a). The peak of the epidemic is preceded by high *V. cholerae* prevalence in the water and is followed by high levels of lytic choleraphages to which the epidemic strain is sensitive. Phage amplification occurs in the intestines of cholera victims, and eventually the build up of phage concentration in the environment might derive the collapse of an epidemic, thus causing cholera epidemics to be self-limiting in nature. Phages lead to the collapse of epidemics by modulating the required infectious dose of the bacteria, and interrupting transmission (Nelson et al. 2008; Zahid et al. 2008). Furthermore, although phage-resistant strains emerge in the process, these derivatives are often less virulent, and hence the dominance of phage-resistant variants due to bactericidal selective mechanism occurs rarely under natural settings, and the emerging variants are thus unable to sustain the ongoing epidemic. However, phages contribute to the evolution of *V. cholerae* in a variety of ways (Seed et al. 2012, 2013), and the occasional emergence of new or altered pathogenic strains may in a large part be driven directly or indirectly by diverse phages. On the other hand, phages also undergo co-evolution to adapt to the genetic changes in the host *V. cholerae* strains, and maintain the ability to multiply on the host strains.

Acknowledgments Research in the laboratory of SMF were funded in part by National Institutes of Health grants 2RO1-GM068851, under a subagreement between the Harvard Medical School, and the International Centre for Diarrhoeal Disease Research, Bangladesh (Icddr, b). The Icddr, b is supported by countries and agencies which share its concern for the health problems of developing countries.

References

Bari SM, Roky MK, Mohiuddin M, Kamruzzaman M, Mekalanos JJ, Faruque SM (2013) Quorum-sensing autoinducers resuscitate dormant *Vibrio cholerae* in environmental water samples. Proc Natl Acad Sci USA 110:9926–9931

Basu S, Mukerjee S (1968) Bacteriophage typing of *Vibrio ElTor*. Experientia 24:299–300

Brussow H, Canchaya C, Hardt W (2004) Phages and the evolution of bacterial pathogens: from genomic rearrangements to lysogenic conversion. Microb Mol Biol Rev 68:560–562

Boyd F (2008) Filamentous phages of *Vibrio cholerae*. In: Faruque SM, Nair GB (eds) *Vibrio cholerae*: genomics and molecular biology. Caister Academic Press, Norfolk

Chakrabarti AK, Ghosh AN, Nair GB, Niyogi SK, Bhattacharya SK, Sarkar BL (2000) Development and evaluation of a phage typing scheme for Vibrio cholerae O139. J Clin Microbiol 38:44–49

Chattopadhyay DJ, Sarkar BL, Ansari MQ, Chakrabarti BK, Roy MK, Ghosh AN, Pal SC (1993) New phage typing scheme for *Vibrio cholerae* O1 biotype E1 Tor strains. J Clin Microbiol 31:1579–1585

D'Herelle F (1917) Sur un microbe invisible antagoniste des bacilles dysentériques. C R Acad Sci (Paris) 165:373–375

D'Herelle F (1930) The bacteriophage and its clinical applications. Charles C Thomas, Springfield

Faruque SM, Naser IB, Islam MJ, Faruque ASG, Ghosh AN, Nair GB, Sack DA, Mekalanos JJ (2005a) Seasonal epidemics of cholera inversely correlate with the prevalence of environmental cholera phages. Proc Natl Acad Sci USA 102:1702–1707

Faruque SM, Albert MJ, Mekalanos JJ (1998) Epidemiology, genetics and ecology of toxigenic *Vibrio cholerae*. Microbiol Mol Biol Rev 62:1301–1314

Faruque SM, Mekalanos JJ (2008) Molecular ecology of *Vibrio cholerae*. In: Faruque SM, Nair GB (eds) *Vibrio cholerae*: genomics and molecular biology. Caister Academic Press, Norfolk

Faruque SM, Mekalanos JJ (2003) Pathogenicity islands and phages in *Vibrio cholerae* evolution. Trends Microbiol 11:505–510

Faruque SM, Mekalanos JJ (2012) Phage bacterial interactions in the evolution of toxigenic *Vibrio cholerae*. Virulence 3:1–10

Faruque SM, Biswas K, Udden SN, Ahmad QS, Sack DA, Nair GB, Mekalanos JJ (2006) Transmissibility of cholera: in vivo-formed biofilms and their relationship to infectivity and persistence in the environment. Proc Natl Acad Sci USA 103:6350–6355

Faruque SM, Islam MJ, Ahmad QS, Faruque ASG, Sack DA, Nair GB, Mekalonas JJ (2005b) Self-limiting nature of seasonal cholera epidemics: role of host-mediated amplification of phage. Proc Natl Acad Sci USA 102:6119–6124

Hankin EH (1896) L'action bactericide des eaux de la Jumna et du Gange sur le vibrion du cholera. Ann Inst Pasteur 10:511

Hassan F, Kamruzzaman M, Mekalanos JJ, Faruque SM (2010) Satellite phage TLCϕ enables toxigenic conversion by CTX phage through dif site alteration. Nature 467:982–985

Jensen MA, Faruque SM, Mekalanos JJ, Levin BR (2006) Modeling the role of bacteriophage in the control of cholera outbreaks. Proc Natl Acad Sci USA 103:4652–4657

Kaper JB, Morris JG, Levine MM (1995) Cholera. Clin Microbiol Rev 8:48–86

Khan MU, Shahidullah M, Haque MS, Ahmed WU (1984) Presence of vibrios in surface water and their relation with cholera in a community. Trop Geogr Med 36:335–340

Meibom KL, Blokesch M, Dolganov NA, Wu C, Schoolnik GK (2005) Chitin induces natural competence in *Vibrio cholerae*. Science 310:1824–1827

Merrell DS, Butler SM, Qadri F, Dolganov NA, Alam A, Cohen MB, Calderwood SB, Schoolnik GK, Camilli A (2002) Host-induced epidemic spread of the cholera bacterium. Nature 417:642–645

Nelson EJ, Chowdhury A, Flynn J, Schild S, Bourassa L, Shao Y, LaRocque RC, Calderwood SB, Qadri F, Camilli A (2008) Transmission of *Vibrio cholerae* is antagonized by lytic phage and entry into the aquatic environment. PLoS Pathog 10:e1000187

Nelson EJ, Harris JB, Morris JG Jr, Calderwood SB, Cammilli A (2009) Cholera transmission: the host, pathogen and bacteriophage dynamic. Nat Rev Microbiol 10:693–702

Seed KD, Faruque SM, Mekalanos JJ, Calderwood SB, Qadri F, Camilli A (2012) Phase variable O antigen biosynthetic genes control expression of the major protective antigen and bacteriophage receptor in *Vibrio cholerae* O1. PLoS Pathog 8:e1002917

Seed KD, Lazinski DW, Calderwood SB, Camilli A (2013) A bacteriophage encodes its own CRISPR/Cas adaptive response to evade host innate immunity. Nature 494:489–491

Siddique AK, Nair GB, Alam M, Sack DA, Huq A, Nizam A, Longini IM, Qadri F, Faruque SM, Colwell RR, Ahmed S, Iqbal A, Bhuiyan NA, Sack RB (2009) El Tor cholera with severe disease: a new threat to Asia and beyond. Epidemiol Infect 14:1–6

Sulakvelidze A, Alavidze Z, Morris Jr JG (2001) Bacteriophage therapy. Antimicrob Agents Chemother 45: 649–659

Twort FW (1915). An investigation on the nature of ultramicroscopic viruses. Lancet 2:1241–1243

Udden SMN, Zahid MSH, Biswas K, Ahmad QS, Cravioto A, Nair GB, Mekalanos JJ, Faruque SM (2008) Acquisition of classical CTX prophage from *Vibrio cholerae* O141 by El Tor strains aided by lytic phages and chitin-induced competence. Proc Natl Acad Sci USA 23:11951–11958

Waldor MK, Mekalanos JJ (1996) Lysogenic conversion by a filamentous bacteriophage encoding cholera toxin. Science 272:1910–1914

World Health Organization (2010) Cholera vaccines. A brief summary of the March 2010 position paper. http://www.who.int/immunization/Cholera_PP_Accomp_letter_Mar_ 10_2010.pdf

Zahid MSH, Waise Z, Kamruzzaman M, Ghosh AN, Nair GB, Bashar SAMK, Mekalanos JJ, Faruque SM (2011) An experimental study of phage mediated bactericidal selection and emergence of the El Tor *Vibrio cholerae*. Indian J Med Res 133:218–224

Zahid MSH, Waise TM, Kamruzzaman M, Ghosh AN, Nair GB, Mekalanos JJ, Faruque SM (2010) The cyclic AMP (cAMP)-cAMP receptor protein signaling system mediates resistance of *Vibrio cholerae* O1 strains to multiple environmental bacteriophages. Appl Environ Microbiol 76:4233–4240

Zahid MSH, Udden SM, Faruque ASG, Calderwood SB, Mekalanos JJ, Faruque SM (2008) Effect of phage on the infectivity of *Vibrio cholerae* and emergence of genetic variants. Infect Immun 76:5266–5273

Circulation and Transmission of Clones of *Vibrio cholerae* During Cholera Outbreaks

O. Colin Stine and J. Glenn Morris Jr.

Abstract Cholera is still a major public health problem. The underlying bacterial pathogen *Vibrio cholerae* (*V. cholerae*) is evolving and some of its mutations have set the stage for outbreaks. After *V. cholerae* acquired the mobile elements VSP I & II, the El Tor pandemic began and spread across the tropics. The replacement of the O1 serotype encoding genes with the O139 encoding genes triggered an outbreak that swept across the Indian subcontinent. The sxt element generated a third selective sweep and most recently a fourth sweep was associated with the exchange of the El Tor ctx allele for a classical ctx allele in the El Tor background. In Kenya, variants of this fourth selective sweep have differentiated and become endemic residing in and emerging from environmental reservoirs. On a local level, studies in Bangladesh have revealed that outbreaks may arise from a nonrandom subset of the genetic lineages in the environment and as the population of the pathogen expands, many novel mutations may be found increasing the amount of genetic variation, a phenomenon known as a founder flush. In Haiti, after the initial invasion and expansion of *V. cholerae* in 2010, a second outbreak occurred in the winter of 2011–2012 driven by natural selection of specific mutations.

Contents

O. C. Stine (✉)
Department of Epidemiology and Public Health, University of Maryland, 596 Howard Hall, 660 W. Redwood St., Baltimore, MD 21201, USA
e-mail: ostin001@umaryland.edu

J. G. Morris Jr.
Emerging Pathogens Institute, University of Florida, 2055 Mowry Road, Gainesville, FL 32610, USA

Current Topics in Microbiology and Immunology (2014) 379: 181–193 181
DOI: 10.1007/82_2013_360

Published Online: 11 January 2014

1 Background

Cholera outbreaks have historically represented major public health events, with the potential for large numbers of cases and deaths. The largest outbreaks have moved across multiple continents (meeting the definition of pandemics), with case counts in the millions. Pandemics are traditionally referred to on the basis of the year in which they commenced: the first started in 1817, the second in 1829, with subsequent ones starting in 1852, 1861, 1881, 1899, and the seventh and most recent (still ongoing) in 1961. More localized outbreaks are known by the location and the year: Orissa 1999, Dhaka 2006, Zimbabwe 2008, Haiti 2010, and Kenya 2010. Left undefined by the term outbreak is the source, the mode of transmission, and the genetic diversity of the causative bacterium, *V. cholerae*.

On the broadest scale there are two modes of transmission, emergence of an endemic strain from environmental reservoirs and/or introduction of strain from a visitor. Multiple port cities, such as New York, Hamburg, St. Petersburg, Alexandria, and Gran Canaria, can trace introductions to specific ships arriving from ports with ongoing outbreaks. More recently, the 2010 outbreak in Haiti has been traced to the UN peacekeeping troops from Nepal. In each of these cases, there is a single source and the tracing of the outbreak involves finding the common origin.

V. cholerae is a very diverse species, including virulent and avirulent strains. The disease cholera is caused by strains that produce cholera toxin, and which, traditionally, have been in a limited number of serotypes, including serotypes O1 and O139. The avirulent strains do not produce cholera toxin, and usually fall into one of the over 200 other *V. cholerae* serotypes recognized to date. There are no data about the strains in the first five pandemics because the discovery that cholera was caused by a bacterium (by Pacini 1855), its isolation (by Koch 1884), and its preservation did not occur until the twentieth century and after the start of the sixth pandemic. Numerous isolates are available from the seventh pandemic. All of the isolates in the sixth and seventh pandemics appear to be derived from a single ancestor: that is, they are clonally related. They differ from each other by nucleotide variants, some of which are de novo mutations, and others the result of recombination events (Garg, Aydanian et al. 2003; Salim, Lan et al. 2005).

2 Genetic Variation and Selective Sweeps

In addition to the point mutations, there are numerous mobile elements that have been incorporated into the genome of some of the sublineages (Chun, Grim et al. 2009). Among the mobile elements are pathogenic islands (described below) and the serotype: although often thought as a phylogenetic marker and by definition not subject to lateral gene transfer, the first evidence that it might be mobile came from the discovery of the O139 morph of the O1–O139 lineage. It has been shown by three groups that the O1 encoding genes were replaced by O139 encoding genes (Bik, Bunschoten et al. 1995; Comstock, Johnson et al. 1996; Mooi and Bik 1997). Subsequently, the O1 encoding genes were shown to transfer between SNP-defined lineages, and furthermore the "jump start" sequence (Hobbs and Reeves 1994) was identified as the junction point and shown to be similar to a DNA uptake sequence leading to the suggestion that serotype genes are mechanistically prone to being mobile (Gonzalez-Fraga, Pichel et al. 2008). After the unprecedented epidemic caused by serotype O139 strains, considerable attention has been paid to non O1–O139 serotypes in the O1–O139 lineage: this includes two serotypes that have caused significant outbreaks of O37 in Czechoslovakia in 1965 and in Sudan in 1968. Other serotypes that have been reported in the O1–O139 lineage include O10, O26, O27, O53, O65, O75, and O141 (Rudra, Mahajan et al. 1996; Dalsgaard, Serichantalergs et al. 2001; Li, Shimada et al. 2002; Octavia, Salim et al. 2013). While these have been associated with disease usually found in patients and occasionally in small outbreaks, they have not caused a major outbreak.

When *V. cholerae*, or any bacteria, acquires a novel genetic element(s) that increases its fitness, a selective sweep will occur. The first selective sweep to be identified was the emergence of O139. Isolates with the serotype O139 did not cross-react serologically with O1 *V. cholerae* and so older persons who were immune to O1 fell ill to O139. The sweep appears to have started near Madras (now known as Chennai) and spread across the Indian subcontinent over the next 2 years. Tracking the epidemic was easy because of its unique serotype and its propensity to strike older individuals (Nair et al. 1994). As shown in Fig. 1, the new serotype spread from Madras south to Madurai and north to Kolkata and then west to Lucknow and eventually to Delhi. Each of these cities represents introduction of the new O139 form of *V. cholerae* to a new geographic region.

Among the O1 strains, the O1 classical strains associated with the sixth pandemic (collected during the first quarter of the twentieth century) are the ancestral isolates (Salim, Lan et al. 2005). The seventh pandemic has been characterized by four selective sweeps. The first sweep chronologically coincided with the emergence of the El Tor strains in 1961. The ancestor of the O1 El Tor strains acquired two major pathogenic islands: *Vibrio* Seventh Pandemic (VSP) I & II that have 11 and 7 genes, respectively (Dziejman, Balon et al. 2002). Additional genes were also acquired, however, the selective advantage conferred by VSP I & II and the other genes is not known. The second selective sweep began when the novel element sxt was acquired around 1981. The sxt element is an integrating conjugative element and in addition to the core region of about two dozen genes that encode its ability to transfer and to be regulated, there are several antibiotic resistance genes. These latter genes are considered to confer the selective advantage on the genomes containing them (Waldor, Tschape et al. 1996). This second selective sweep is referred to as wave two (see Fig. 2) that spread around the world. The third selective sweep was the O139 sweep mentioned above. The fourth and the most

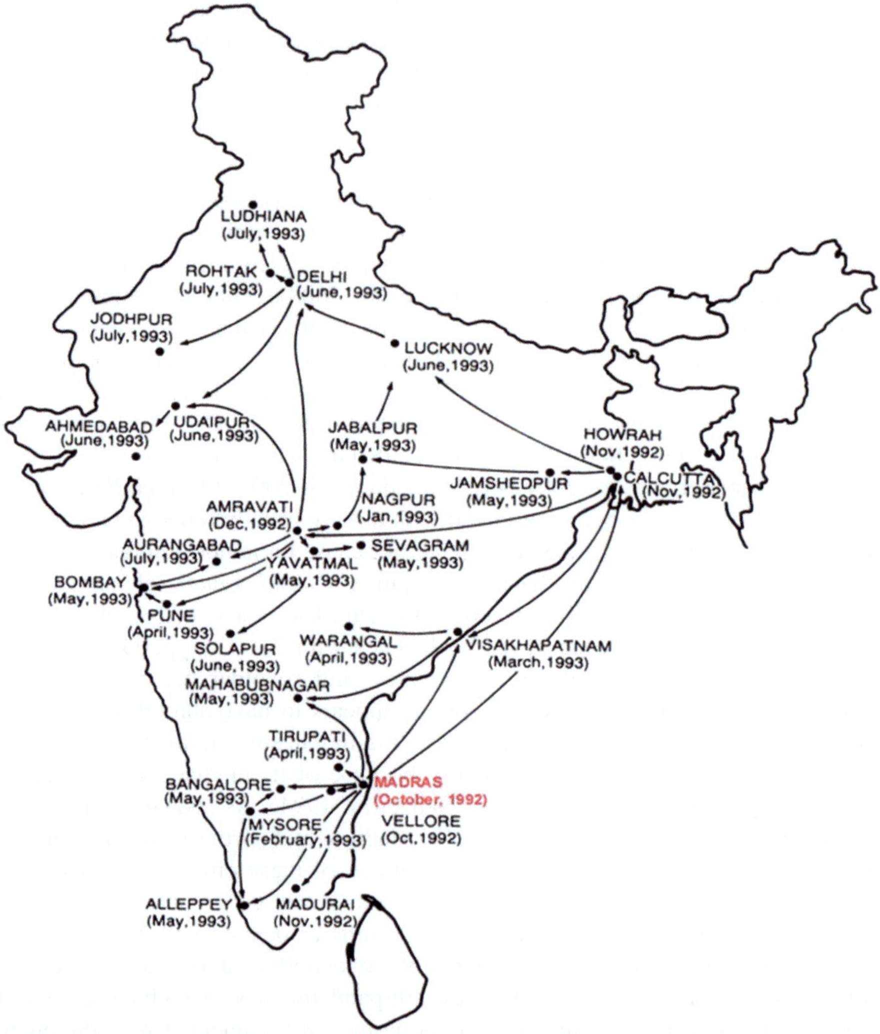

Fig. 1 Map of India detailing the spread of O139 *V. cholerae*. The *dates* indicate the first observation of O139 in that city and the *arrows* represent the likely directions of the spread. From Nair et al. 1994

recent selective sweep was initiated after an sxt-positive El Tor strain acquired the classical allele of the cholera toxin gene. The classical cholera toxin allele isolates selectively replaced the El Tor ctx allele carrying isolates (Raychoudhuri, Patra et al. 2009) and may be associated with more severe disease (Nair, Faruque et al. 2002). This fourth wave expanded in Asia and across the world including Kenya and Haiti (Mutreja, Kim et al. 2011). During each selective sweep, the common ancestor differentiates with the acquisition of many novel variant nucleotides that produce a radiation of different but closely related genotypes. While the nucleotide

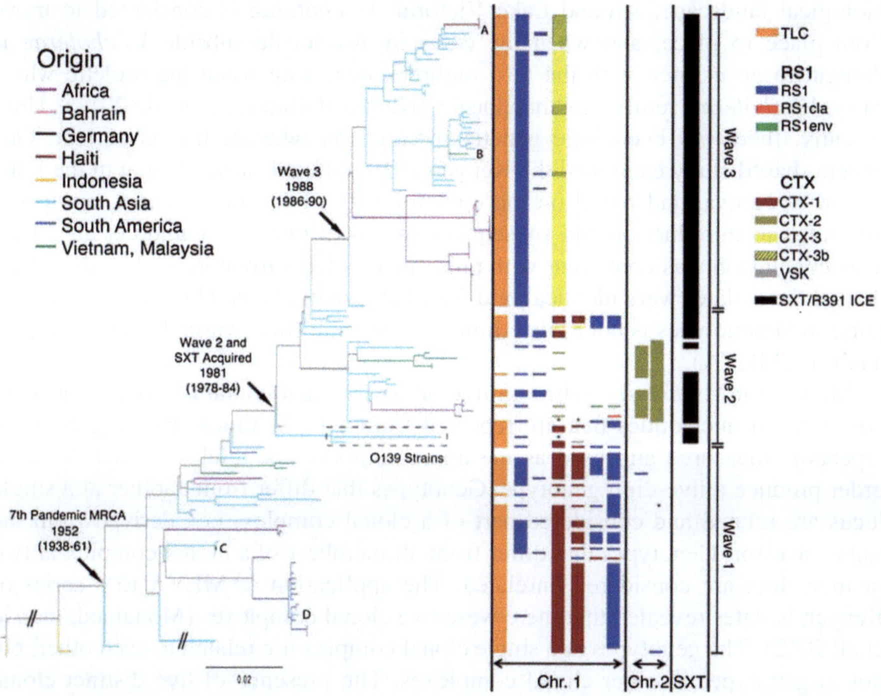

Fig. 2 Phylogenetic tree based on variable nucleotides. Points at which selective sweeps begin are indicated by the *arrows*. The *right side* of the figure indicates the presence of various mobile elements. From Mutreja et al. 2011

changes may be fit neatly into a "phylogenetic" tree, the bacteria are also differentiating by the gain and loss of mobile elements (Chun, Grim et al. 2009). It should be noted that while the selected variants in these expansions become the most frequent type, there is no reason to expect they entirely outcompete the previous forms. Despite claims of the extinction of earlier types, evidence of their existence continues to appear. Classical strains (sixth pandemic) have been identified in the last 20 years (Boyd, Heilpern et al. 2000; Alam, Islam et al. 2012) and typical El Tor strains in the last five (Rashed et al. 2013), though they were competitively swept aside by the most recent variant 10 or more years ago. Although there is no way to predict where or when the next acquisition of a novel element or novel mutations will occur, it is a safe prediction that such an event will occur and it will be selectively spread wherever there is cholera.

3 *V. cholerae* is Endemic in Kenya

In Africa, an open question is whether or not *V. cholerae* is endemic. Although all three waves of O1 have invaded the continent (Mutreja, Kim et al. 2011), one working hypothesis is that *V. cholerae* has not become an endemic part of the biological landscape. Around Lake Victoria, *V. cholerae* is considered to move from place to place, and when the cases in any locale subside *V. cholerae* is thought to go extinct, with the next outbreak occurring when the roulette wheel carry *V. cholerae* returns to that locale (Nkoko, Giraudoux et al. 2011). Until recently, there has been little genetic research on whether this is correct. One genetic-based study examined the Kenyan 2010 outbreak which began in the Lake region of Kenya, and based on the epidemiology of the initial cases, onset was attributed to introduction and subsequent spread (Mohamed, Oundo et al. 2012). This conclusion was consistent with pulse field gel electrophoretic data that show that all the isolates were identical or differed at a single band. However, analysis of pulse field genotypes is not as discriminatory as multilocus variable tandem repeat analysis (MLVA).

MLVA for *V. cholerae* relies on five or six loci that contain tandem repeats of six or seven nucleotides that are repeated from 4 to 31 times. The length of the repeats is measured and used as the allele number. The alleles at each locus in order produce a five-digit genotype. Genotypes that differ from another at a single locus are related and considered part of a clonal complex, i.e., derived from the same ancestor. Genotypes that differ from all members of a clonal complex at two or more loci are considered unrelated. The application of MLVA to a series of Kenyan isolates revealed that there were five clonal complexes (Mohamed, Oundo et al. 2012). The genotypes in a single clonal complex are related to each other, but not to genotypes in other clonal complexes. The presence of five distinct clonal complexes rejects unequivocally the hypothesis that this outbreak is the result of introduction and spread of a clone. More recent data using nucleotide variants from whole genome sequencing also showed that there are multiple genetic lineages within the 2010 outbreak (Kiiru, Mutreja et al. 2013). In Kenya, as in other countries, when a selective sweep occurs, the isolates may diverge. In this case there are two large well-separated groups by SNP analysis, from an earlier introduction (estimated to be about 1990), confirming that some of these strains have resided in Kenya for at least a decade. Thus both MLVA and whole genome sequencing data lead to the same conclusion that, in Kenya, the only African country with data, the question is settled, *V. cholerae* is endemic (Fig. 3).

4 Molecular Epidemiology in Local Outbreaks

Tracking *V. cholerae* when it is endemic presents a more difficult problem because *V. cholerae* can alter its physiological state and the question of transmission includes whether novel isolates are introduced into the region or native isolates are emerging from the environment into the human population. Throughout south Asia, especially around the Bay of Bengal, *V. cholerae* is endemic. *V. cholerae* survive in ponds, streams, and estuaries (Huq, Colwell et al. 1990; Huq, Parveen et al. 1993). The disease-causing strains are rare in the environment being heavily outnumbered by avirulent strains of *V. cholerae*. Although unusual in the

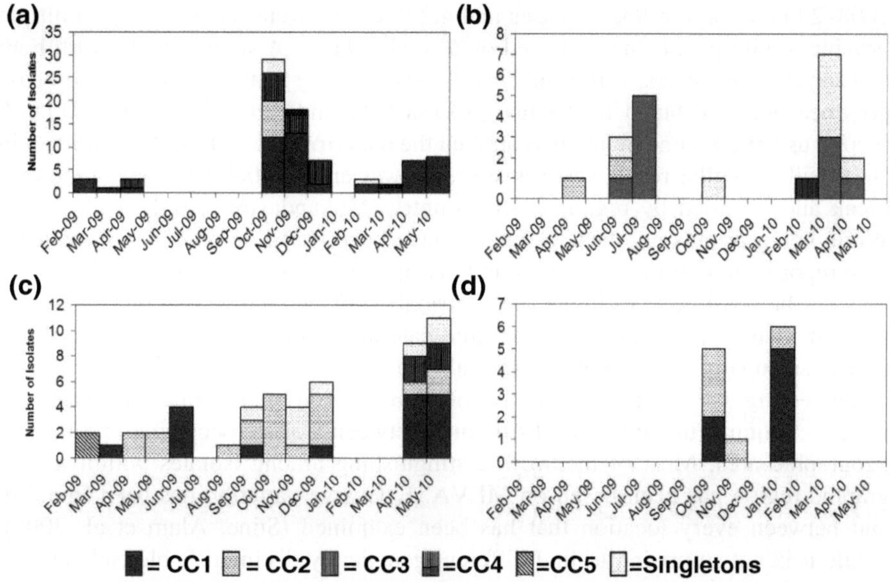

Fig. 3 Months in which various clonal complexes appeared in **a** Highland region including Nairobi, **b** coastal region, **c** Semi-arid Northern region, and **d** Lower Eastern region. Distinct clonal complexes occur simultaneously in different regions, thus the isolates could not have been transported between regions. From Mohamed et al. 2012

environment, the O1–O139 s can survive long periods in the environment either attached to copepods or in an altered physiological state: viable but nonculturable state (VBNC) (Huq, Grim et al. 2006), or possibly a newly described "persister" state (Jubair, Morris et al. 2012). The VBNC state may be associated with biofilms in which *V. cholera* can survive months in sterilized water. *V. cholerae* reside in the environment and their numbers fluctuate with the seasons. When they reach sufficient numbers and densities to provide an infectious dose, they emerge from their environmental refuge and wreak havoc among the human population (Huq, Colwell et al. 1990). At this stage there are many potential sources, the affected humans and the environmental refuge. The relative proportion that these two sources contribute to the outbreak has been disputed. The extreme position is that all cases result from the bacteria emerging from the environment. Complicating the issue, is the recent observation that after traveling through either a mouse or a human intestine, *V. cholerae* enters a second altered physiological state referred to as "hyperinfective." When it is hyperinfective, the infectious dose is decreased to 10^4, and after ~ 18 h in water, *V. cholerae* reverts to normal infectiveness ($\sim 10^6$) (Merrell et al. 2002).

Mathematical modeling of incidence data from outbreaks has been used to estimate the contribution of "fast" and "slow" transmission. The initial slow transmission is from the environment to humans, while the accelerated fast transmission occurs when *V. cholerae* is hyperinfective. In the outbreak in Zimbabwe in

2008–2009, a total of 98,585 cases and 4,285 deaths were reported from multiple provinces with data being collected on a weekly basis. A simple model with both fast and slow transmission revealed that 41–95 % of the transmission, depending on province, was attributed to the fast process (Mukandavire, Liao et al. 2011). A second use of the same model was applied the data from the 2010–2011 outbreak in Haiti with a similar result, fast transmission was an essential amplifier in the outbreak and it varied by region of the country (Mukandavire, Smith et al. 2013). While being promising, these estimates have been based on official symptomatic case reports without more detailed underlying epidemiologic data. Furthermore, it may not be possible to estimate the contribution of two transmission mechanisms from incidence data alone when the timescale of the slow is similar to that of fast transmission (Eisenberg, Robertson et al. 2013).

Dissecting the alternative routes of transmission in seasonal outbreaks in endemic requires the ability to distinguish between isolates occurring in a limited geographic area. Most of the work distinguishing among isolates within a geographic region has been based on MLVA. Extensive variation has been found in and between every location that has been examined (Stine, Alam et al. 2008). While it is not surprising to find different genetically distinguishable isolates in a geographically restricted area because O1 Inaba and Ogawa (the two common biotypes of O1) and O139 isolates are occasionally observed in a single sampling location, it was completely unexpected to find multiple genetic lineages of *V. cholerae* within a single individual (Kendall, Chowdhury et al. 2010). Interestingly, the three loci on the first large chromosome seem to vary at a slower rate than those on the second or small chromosome (Kendall, Chowdhury et al. 2010). Even if the analysis is limited to the slower evolving loci, multiple genetic lineages were found in a single stool. Whether this increases the difficultly of tracking, *V. cholerae* as it spreads because tracking needs to account for all the lineages, or narrows the sources because of having greater genetic differentiation between samples, remains to be seen.

5 Genetic Variation and Founder Flush Events

Notably missing from the above discussion is any consideration of the number of bacteria. The numbers are enormous. A single case represents the growth of an infectious dose ($\sim 10^6$) to 10^{14} (100 trillion) bacteria that are excreted. Multiplying a single case ten million times and the number reaches 10^{21}, a sextillion. The sixth pandemic caused an estimated 1.5 million deaths in India (800,000), Russia (500,000), and the Philippines (200,000) and it devastated other numerous countries.

Each case, outbreak, and pandemic represents an exponential expansion of the population of *V. cholerae* and then an exponential decrease. Yet the implications of these fluctuations on the genetics of *V. cholerae* have seldom been discussed. Multilocus sequence typing of O139 isolates from Kolkata demonstrated that although one allele was the most frequently found allele (77–99 % depending on the locus), alternative alleles were observed and the same alternative allele could be found in multiple years implying a persistence of the minor alleles. The authors (Garg, Aydanian et al. 2003) suggested the founder flush phenomenon might be why novel alleles were seen. Founder flush, initially described by H.D. and E.B. Ford (1930) and recounted by Wallace (1981), posits that as a population expands, variants that otherwise would not survive, do survive and expand in number along with the rest of the population.

The founder flush phenomenon may also apply in short seasonal outbreaks. In October and November of 2010, 138 isolates from Chhatak, Bangladesh were genotyped using MLVA (Rashed et al. 2014). Twenty-six genotypes were found in a single clonal complex. A "founder" genotype defined as the genotype with the most single locus variants related to it was identified. It was one of several genotypes observed on the first day of sampling clinic patients. Of the 25 derived genotypes, 23 were observed temporally after the genotype closer to the founder than from which they were derived. This observation is consistent with successive mutations occurring during the expansion. Although these polymorphic alleles occur within coding sequences (thus increasing the size of the protein by two amino acids for each additional repeat) in four of the five loci, whether or not these have a selective value is not known. In Haiti in 2010, the founder genotype radiated into eight additional MLVA genotypes (Ali, Chen et al. 2011). In Dhaka from 2004–2006, the three major clonal complexes all included additional genotypes as the years progressed (Kendall, Chowdhury et al. 2010). Thus, it is clear that during an expansion, novel MLVA alleles can be detected (Fig. 4).

Apropos to the discussion of the role of the environment in the transmission of the *V. cholerae*, the outbreaks in Chhatak 2010 and Mathbaria 2011 revealed that the genotypes in the patients were a nonrandom subset of the genotypes in the environment (Rashed et al. 2014). In both outbreaks, multiple genotypes were observed in the environment whether the analysis included the second chromosome loci or not and a single genotype or if the second chromosome loci were included a single clonal complex or genetic lineage was found in the patients. This is very strong support for an accelerated mode of transmission. However, whether the accelerated mode incorporates the hyperinfective state or involves massive numerical increases of a genetic lineage from the earliest cases cannot be distinguished from these analyses.

V. cholerae readily accepts novel DNA elements. It has been shown to recombine in the presence of chitin (Blokesch and Schoolnik 2007). It may have a mechanism for the uptake of specific DNA sequences. Serotype encoding genes (Gonzalez-Fraga, Pichel et al. 2008) and housekeeping genes have been shown to recombine (Garg, Aydanian et al. 2003; Salim, Lan et al. 2005; Octavia, Salim et al. 2013). The incorporation of these novel elements is an ongoing process and numerous novel combinations have been detected recently with the advent of genomic sequencing. However, the key for these variants is whether or not they are favored by natural selection. If not, they will eventually disappear, but if so they will be swept into the population causing disease as new variant expands in frequency.

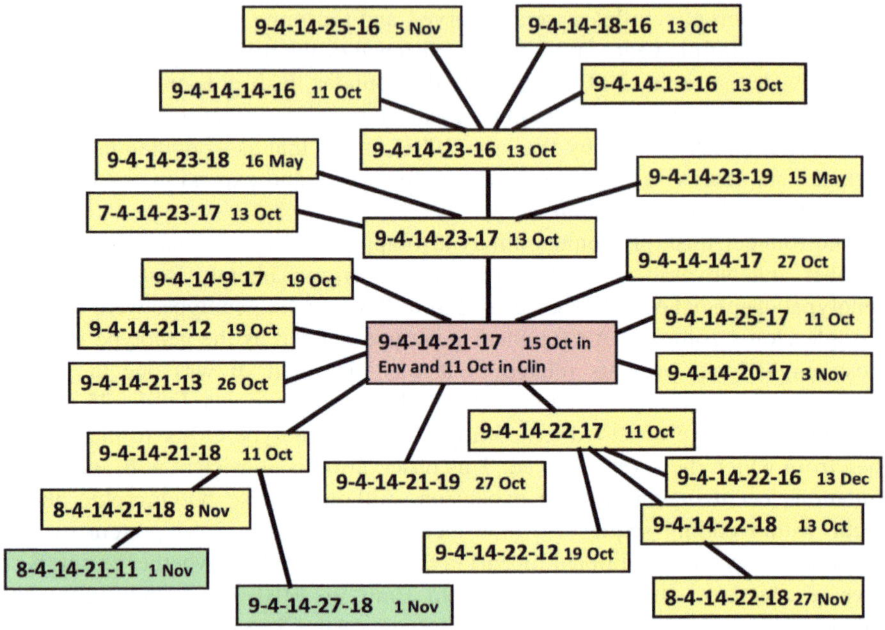

Fig. 4 Clonal complex found in Chhatak 2010. The *dates* of the first observation of each isolate are indicated. Genotypes seen only in isolates from clinic patients have a *yellow background*, while those in environmental isolates only have a *green background* and when the genotype was isolated from both patient and environmental sources it had a *blue background*. From Rashed et al. 2014

One example of natural selection for SNPs comes from *V. cholerae* in Haiti. Consistent with a founder flush event, as the pathogen population expands, the number of polymorphic sites expands from approximately 0 in 2010 to 195 SNPs in 2012 (Fig. 5) (Salemi et al. 2014). For these SNPs, the presumptive role of selection can be ascertained. The number of nonsynonymous substitutions (those that change the amino acid) continues to increase and at a rate exceeding that of synonymous substitutions. The excess of nonsynonymous to synonymous substitutions (a 2:1 ratio, in this case) is a hallmark of positive selection. Although the precise selective force is not known, it may be the pathogen adapting to expand the number of individuals that it successfully infects. In Fig. 5b, the bars labeled I, II, and III mark periods of increased incidence of cases, a pattern consistent of the selective sweeps described above and the radiation or expansion of genetic variation often found during a flush.

In summary, *V. cholerae* is evolving. The circulating clones are expected to vary over time. Genetic changes, both mutations and acquisitions of new genetic sequences, provide the substrate for natural selection to shape the population. Unfortunately for us, a major selected path is to increase the spread of *V. cholerae*, so in the foreseeable future, there will be an increasing number of cases of cholera.

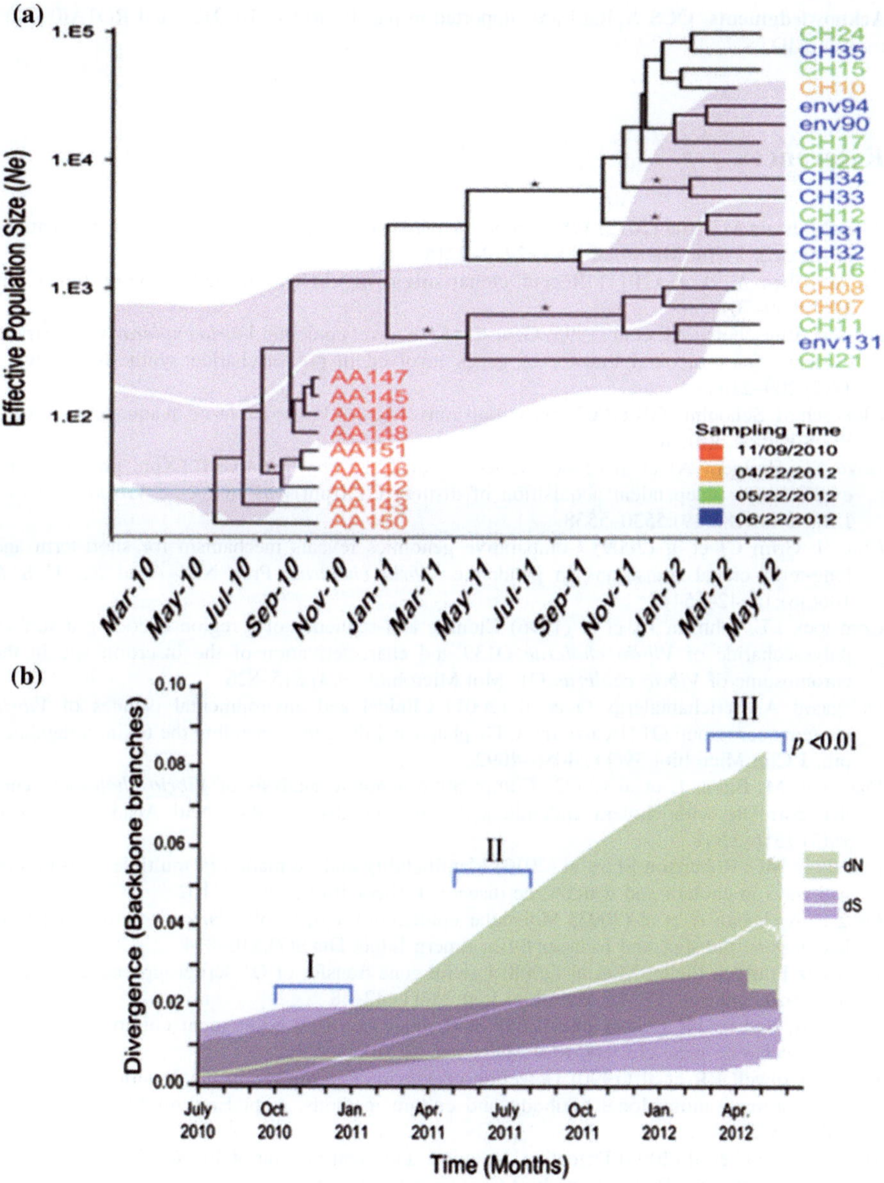

Fig. 5 Genetic and population variation in Haiti 2010–2012. Panel **a** graphs the effective population size with its 95 % confidence limits over time with an overlay of the phylogram reflecting the genetic variation. Panel **b** graphs the proportion of SNPs that are synonymous (*purple*) versus those that nonsynonymous (*green*). In each case, the *white line* is the mean and the *colored area* represents the 95 % confidence limits. From Salemi et al. 2014

Acknowledgments OCS & JGM are supported in part by RO-1A1039129 and RO1AI097405 from NIAID.

References

Alam M, Islam MT et al (2012) *Vibrio cholerae* classical biotype strains reveal distinct signatures in Mexico. J Clin Microbiol 50(7):2212–2216

Ali A, Chen Y et al (2011) Recent clonal origin of cholera in Haiti. Emerg Infect Dis 17(4):699–701

Bik EM, Bunschoten AE et al (1995) Genesis of the novel epidemic *Vibrio cholerae* O139 strain: evidence for horizontal transfer of genes involved in polysaccharide synthesis. EMBO J 14(2):209–216

Blokesch M, Schoolnik GK (2007) Serogroup conversion of *Vibrio cholerae* in aquatic reservoirs. PLoS Pathog 3(6):e81

Boyd EF, Heilpern AJ et al (2000) Molecular analyses of a putative CTXphi precursor and evidence for independent acquisition of distinct CTX(phi)s by toxigenic *Vibrio cholerae*. J Bacteriol 182(19):5530–5538

Chun J, Grim CJ et al (2009) Comparative genomics reveals mechanism for short-term and long-term clonal transitions in pandemic *Vibrio cholerae*. Proc Natl Acad Sci U S A 106(36):15442–15447

Comstock LE, Johnson JA et al (1996) Cloning and sequence of a region encoding a surface polysaccharide of *Vibrio cholerae* O139 and characterization of the insertion site in the chromosome of *Vibrio cholerae* O1. Mol Microbiol 19(4):815–826

Dalsgaard A, Serichantalergs O et al (2001) Clinical and environmental isolates of *Vibrio cholerae* serogroup O141 carry the CTX phage and the genes encoding the toxin-coregulated pili. J Clin Microbiol 39(11):4086–4092

Dziejman M, Balon E et al (2002) Comparative genomic analysis of *Vibrio cholerae*: genes that correlate with cholera endemic and pandemic disease. Proc Natl Acad Sci U S A 99(3):1556–1561

Eisenberg MC, Robertson SL et al (2013) Identifiability and estimation of multiple transmission pathways in cholera and waterborne disease. J Theor Biol 324C:84–102

Garg P, Aydanian A et al (2003) Molecular epidemiology of O139 *Vibrio cholerae*: mutation, lateral gene transfer, and founder flush. Emerg Infect Dis 9(7):810–814

Gonzalez-Fraga S, Pichel M et al (2008) Lateral gene transfer of O1 serogroup encoding genes of *Vibrio cholerae*. FEMS Microbiol Lett 286(1):32–38

Hobbs M, Reeves PR (1994) The JUMP start sequence: a 39 bp element common to several polysaccharide gene clusters. Mol Microbiol 12(5):855–856

Huq A, Colwell RR et al (1990) Detection of *Vibrio cholerae* O1 in the aquatic environment by fluorescent-monoclonal antibody and culture methods. Appl Environ Microbiol 56(8): 2370–2373

Huq A, Grim C et al (2006) Detection, isolation, and identification of *Vibrio cholerae* from the environment. Curr Protoc Microbiol Chapter 6(Unit6A):5

Huq A, Parveen S et al (1993) Comparison of *Vibrio cholerae* serotype 01 strains isolated from patients and the aquatic environment. J Trop Med Hyg 96(2):86–92

Jubair M, Morris JG Jr et al (2012) Survival of *Vibrio cholerae* in nutrient-poor environments is associated with a novel "persister" phenotype. PLoS ONE 7(9):e45187

Kendall EA, Chowdhury F et al (2010) Relatedness of *Vibrio cholerae* O1/O139 isolates from patients and their household contacts, determined by multilocus variable-number tandem-repeat analysis. J Bacteriol 192(17):4367–4376

Kiiru J, Mutreja A et al (2013) A Study on the geophylogeny of clinical and environmental *Vibrio cholerae* in Kenya. PLoS ONE 8(9):e74829

Koch R (1884) Funfter Bericht Leiters der Deutschen wissenschaftlichen Commission zur Erforschung der Cholera, Geheimen Regierungsraths Dr Koch. Dtsch Med Wochenschr 10:221–222

Li M, Shimada T et al (2002) Evidence for the emergence of non-O1 and non-O139 *Vibrio cholerae* strains with pathogenic potential by exchange of O-antigen biosynthesis regions. Infect Immun 70(5):2441–2453

Merrell DS, Butler SM, Qadri F, Dolganov NA, Alam A, Cohen MB, Calderwood SB, Schoolnik GK, Camilli A (2002) Host-induced epidemic spread of the cholera bacterium. Nature 417(6889):642–645

Mohamed AA, Oundo J et al (2012) Molecular epidemiology of geographically dispersed *Vibrio cholerae*, Kenya, Jan 2009–May 2010. Emerg Infect Dis 18(6):925–931

Mooi FR, Bik EM (1997) The evolution of epidemic *Vibrio cholerae* strains. Trends Microbiol 5(4):161–165

Mukandavire Z, Liao S et al (2011) Estimating the reproductive numbers for the 2008–2009 cholera outbreaks in Zimbabwe. Proc Natl Acad Sci U S A 108(21):8767–8772

Mukandavire Z, Smith DL et al (2013) Cholera in Haiti: reproductive numbers and vaccination coverage estimates. Sci Rep 3:997

Mutreja A, Kim DW et al (2011) Evidence for several waves of global transmission in the seventh cholera pandemic. Nature 477(7365):462–465

Nair GB, Faruque SM et al (2002) New variants of *Vibrio cholerae* O1 biotype El Tor with attributes of the classical biotype from hospitalized patients with acute diarrhea in Bangladesh. J Clin Microbiol 40(9):3296–3299

Nair GB, Ramamurthy T, Bhattacharya SK, Mukhopadhyay AK, Garg S, Bhattacharya MK, Takeda T, Shimada T, Takeda Y, Deb BC (1994) Spread of *Vibrio cholerae* O139 Bengal in India. J Infect Dis 169(5):1029–1034

Nkoko DB, Giraudoux P et al (2011) Dynamics of cholera outbreaks in great lakes region of Africa, 1978–2008. Emerg Infect Dis 17(11):2026–2034

Octavia S, Salim A et al (2013) Population structure and evolution of non-O1/non-O139 *Vibrio cholerae* by multilocus sequence typing. PLoS ONE 8(6):e65342

Pacini (1855) http://en.wikipedia.org/wiki/Filippo_Pacini

Rashed SM, Iqbal A, Mannan SB, Islam T, Rashid MU, Johura FT, Watanabe H, Hasan NA, Huq A, Stine OC, Sack RB, Colwell RR, Alam M (2013) *Vibrio cholerae* O1 El Tor and O139 Bengal strains carrying ctxB(ET). Emerg Infect Dis 19(10):1713–1715

Rashed, SM, Azman AS, Alam M, Li S, Sack DA, Morris JG, Longini I, Siddique AK, Iqbal A, Huq A, Colwell RR, Sack RB, Stine OC (2014) Genetic analysis of *Vibrio cholerae* in the human population of two rural communities in Bangladesh during outbreaks. Emerg Infect Dis 20(1)

Raychoudhuri A, Patra T et al (2009) Classical ctxB in *Vibrio cholerae* O1, Kolkata, India. Emerg Infect Dis 15(1):131–132

Rudra S, Mahajan R et al (1996) Cluster of cases of clinical cholera due to *Vibrio cholerae* 010 in east Delhi. Indian J Med Res 103:71–73

Salemi M, Ali A, Azarian T, Johnson JA, Mohr D, Prosperi M, Veras NM, Jubair M, Strickland S, Allem MT, Weppelmann TA, Morris JG (2014) Phylodynamics of *Vibrio cholerae* O1 in haiti demonstrates evidence of sequential population bottlenecks driven by positive selection. Proc Nat Acad Sci USA

Salim A, Lan R et al (2005) *Vibrio cholerae* pathogenic clones. Emerg Infect Dis 11(11):1758–1760

Stine OC, Alam M et al (2008) Seasonal cholera from multiple small outbreaks, rural Bangladesh. Emerg Infect Dis 14(5):831–833

Waldor MK, Tschape H et al (1996) A new type of conjugative transposon encodes resistance to sulfamethoxazole, trimethoprim, and streptomycin in *Vibrio cholerae* O139. J Bacteriol 178(14):4157–4165

Wallace B (1981) Basic population genetics. Columbia University Press, New York

[illegible] (2013) [illegible]

Modeling Cholera Outbreaks

Dennis L. Chao, Ira M. Longini Jr. and J. Glenn Morris Jr.

Abstract Mathematical modeling can be a valuable tool for studying infectious disease outbreak dynamics and simulating the effects of possible interventions. Here, we describe approaches to modeling cholera outbreaks and how models have been applied to explore intervention strategies, particularly in Haiti. Mathematical models can play an important role in formulating and evaluating complex cholera outbreak response options. Major challenges to cholera modeling are insufficient data for calibrating models and the need to tailor models for different outbreak scenarios.

Contents

D. L. Chao (✉)
Center for Statistics and Quantitative Infectious Diseases, Vaccine and Infectious Disease Division, Fred Hutchinson Cancer Research Center, Seattle, WA 98109, USA
e-mail: dchao@fhcrc.org

I. M. Longini Jr.
Department of Biostatistics, Colleges of Public Health and Health Professions, and Medicine, and Emerging Pathogens Institute, University of Florida, Gainesville, FL 32611, USA

J. G. Morris Jr.
Emerging Pathogens Institute, University of Florida, Gainesville, FL 32610, USA

Current Topics in Microbiology and Immunology (2014) 379: 195–209
DOI: 10.1007/82_2013_307

Published Online: 15 February 2013

1 Introduction

Although early studies of cholera have become exemplars of modern epidemiology (e.g., Snow 1855; Koch 1886, 1893), predicting and managing cholera outbreaks is still a major challenge in the developing world. Improvements in sanitation and the use of oral rehydration therapy have greatly reduced the burden of disease, but we lack a predictive framework for anticipating outbreaks and planning for interventions. Mathematical modeling is one approach to synthesizing our knowledge of cholera into a quantitative framework. Mathematical models have been used to study the dynamics of disease outbreaks and predict the effectiveness of potential intervention strategies (Garnett et al. 2011; Hutubessy et al. 2011).

Recommendations for the response to cholera outbreaks have evolved over the past decade. Earlier guidelines emphasized case management and discouraged the use of vaccines until post-emergency (Connolly 2005). Later, pre-emptive vaccination was proposed for use during complex emergencies (Chaignat and Monti 2007), and mass vaccination was being considered for containing outbreaks (Global Task Force on Cholera Control 2010). However, vaccination is usually not a practical option because of the small global supply of cholera vaccine. Recent massive and prolonged outbreaks of cholera in Haiti and several countries in Africa renewed interest in creating a global cholera vaccine stockpile, which would increase availability of the vaccine for emergency use as well as for seasonal epidemics (Waldor et al. 2010; World Health Organization 2010, 2012; Holmgren 2012; International Vaccine Institute 2012; Martin et al. 2012). But even if more vaccine were available, there is a lack of guidance for its use. Mathematical modeling can help fill this gap.

As the options for cholera outbreak responses become more complex, there is a greater need for quantitative frameworks such as mathematical modeling to both evaluate and help formulate them (Clemens 2011). In particular, the ongoing multi-year epidemic in Haiti has challenged us to plan for more comprehensive, integrated, and long-term strategies for cholera outbreaks that would involve improved identification and treatment of cases, increased access to clean water, and vaccine (Ivers et al. 2010; Farmer et al. 2011). Because cholera vaccine has rarely been used *during* an outbreak, modeling may be needed to extrapolate what little *has* been observed. Because there are many competing needs for scarce resources during complex emergencies, modeling may be required to help weigh the costs and benefits of different options (Miller Neilan et al. 2010). In this chapter, we describe how mathematical models have been applied to study cholera.

2 Mathematical Models of Cholera Transmission

Here, we describe basic mathematical models of cholera transmission, then we discuss approaches to making more detailed cholera outbreaks models, including the addition of contaminated water supplies, spatial effects, within-household transmission, and interventions.

2.1 Modeling Cholera Transmission Within a Well-Mixed Population

Basic mathematical models of infectious disease transmission describe the transitions of individuals among susceptible, infectious, and recovered states. In a susceptible-infected-recovered (SIR) model, susceptible individuals become infected at a rate proportional to the number of infected individuals, infected individuals recover at a constant rate, and recovered individuals are immune to infection (Kermack and McKendrick 1927). To account for the incubation period of a disease, one may introduce a transient "exposed" state for infected individuals before they become infectious (e.g., an SEIR model). This basic model generates a single epidemic peak, but variants that include the waning of immunity or the introduction of new susceptibles can produce cyclical dynamics (Hethcote 2000).

This basic modeling framework can be adapted to specific infectious agents by tuning infectiousness and recovery rate parameters to match the known natural history parameters or outbreak dynamics of a pathogen. A mathematical model of cholera could include an incubation period of a few hours to a few days and an infectious period of one or two weeks (Longini et al. 2007; Chao et al. 2011). To include multi-season dynamics, waning immunity can be added to the model (e.g., an SIRS model) (Koelle and Pascual 2004; Koelle et al. 2005; Rinaldo et al. 2012). One may also add symptomatic and asymptomatic infections, which could play different roles in disease transmission and surveillance (Longini et al. 2007; King et al. 2008; Nelson et al. 2009; Andrews and Basu 2011).

Many cholera models assume that individuals become infected by consumption of *V. cholerae* from the environment and therefore include an explicit environmental compartment (Codeço 2001; Tien and Earn 2010). A susceptible individual's risk of infection, λ, at time t can be expressed as $\lambda(t) = \mu I(t) + \beta B(t)$, where μ is the rate of exposure between individuals, $I(t)$ is the number of infectious individuals at time t, β is the rate of exposure to the environment, and $B(t)$ is the level of contamination of the environment. Note that the first term is proportional to the number of infectious individuals, and we refer to this as the *ciclo corto* ("short cycle") transmission pathway. This route is also known as "person-to-person" transmission and accounts for infections occurring during the short time window of an infected close contact's infectious period. The second term is proportional to the level of contamination in the environment and is also known as *ciclo largo* ("long cycle") transmission, which could be caused by exposure to sewage or contaminated water not necessarily traceable to an infected contact. A cholera model can include either or both of these terms. Inserting the environment into the chain of cholera transmission can create a lag in the generation time and allows for cholera transmission to occur in the absence of infected individuals, which can help the disease persist in a population. Figure 1 diagrams a modeling framework that includes both *ciclo corto* and *ciclo largo* transmission.

Different models based on alternative sets of assumptions may be able to fit observations equally well. For example, simple SIR models of cholera can produce

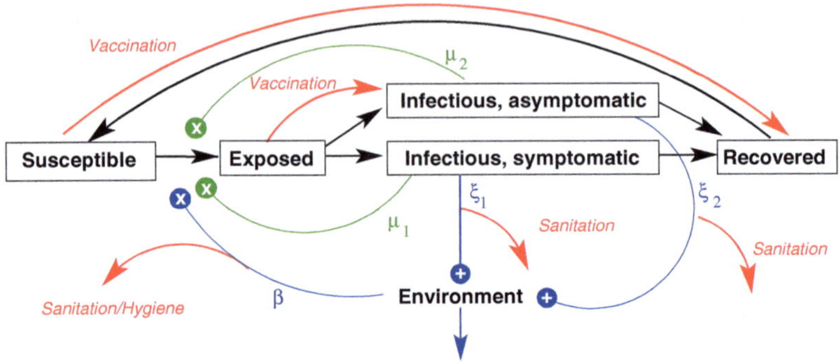

Fig. 1 Basic cholera model diagram. Individuals can be Susceptible to cholera, Exposed, Infectious (either symptomatically or asymptomatically), or Recovered (and immune to infection). *Black arrows* indicate transitions between these states. Infectious individuals shed cholera into the environment (indicated by the "+"s). Susceptible individuals become infected by exposure to *Vibrio cholerae* from the Environment (the *ciclo largo* route indicated by *blue* "*x*") at the rate of β or "directly" from Infectious individuals at the rate of μ (the *ciclo corto* route indicated by *green* "*x*"s). After an incubation period, individuals transition from the Exposed to the Infectious state. Infectious individuals shed vibrios into the environment at rate ξ. Symptomatic and asymptomatic may have different levels of infectiousness, indicated by the subscripts following ξ and μ. *Red arrows* indicate possible effects of interventions labeled in italics, including vaccination, sanitation, and improved hygiene

outbreak dynamics nearly indistinguishable from those that include *ciclo largo* transmission. However, a particular intervention may target one of these routes of transmission more than the other. Therefore, to accurately predict the effectiveness of interventions, one should include the major routes of exposure.

With high quality surveillance data, models might be used to determine the relative contribution of *ciclo corto* and *ciclo largo* transmission. In regions with seasonal cholera epidemics, outbreaks may be triggered by *V. cholerae* in the aquatic reservoir while secondary transmission (*ciclo corto*) drives dramatic local outbreaks (Franco et al. 1997; Ruiz-Moreno et al. 2010). King et al. (2008) used over 50 years of cholera mortality data from Bengal to test alternative models of disease transmission and found support for a large role for *ciclo largo* transmission in certain districts. Mukandavire et al. (2011) used weekly surveillance data to estimate the relative contributions of *ciclo corto* and *ciclo largo* transmission of a major outbreak in Zimbabwe that started in 2008. They concluded that the relative contributions of these two routes of transmission were different by province, which may be due to differences in the modes of transmission. Studies such as these reveal spatial heterogeneities in cholera transmission.

2.2 Spatial Modeling and Pathogen Movement

For disease outbreaks in small, tightly connected communities, models of single well-mixed populations may be the most appropriate and parsimonious approach.

However, if an outbreak encompasses a large population or if the geographic region includes heterogeneities relevant to disease transmission, such as population density, socioeconomic differences, or geographic features that could block or enhance transmission, then models may need to include multiple interacting populations.

There are several options for geographically subdividing a population for modeling purposes. An obvious choice would be to match the spatial resolution of available surveillance data, so that each reporting area is a single subpopulation within a "metapopulation" or "patch" model (Tuite et al. 2011; Andrews and Basu 2011). However, surveillance data may be coarse, and disease outbreaks may occur on a much finer scale. One could instead use finer political boundaries [e.g., districts or other administrative boundaries (Bertuzzo et al. 2011)], geographical/geological features [e.g., watersheds (Rinaldo et al. 2012)], or a fine regular grid (Longini et al. 2007; Chao et al. 2011). Using smaller geographic units may better capture spatial heterogeneity relevant to cholera transmission, but can complicate the model with excessive parameters and lead to a loss of generality of modeling results.

Perhaps the spatial resolution of the model should not be determined by convenient political boundaries, but instead by the "natural scale" of cholera outbreaks. Cholera outbreaks are known to be fast and produce sharply peaked epidemic curves, but when case reporting is aggregated by large geographic regions, such as at the country-level, sharp epidemic spikes and outbreak dynamics in general can be masked. Trying to fit a single epidemic curve that is actually the aggregate of multiple spatially separated outbreaks will result in misleading results (Grad et al. 2012). Unfortunately, the scale of an outbreak probably depends on local environmental and sociological factors. Spatial analyses and sequencing of cholera isolates may help identify distinct outbreaks in endemic settings (Stine et al. 2008), which could help modelers dis-aggregate concurrent but distinct outbreaks.

Metapopulation models include mechanisms governing the flow of the infectious agent among the populations. Many models assume that pathogens are transported primarily by infectious people. In such models, susceptible people in one community can be infected by infectious people in neighboring communities. This is usually implemented by setting the force of infection in a community to be a function of both the number of infectious individuals residing in the community and the number of infectious individuals in neighboring communities. Thus, an infectious person contributes to infections in co-located susceptibles and in neighboring populations, often with a force of infection inversely proportional to distance (Bertuzzo et al. 2011; Tuite et al. 2011; Mari et al. 2012). In addition to using geographic distance, one can assume that individuals living along major transportation routes are more mobile and can spread disease farther than those who are more isolated (Chao et al. 2011). In agent-based, or individual-based, models in which each person is individually represented, infectious individuals can move from location to location, infecting individuals as they travel (Longini et al. 2007; Chao et al. 2011). Eventually, studies that track cell phones and other mobile devices might tell us how people actually move during an outbreak (Chunara et al. 2012; Bengtsson et al. 2011; Khan et al. 2012).

Alternatively, models can assume that the pathogen moves via the environment. The environmental reservoirs of adjacent populations can be linked, which would cause *V. cholerae* shed by one population to diffuse to neighboring populations (Bertuzzo et al. 2010, 2011; Mari et al. 2012), or hydrology can be modeled so that communities can infect populations that are downstream (Chao et al. 2011; Rinaldo et al. 2012). Including realistic hydrology may be important when rivers play a major role in cholera transmission. Some cholera models include the transport of the pathogen through both people and the environment (Chao et al. 2011; Rinaldo et al. 2012).

2.3 Transmission Within Households and Hyperinfectivity

High secondary attack rates have been observed within households of cases (Mosley et al. 1965, 1968; McCormack et al. 1968; Harris et al. 2008; Weil et al. 2009; Kendall et al. 2010). Although a common source of exposure could account for many of these heavily infected households, studies of the time intervals between cases or that genotype infecting strains have found patterns of transmission consistent with *ciclo corto* transmission (Snow 1855; Tamayo et al. 1965; Kendall et al. 2010). A tell tale sign of *ciclo corto* transmission would be the rapid appearance of secondary cases consistent with the incubation period of cholera.

A large inoculum of *V. cholerae* is required to infect an individual (Cash et al. 1974; Levine et al. 1979; Suntharasamai et al. 1992), which makes *ciclo corto* transmission appear to be physiologically challenging. There are several possible mechanisms for transmission within a household. For example, a household's food or water supply could be contaminated by an infected individual (St Louis et al. 1990; Albert et al. 1997; Rabbani and Greenough 1999; Roberts et al. 2001; Palit et al. 2012). Another possibility is that *V. cholerae* "hyperinfectious" state facilitates *ciclo corto* transmission. *V. cholerae* can be orders of magnitude more infectious within the first several hours after excretion from its host (Merrell et al. 2002). This *hyperinfectious* state of the pathogen would have a much lower infectious dose, which could allow for rapid transmission among close contacts.

Hartley et al. (2006) modeled the effects of hyperinfectivity by including two environmental reservoirs; infectious individuals contribute to a highly infectious environmental reservoir, which transitions to a second, less infectious reservoir. Including the hyperinfectious reservoir allowed the model to replicate the "explosive" dynamics of outbreaks (Hartley et al. 2006; Morris 2011). However, rapid cholera outbreaks can also be modeled using simple SIR models without explicitly including hyperinfectivity (Pascual et al. 2006). It may be impossible to resolve the role of hyperinfectivity in actual outbreaks using models alone—careful epidemiological studies are required. Conversely, it is not obvious which modeling framework should be used, and it may depend on the particular scenario and possible interventions being considered.

Regardless of the actual mechanism invoked, models can include cholera transmission within households in order to capture the elevated attack rates within households with index cases (Chao et al. 2011). Including within-household transmission may be necessary to model certain household-level interventions, such as targeting certain individuals for vaccination in order to protect their families (Ali et al. 2008).

2.4 Modeling Interventions

Models can be used to estimate the effectiveness of intervention strategies. Interventions in the cholera modeling literature have included vaccination and improvements in sanitation and hygiene.

The effect of vaccines can be modeled in several ways, depending on assumptions about the vaccine's mode of protection (Halloran et al. 1999). Most cholera models assume that vaccination has the same protective effect as natural infection, so vaccinated susceptibles are simply treated as resistant individuals (Miller Neilan et al. 2010; Bertuzzo et al. 2011; Tuite et al. 2011; Andrews and Basu 2011; Azman et al. 2012), as shown in Fig. 1. However, vaccination may have immunological consequences different from natural infection (Leung et al. 2012; Arifuzzaman et al. 2012). In one challenge study, vaccine appears to protect against symptomatic illness but not necessarily against infection (Black et al. 1987). If one assumes that asymptomatically infected individuals are infectious, then those protected by vaccine could still transmit disease. The model described in Chao et al. (2011) assumes that vaccinees are not protected against infection but have a lower probability of becoming symptomatic upon infection, as shown in Fig. 1.

Unvaccinated individuals may be indirectly protected when a sufficient number of their contacts are vaccinated (Fox et al. 1971). Models can be used to compute the critical vaccination fraction, or the fraction of the population that needs to be vaccinated to essentially stop local transmission (Hill and Longini 2003). If the basic reproductive number, R_0 is known, then the critical vaccination fraction is approximately $(1/\mathrm{VE})(1 - 1/R_0)$, where VE is the vaccine efficacy against infection. More detailed transmission models can be used to make more refined estimates for the critical vaccination fraction and other measures of indirect protection. In a large cholera vaccine trial, herd immunity was observed (Ali et al. 2005), and a modeling study used these results to explore the effectiveness of different levels of vaccine coverage (Longini et al. 2007). The Longini et al. (2007) study estimated that the critical vaccination fraction of the study population was about 70 %.

Improvements in sanitation and hygiene are essential non-pharmaceutical measures for cholera outbreak control. Interventions that reduce the consumption of contaminated water, such as the provision of clean water or the promotion of chlorination, can be modeled as a reduction in the exposure to cholera from the environment (Miller Neilan et al. 2010; Tuite et al. 2011; Chao et al. 2011; Mari et al. 2012). Interventions that better manage the waste of infected individuals, such as the cleaning or building of latrines, could be modeled as a reduction in the contribution of infected individuals to the environmental reservoir (Chao et al. 2011; Mari et al. 2012). Both of these approaches to modeling improved sanitation and hygiene are depicted in Fig. 1.

3 Modeling the 2010 Cholera Outbreak in Haiti

In October 2010, cases of cholera began appearing in central Haiti, the start of a massive and prolonged epidemic that spread across the country and sickened over half a million people within a year (Walton and Ivers 2011; Cravioto et al. 2011). The conditions in Haiti seemed perfect for cholera transmission, with unrepaired damage from a major earthquake earlier in the year and Hurricane Tomas striking soon after the first cases of cholera were identified. Public health workers were trained to treat cases, and temporary cholera treatment centers were quickly established. Haiti's Ministère de la Santé Publique et de la Population (MSPP) launched a media campaign to promote better sanitation and hygiene (Centers for Disease Control and Prevention (CDC) 2010).

Several modeling efforts began soon after the first cases were reported (Bertuzzo et al. 2011; Tuite et al. 2011; Andrews and Basu 2011; Chao et al. 2011; Abrams et al. 2012). All of these studies attempted to reproduce the dynamics of the epidemic for a single season at the department level, the spatial resolution of reported case and hospitalization counts publicly released by MSPP. Two modeling groups divided the departments into much smaller regions to implement more realistic cholera transmission dynamics (Bertuzzo et al. 2011; Chao et al. 2011). All of these modeling studies focused on the size and duration of the first, and largest, wave of the epidemic, but the first were published in March of 2011, months after the peak actually occurred.

What emerged from the modeling community was a set of models and a small body of literature on modeling cholera during an outbreak. Common themes were the spatial coarseness of the surveillance data, the limited impact a small supply of vaccine would have on a nationwide outbreak, and the need for better surveillance. Most of the modeling groups used the case and hospitalization estimates from the MSPP, but one of the studies attempted to estimate and correct for the different reporting rates by department (Andrews and Basu 2011).

Chao et al. (2011) modeled scenarios in which there was much more vaccine than was actually available at the time. The study suggested that achieving high levels of coverage in regions with high exposure to cholera, particularly along rivers, could have had a major impact on the course of the epidemic. However, the study found that mass vaccination alone would have been insufficient to stop the

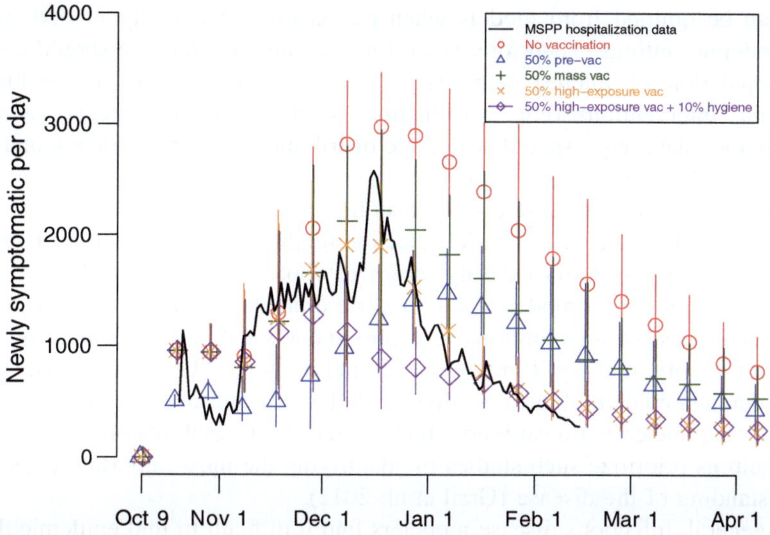

Fig. 2 Simulated effects of interventions during the first wave of the 2010 cholera epidemic in Haiti. The stochastic model described in Chao et al. (2011) was run 50 times per scenario, and the points plot the median attack rates for the stochastic simulations and the lines represent the range of the minimum and maximum attack rates. Several intervention scenarios were modeled: no intervention (in *red*), vaccination well before the epidemic (pre-vaccination, in *blue*), vaccination after the first cholera cases were confirmed (mass vaccination, in *green*), vaccination targeted to communities near rivers after the first cholera cases were confirmed (high-exposure vaccination, in *yellow*), and prioritizing vaccination and educational campaigns to improve hygiene and sanitation to communities near rivers after the first cholera cases were confirmed (in *purple*). Note that pre-vaccination delays the epidemic peak, while reactive strategies tend to reduce but not delay the peak

spread of cholera—improving sanitation and hygiene to reduce the public's exposure to the pathogen was also necessary to greatly reduce cholera transmission in Haiti (Fig. 2). The results highlight the need to target vaccination campaigns and other interventions efficiently when resources are scarce.

4 Discussion and Conclusions

We have described a variety of approaches to modeling cholera outbreaks. The same modeling frameworks can be used to describe both epidemic and endemic cholera, but the modeler must make the appropriate choices of initial conditions, parameterization, and possibly model structure. For cholera outbreaks in non-endemic regions, there may be little prior immunity, a high attack rate, similar attack rates among age groups, and high symptomatic fractions (Sack 2003; Sack et al. 2004). The issues more important in endemic regions, such as drivers of seasonality and environmental predictors of outbreaks, may be of little concern and can be omitted from models when one is interested solely in outbreaks in non-endemic settings. Therefore, when formulating a model, one should consider the population of interest (e.g., size, heterogeneity, prior exposure history), available interventions (e.g., vaccination, sanitation improvements), available surveillance data (e.g., spatial scale, age distributions, reporting rates), and time-scale (e.g., days, months, or years).

Models with different assumptions may fit the dynamics of a particular outbreak equally well. In some cases, model selection might not be an important issue. But when one wants to perturb the dynamics of cholera transmission by simulating interventions, different models could produce dramatically different projections of the effectiveness of interventions. Complex models will also encounter problems of identifiability, making it impossible to find a unique "best" set of parameters. More detailed epidemiological studies of cholera transmission are needed in order to better parameterize transmission models. Sensitivity analyses of cholera models may help us prioritize such studies by identifying the most important gaps in our understanding of the disease (Grad et al. 2012).

In general, infectious disease modelers find it difficult to find epidemic data of sufficient quality for model-fitting. Public health departments generally release surveillance data aggregated over large spatial scales. More detailed outbreak data is usually obtainable only through direct collaborations with the outbreak investigators, which is rare in the modeling world. Therefore, there are few modeling studies of real outbreaks and many studies of the properties of the models themselves. The dearth of data and well-parameterized models may lead to the overgeneralization of modeling results. There is a clear need for more modeling studies of actual outbreaks, which would require either more direct collaborations between modelers and surveillance groups or more receptiveness to sharing outbreak data with modelers and other analysts.

Modeling studies can be a valuable source of information for public health officials evaluating potential interventions for cholera outbreaks (Garnett et al. 2011; Hutubessy et al. 2011). Most published studies that evaluate the cost-effectiveness of cholera vaccination do not include a dynamic model of disease transmission (Sack 2003; Jeuland et al. 2009; Cook et al. 2009; Kim et al. 2011; Reyburn et al. 2011). Dynamic transmission models such as those described here capture indirect protection, which increases the estimated effectiveness of mass vaccination and other interventions (Brisson and Edmunds 2003). Based on earlier studies, many concluded that reactive vaccination would not be helpful during outbreaks (Sommer and Mosley 1973; Naficy et al. 1998). However, large and prolonged outbreaks could be mitigated using reactive vaccination, particularly if interventions target key populations (Chao et al. 2011; Azman et al. 2012). Models could and should be used to weigh the costs and benefits of different interventions for a range of scenarios, from seasonal endemic cholera outbreaks to epidemics exacerbated by natural disasters (Legros et al. 1999; Calain et al. 2004; Jeuland et al. 2009; Chaignat and Monti 2007; Global Task Force on Cholera Control 2010).

References

Abrams JY, Copeland JR, Tauxe RV, Date KA, Belay ED, Mody RK, Mintz ED (2012) Real-time modelling used for outbreak management during a cholera epidemic, Haiti, 2010–2011. Epidemiol Infect, pp 1–10 (in press)

Albert MJ, Neira M, Motarjemi Y (1997) The role of food in the epidemiology of cholera. World Health Stat Q 50(1–2):111–118

Ali M, Emch M, von Seidlein L, Yunus M, Sack DA, Rao M, Holmgren J, Clemens JD (2005) Herd immunity conferred by killed oral cholera vaccines in Bangladesh: a reanalysis. Lancet 366(9479):44–49

Ali M, Emch M, Yunus M, Sack D, Lopez AL, Holmgren J, Clemens J (2008) Vaccine protection of Bangladeshi infants and young children against cholera: implications for vaccine deployment and person-to-person transmission. Pediatr Infect Dis J 27(1):33–37. doi:00006454-200801000-00007[pii]

Andrews JR, Basu S (2011) Transmission dynamics and control of cholera in Haiti: an epidemic model. Lancet 377(9773):1248–1255. doi:10.1016/S0140-6736(11)60273-0

Arifuzzaman M, Rashu R, Leung DT, Hosen MI, Bhuiyan TR, Bhuiyan MS, Rahman MA, Khanam F, Saha A, Charles RC, Larocque RC, Weil AA, Clements JD, Holmes RK, Calderwood SB, Harris JB, Ryan ET, Qadri F (2012) Antigen-specific memory T cell responses after vaccination with an oral killed cholera vaccine in Bangladeshi children and comparison to responses in patients with naturally acquired cholera. Clin Vaccine Immunol 19(8):1304–1311. doi:10.1128/CVI.00196-12

Azman AS, Luquero FJ, Rodrigues A, Palma PP, Grais RF, Banga CN, Grenfell BT, Lessler J (2012) Urban cholera transmission hotspots and their implications for reactive vaccination: Evidence from Bissau City, Guinea Bissau.. PLoS Negl Trop Dis 6(11):e1901. doi:10.1371/journal.pntd.0001901

Bengtsson L, Lu X, Thorson A, Garfield R, von Schreeb J (2011) Improved response to disasters and outbreaks by tracking population movements with mobile phone network data: a post-earthquake geospatial study in Haiti. PLoS Med 8(8):e1001,083. doi:10.1371/journal.pmed.1001083

Bertuzzo E, Casagrandi R, Gatto M, Rodriguez-Iturbe I, Rinaldo A (2010) On spatially explicit models of cholera epidemics. J R Soc Interf 7(43):321–333. doi:10.1098/rsif.2009.0204

Bertuzzo E, Mari L, Righetto L, Gatto M, Casagrandi R, Blokesch M, Rodriguez-Iturbe I, Rinaldo A (2011) Prediction of the spatial evolution and effects of control measures for the unfolding Haiti cholera outbreak. Geophys Res Lett 38:L06,403

Black RE, Levine MM, Clements ML, Young CR, Svennerholm AM, Holmgren J (1987) Protective efficacy in humans of killed whole-vibrio oral cholera vaccine with and without the B subunit of cholera toxin. Infect Immun 55(5):1116–1120

Brisson M, Edmunds WJ (2003) Economic evaluation of vaccination programs: the impact of herd-immunity. Med Decis Making 23(1):76–82

Calain P, Chaine JP, Johnson E, Hawley ML, O'Leary MJ, Oshitani H, Chaignat CL (2004) Can oral cholera vaccination play a role in controlling a cholera outbreak? Vaccine 22(19):2444–2451

Cash RA, Music SI, Libonati JP, Snyder MJ, Wenzel RP, Hornick RB (1974) Response of man to infection with *Vibrio cholerae*. I. clinical, serologic, and bacteriologic responses to a known inoculum. J Infect Dis 129(1):45–52

Centers for Disease Control and Prevention (CDC) (2010) Update: cholera outbreak—Haiti, 2010. MMWR Morb Mortal Wkly Rep 59(45):1473–1479

Chaignat CL, Monti V (2007) Use of oral cholera vaccine in complex emergencies: what next? Summary report of an expert meeting and recommendations of WHO. J Health Popul Nutr 25(2):244–261

Chao DL, Halloran ME, Longini IM Jr (2011) Vaccination strategies for epidemic cholera in Haiti with implications for the developing world. Proc Natl Acad Sci U S A 108(17):7081–7085. doi:10.1073/pnas.1102149108

Chunara R, Andrews JR, Brownstein JS (2012) Social and news media enable estimation of epidemiological patterns early in the 2010 Haitian cholera outbreak. Am J Trop Med Hyg 86(1):39–45. doi:10.4269/ajtmh.2012.11-0597

Clemens JD (2011) Vaccines in the time of cholera. Proc Natl Acad Sci U S A 108(21):8529–8530. doi:10.1073/pnas.1105807108

Codeço CT (2001) Endemic and epidemic dynamics of cholera: the role of the aquatic reservoir. BMC Infect Dis 1:1

Connolly, MA (eds) (2005) Communicable disease control in emergencies: a field manual. World Health Organization, Geneva

Cook J, Jeuland M, Maskery B, Lauria D, Sur D, Clemens J, Whittington D (2009) Using private demand studies to calculate socially optimal vaccine subsidies in developing countries. J Policy Anal Manage 28(1):6–28

Cravioto A, Lanta CF, Lantagne DS, Nair GB (2011) Final report of the independent panel of experts on the cholera outbreak in Haiti. United Nations, New York

Farmer P, Almazor CP, Bahnsen ET, Barry D, Bazile J, Bloom BR, Bose N, Brewer T, Calderwood SB, Clemens JD, Cravioto A, Eustache E, Jérôme G, Gupta N, Harris JB, Hiatt HH, Holstein C, Hotez PJ, Ivers LC, Kerry VB, Koenig SP, LaRocque RC, Léandre F, Lambert W, Lyon E, Mekalanos JJ, Mukherjee JS, Oswald C, Pape JW, Gretchko Prosper A, Rabinovich R, Raymonville M, Réjouit JR, Ronan LJ, Rosenberg ML, Ryan ET, Sachs JD, Sack DA, Surena C, Suri AA, Ternier R, Waldor MK, Walton D, Weigel JL (2011) Meeting cholera's challenge to Haiti and the world: A joint statement on cholera prevention and care. PLoS Negl Trop Dis 5(5):e1145. doi:10.1371/journal.pntd.0001145

Fox JP, Elveback L, Scott W, Gatewood L, Ackerman E (1971) Herd immunity: basic concept and relevance to public health immunization practices. Am J Epidemiol 94(3):179–189

Franco AA, Fix AD, Prada A, Paredes E, Palomino JC, Wright AC, Johnson JA, McCarter R, Guerra H, Morris JG Jr (1997) Cholera in Lima, Peru, correlates with prior isolation of *Vibrio cholerae* from the environment. Am J Epidemiol 146(12):1067–1075

Garnett GP, Cousens S, Hallett TB, Steketee R, Walker N (2011) Mathematical models in the evaluation of health programmes. Lancet 378(9790):515–525. doi:10.1016/S0140-6736(10)61505-X

Global Task Force on Cholera Control (2010) Oral cholera vaccines in mass immunization campaigns: Guidance for planning and use. World Health Organization, Geneva, http://whqlibdoc.who.int/publications/2010/9789241500432_eng.pdf

Grad YH, Miller JC, Lipsitch M (2012) Cholera modeling: challenges to quantitative analysis and predicting the impact of interventions. Epidemiology 23(4):523–530. doi:00001648-201207000-00004

Halloran ME, Longini IM Jr, Struchiner CJ (1999) Design and interpretation of vaccine field studies. Epidemiol Rev 21(1):73–88

Harris JB, LaRocque RC, Chowdhury F, Khan AI, Logvinenko T, Faruque ASG, Ryan ET, Qadri F, Calderwood SB (2008) Susceptibility to *Vibrio cholerae* infection in a cohort of household contacts of patients with cholera in Bangladesh. PLoS Negl Trop Dis 2(4):e221

Hartley DM, Morris JG Jr, Smith DL (2006) Hyperinfectivity: a critical element in the ability of *V cholerae* to cause epidemics. PLoS Med 3(1):e7

Hethcote HW (2000) The mathematics of infectious diseases. SIAM Rev 42(4):599–653

Hill AN, Longini IM Jr (2003) The critical vaccination fraction for heterogeneous epidemic models. Mathematical Biosciences 181:85–106

Holmgren J (2012) A case for control of cholera in Africa by vaccination. Lancet Infect Dis 12(11):818–819. doi:10.1016/S1473-3099(12)70204-9

Hutubessy R, Henao AM, Namgyal P, Moorthy V, Hombach J (2011) Results from evaluations of models and cost-effectiveness tools to support introduction decisions for new vaccines need critical appraisal. BMC Med 9:55. doi:10.1186/1741-7015-9-55

International Vaccine Institute (2012) An investment case for the accelerated introduction of oral cholera vaccines. International Vaccine Institute, Seoul. http://www.ivi.int/publication/IVI_Global_cholera_case.pdf

Ivers LC, Farmer P, Almazor CP, Léandre F (2010) Five complementary interventions to slow cholera: Haiti. Lancet 376(9758):2048–2051. doi:10.1016/S0140-6736(10)62243-X

Jeuland M, Cook J, Poulos C, Clemens J, Whittington D (2009) Cost-effectiveness of new-generation oral cholera vaccines: a multisite analysis. Value Health 12(6):899–908

Kendall EA, Chowdhury F, Begum Y, Khan AI, Li S, Thierer JH, Bailey J, Kreisel K, Tacket CO, LaRocque RC, Harris JB, Ryan ET, Qadri F, Calderwood SB, Stine OC (2010) Relatedness of *Vibrio cholerae* O1/O139 isolates from patients and their household contacts, determined by multilocus variable-number tandem-repeat analysis. J Bacteriol 192(17):4367–4376. doi:10.1128/JB.00698-10

Kermack WO, McKendrick AG (1927) A contribution to the mathematical theory of epidemics. Proc Roy Soc Lon Ser A 115:700–721

Khan K, McNabb SJ, Memish ZA, Eckhardt R, Hu W, Kossowsky D, Sears J, Arino J, Johansson A, Barbeschi M, McCloskey B, Henry B, Cetron M, Brownstein JS (2012) Infectious disease surveillance and modelling across geographic frontiers and scientific specialties. Lancet Infect Dis 12(3):222–230

Kim SY, Choi Y, Mason PR, Rusakaniko S, Goldie SJ (2011) Potential impact of reactive vaccination in controlling cholera outbreaks: an exploratory analysis using a Zimbabwean experience. S Afr Med J 101(9):659–664

King AA, Ionides EL, Pascual M, Bouma MJ (2008) Inapparent infections and cholera dynamics. Nature 454(7206):877–880

Koch R (1886) Further researches on cholera. Br Med J 1(1306):62–66

Koch R (1893) Ueber den augenblicklichen Stand der bakteriologischen Choleradiagnose. Medical Microbiology and Immunology 14:319–338

Koelle K, Pascual M (2004) Disentangling extrinsic from intrinsic factors in disease dynamics: a nonlinear time series approach with an application to cholera. Am Nat 163(6):901–913

Koelle K, Rodó X, Pascual M, Yunus M, Mostafa G (2005) Refractory periods and climate forcing in cholera dynamics. Nature 436(7051):696–700

Legros D, Paquet C, Perea W, Marty I, Mugisha NK, Royer H, Neira M, Ivanoff B (1999) Mass vaccination with a two-dose oral cholera vaccine in a refugee camp. Bull World Health Organ 77(10):837–842

Leung DT, Rahman MA, Mohasin M, Patel SM, Aktar A, Khanam F, Uddin T, Riyadh MA, Saha A, Alam MM, Chowdhury F, Khan AI, Charles R, Larocque R, Harris JB, Calderwood SB, Qadri F, Ryan ET (2012) Memory B cell and other immune responses in children receiving two doses of an oral killed cholera vaccine compared to responses following natural cholera infection in Bangladesh. Clin Vaccine Immunol 19(5):690–698. doi:10.1128/CVI.05615-11

Levine MM, Nalin DR, Rennels MB, Hornick RB, Sotman S, Van Blerk G, Hughes TP, O'Donnell S, Barua D (1979) Genetic susceptibility to cholera. Ann Hum Biol 6(4):369–374

Longini IM Jr, Nizam A, Ali M, Yunus M, Shenvi N, Clemens JD (2007) Controlling endemic cholera with oral vaccines. PLoS Med 4(11):e336

Mari L, Bertuzzo E, Righetto L, Casagrandi R, Gatto M, Rodriguez-Iturbe I, Rinaldo A (2012) Modelling cholera epidemics: the role of waterways, human mobility and sanitation. J R Soc Interf 9(67):376–388. doi:10.1098/rsif.2011.0304

Martin S, Costa A, Perea W (2012) Stockpiling oral cholera vaccine. Bull World Health Organ 90(10):714. doi:BLT.12.112433

McCormack WM, Chowdhury AM, Jahangir N, Ahmed AB, Mosley WH (1968) Tetracycline prophylaxis in families of cholera patients. Bull World Health Organ 38(5):787–792

Merrell DS, Butler SM, Qadri F, Dolganov NA, Alam A, Cohen MB, Calderwood SB, Schoolnik GK, Camilli A (2002) Host-induced epidemic spread of the cholera bacterium. Nature 417(6889):642–645

Miller Neilan RL, Schaefer E, Gaff H, Fister KR, Lenhart S (2010) Modeling optimal intervention strategies for cholera. Bull Math Biol 72(8):2004–2018. doi:10.1007/s11538-010-9521-8

Morris JG Jr (2011) Cholera-modern pandemic disease of ancient lineage. Emerg Infect Dis 17(11):2099–2104. doi:10.3201/eid1711.111109

Mosley WH, Alvero MG, Joseph PR, Tamayo JF, Gomez CZ, Montague T, Dizon JJ, Henderson DA (1965) Studies of cholera El Tor in the Philippines. 4. Transmission of infection among neighbourhood and community contacts of cholera patients. Bull World Health Organ 33(5):651–660

Mosley WH, Ahmad S, Benenson AS, Ahmed A (1968) The relationship of vibriocidal antibody titre to susceptibility to cholera in family contacts of cholera patients. Bull World Health Organ 38(5):777–785

Mukandavire Z, Liao S, Wang J, Gaff H, Smith DL, Morris JG Jr (2011) Estimating the reproductive numbers for the 2008–2009 cholera outbreaks in Zimbabwe. Proc Natl Acad Sci U S A 108(21):8767–8772. doi:10.1073/pnas.1019712108

Naficy A, Rao MR, Paquet C, Antona D, Sorkin A, Clemens JD (1998) Treatment and vaccination strategies to control cholera in sub-Saharan refugee settings: a cost-effectiveness analysis. JAMA 279(7):521–525

Nelson EJ, Harris JB, Morris JG Jr, Calderwood SB, Camilli A (2009) Cholera transmission: the host, pathogen and bacteriophage dynamic. Nat Rev Microbiol 7(10):693–702

Palit A, Batabyal P, Kanungo S, Sur D (2012) In-house contamination of potable water in urban slum of Kolkata, India: a possible transmission route of diarrhea. Water Sci Technol 66(2):299–303. doi:10.2166/wst.2012.177

Pascual M, Koelle K, Dobson AP (2006) Hyperinfectivity in cholera: a new mechanism for an old epidemiological model. PLoS Med 3(6):e280

Rabbani GH, Greenough WB 3rd (1999) Food as a vehicle of transmission of cholera. J Diarrhoeal Dis Res 17(1):1–9

Reyburn R, Deen JL, Grais RF, Bhattacharya SK, Sur D, Lopez AL, Jiddawi MS, Clemens JD, von Seidlein L (2011) The case for reactive mass oral cholera vaccinations. PLoS Negl Trop Dis 5(1):e952. doi:10.1371/journal.pntd.0000952

Rinaldo A, Bertuzzo E, Mari L, Righetto L, Blokesch M, Gatto M, Casagrandi R, Murray M, Vesenbeckh SM, Rodriguez-Iturbe I (2012) Reassessment of the 2010–2011 Haiti cholera outbreak and rainfall-driven multiseason projections. Proc Natl Acad Sci U S A 109(17):6602–6607. doi:10.1073/pnas.1203333109

Roberts L, Chartier Y, Chartier O, Malenga G, Toole M, Rodka H (2001) Keeping clean water clean in a Malawi refugee camp: a randomized intervention trial. Bull World Health Organ 79(4):280–287

Ruiz-Moreno D, Pascual M, Emch M, Yunus M (2010) Spatial clustering in the spatio-temporal dynamics of endemic cholera. BMC Infect Dis 10:51

Sack DA (2003) When should cholera vaccine be used in cholera-endemic areas. J Health Popul Nutr 21(4):299–303

Sack DA, Sack RB, Nair GB, Siddique AK (2004) Cholera. Lancet 363(9404):223–233

Snow J (1855) On the mode of communication of cholera. John Churchill, London

Sommer A, Mosley WH (1973) Ineffectiveness of cholera vaccination as an epidemic control measure. Lancet 1(7814):1232–1235

St Louis ME, Porter JD, Helal A, Drame K, Hargrett-Bean N, Wells JG, Tauxe RV (1990) Epidemic cholera in West Africa: the role of food handling and high-risk foods. Am J Epidemiol 131(4):719–728

Stine OC, Alam M, Tang L, Nair GB, Siddique AK, Faruque SM, Huq A, Colwell R, Sack RB, Morris JG Jr (2008) Seasonal cholera from multiple small outbreaks, rural Bangladesh. Emerg Infect Dis 14(5):831–833

Suntharasamai P, Migasena S, Vongsthongsri U, Supanaranond W, Pitisuttitham P, Supeeranan L, Chantra A, Naksrisook S (1992) Clinical and bacteriological studies of El Tor cholera after ingestion of known inocula in Thai volunteers. Vaccine 10(8):502–505

Tamayo JF, Mosley WH, Alvero MG, Joseph PR, Gomez CZ, Montague T, Dizon JJ, Henderson DA (1965) Studies of cholera El Tor in the Philippines. Transmission of infection among household contacts of cholera patients. Bull World Health Organ 33(5):645–649

Tien JH, Earn DJD (2010) Multiple transmission pathways and disease dynamics in a waterborne pathogen model. Bull Math Biol 72(6):1506–1533. doi:10.1007/s11538-010-9507-6

Tuite AR, Tien J, Eisenberg M, Earn DJD, Ma J, Fisman DN (2011) Cholera epidemic in Haiti, 2010: using a transmission model to explain spatial spread of disease and identify optimal control interventions. Ann Intern Med 154(9):593–601. doi:10.1059/0003-4819-154-9-201105030-00334

Waldor MK, Hotez PJ, Clemens JD (2010) A national cholera vaccine stockpile—a new humanitarian and diplomatic resource. N Engl J Med 363(24):2279–2282. doi:10.1056/NEJMp1012300

Walton DA, Ivers LC (2011) Responding to cholera in post-earthquake Haiti. N Engl J Med 364(1):3–5. doi:10.1056/NEJMp1012997

Weil AA, Khan AI, Chowdhury F, Larocque RC, Faruque ASG, Ryan ET, Calderwood SB, Qadri F, Harris JB (2009) Clinical outcomes in household contacts of patients with cholera in Bangladesh. Clin Infect Dis 49(10):1473–1479. doi:10.1086/644779

World Health Organization (2010) Cholera vaccines: WHO position paper. Wkly Epidemiol Rec 85(13):117–128

World Health Organization (2012) Meeting report of the WHO Technical Working Group on creation of an oral cholera vaccine stockpile. World Health Organization, Geneva

Genomic Science in Understanding Cholera Outbreaks and Evolution of *Vibrio cholerae* as a Human Pathogen

William P. Robins and John J. Mekalanos

Abstract Modern genomic and bioinformatic approaches have been applied to interrogate the *V. cholerae* genome, the role of genomic elements in cholera disease, and the origin, relatedness, and dissemination of epidemic strains. A universal attribute of choleragenic strains includes a repertoire of pathogenicity islands and virulence genes, namely the CTXϕ prophage and Toxin Co-regulated Pilus (TCP) in addition to other virulent genetic elements including those referred to as Seventh Pandemic Islands. During the last decade, the advent of Next Generation Sequencing (NGS) has provided highly resolved and often complete genomic sequences of epidemic isolates in addition to both clinical and environmental strains isolated from geographically unconnected regions. Genomic comparisons of these strains, as was completed during and following the Haitian outbreak in 2010, reveals that most epidemic strains appear closely related, regardless of region of origin. Non-O1 clinical or environmental strains may also possess some virulence islands, but phylogenic analysis of the core genome suggests they are more diverse and distantly related than those isolated during epidemics. Like Haiti, genomic studies that examine both the *Vibrio* core and pan-genome in addition to Single Nucleotide Polymorphisms (SNPs) conclude that a number of epidemics are caused by strains that closely resemble those in Asia, and often appear to originate there and then spread globally. The accumulation of SNPs in the epidemic strains over time can then be applied to better understand the evolution of the *V. cholerae* genome as an etiological agent.

W. P. Robins (✉) · J. J. Mekalanos
Department of Microbiology and Immunobiology, Harvard Medical School,
Boston, MA 02115, USA
e-mail: William_Robins@hms.harvard.edu

Current Topics in Microbiology and Immunology (2014) 379: 211–229
DOI: 10.1007/82_2014_366

Published Online: 5 March 2014

Contents

1 Introduction

Even with modern established treatments and preventative measures, *V. cholerae* continues to emerge as a dangerous pathogen. This is especially true in Southeast Asia where the yearly appearance of cholera cases follow predicted patterns or "seasons" (Russell 1925; Pascual et al. 2002). However, cholera epidemics have an unpredictable history of manifesting on a much larger scale and the accounts of global pandemics are well-defined and documented during the last two centuries. The seven recognized cholera pandemics can be traced from Asia and the Indo-Pacific region; the current 7th pandemic manifesting as two waves, one between 1961 and 1966 and the other spreading to much of the world after 1970 (Karaolis et al. 1994). Most pandemic strains possess the lipopolysaccharide antigen groups O1 and to a lesser extent O139. Apart from the antigen, O1/O139 strains are highly conserved at the nucleotide level and possess a number of common-related genetic islands (GIs). The assemblage of GIs and subtle variance at the nucleotide level provides a useful scaffold for determining the genetic relatedness of both epidemic and environmental strains. A key theme in the study of cholera disease is how environmental factors and host-pathogen interactions influence genetic variability in *V. cholerae* genes and GIs and as well as their relatedness to virulence. The current repertoire of genomic tools has begun to answer these questions.

2 Conventional Genomics and Established Virulence Islands

The completion of the El Tor N16961 strain genome sequence in the year 2000 confirmed and identified the positions of the recognized 7th pandemic virulence islands (Heidelberg et al. 2000). Whereas established methods such as ribotyping (Wachsmuth et al. 1993), pulsed field gel electrophoresis (Weber et al. 1994), and multilocus enzyme analysis/sequence typing (Byun et al. 1999; Li et al. 2003; Lam et al. 2012) examined genomic complexity of isolated strains by probing the sequences of individual genes and regions or sizes of generated distinct fragments, the thoroughness of these examinations were limited by their design. Though useful, this level of resolution was still inadequate; for example, it was only recently during the late 1990s when it was discovered that most if not all *Vibrio* species possessed two chromosomes (Trucksis et al. 1998; Yamaichi et al. 1999). In whole, the deciphered genomic sequence of this 7th pandemic strain has paved the way for tools such as microarray analysis (Dziejman et al. 2002) and parallel whole genome sequencing (Grim et al. 2010; Mutreja et al. 2011) to better understand genomic complexity of *V. cholerae* and gene expression at nucleotide resolution (Mandlik et al. 2011). Most recently, the de novo assembly of the closed and complete sequences of both chromosomes I and II by coupling different modern sequencing platforms such as Illumina, Sanger 454, and Pacific Biosciences exemplifies how technology has pushed *Vibrio* genomics past the limits of the basic molecular typing methods (Bashir et al. 2012).

The sequence and assemblage of both virulence-associated GIs and housekeeping genes now provides a highly resolved template that has proved useful for further interrogation. In the approximate 4 Mb of genomic DNA present in the large chromosome I ($\sim$3 Mb) and small chromosome II ($\sim$1 Mb), many of the core genes ($\sim$1,500) are well-conserved in both O1 and non-O1 serotypes (Vesth et al. 2010). However, among these core genes are interspersed GIs and phage-related sequences. Some of these are demonstrated to contribute to pathogenicity. Of the GIs found in various *V. cholerae* serotypes, we know of a handful that exhibit high conservation in more virulent isolates. Some GIs such as toxin co-regulated pilus (TCP) island and the integrated phage CTXϕ together regulate and encode expression of cholera toxin, the protein toxin that causes the most of the cholera diarrheal syndrome.

Using the genome reconstruction of the recent Haitian outbreak strain (H1, 2010) as a reference and comparator, and then mapping the nucleotide and protein identity from a diverse panel of *Vibrio* strains, the GIs specific to 7th pandemic strains are apparent when aligned and illustrated as a Blast Atlas (Fig. 1) (Vesth et al. 2013). Apart from these GIs, the a bulk of the DNA sequence from 7th pandemic El Tor O1 isolates is nearly identical, thus making these islands useful for identification of virulent strains and genomic analysis. These genetic elements include *Vibrio* 7th Pandemic island I and II (VSPI and VSPII), TCP, *Vibrio* pathogenicity island II (VPI-II), CTXϕ and the Toxin linked cryptic (TLC) (Dziejman et al. 2002; Faruque and Mekalanos 2003; Chun et al. 2009). Another mobile element, SXT, was first identified in O139 clinical isolates during the 1990s. SXT is a self-transmissible integrating conjugative element that encodes antibiotic resistance and is now found to be present in almost all O1 clinical isolates post early 1990s (Waldor et al. 1996). In all *Vibrio* species, a large and hyper variable segment of chromosome II called the superintegron (SI) encodes more than 200 open reading frames that exist as individual mobile gene cassettes (MGC). The conservation of the collective GIs in sequenced clinical isolates has facilitated the use of genomic analysis to better elucidate their requisite role in virulence and pathogenesis.

Core and Pan-Genome Collections of genome sequences are used to extrapolate the conserved minimal core and expanded pan genome/pan proteome within

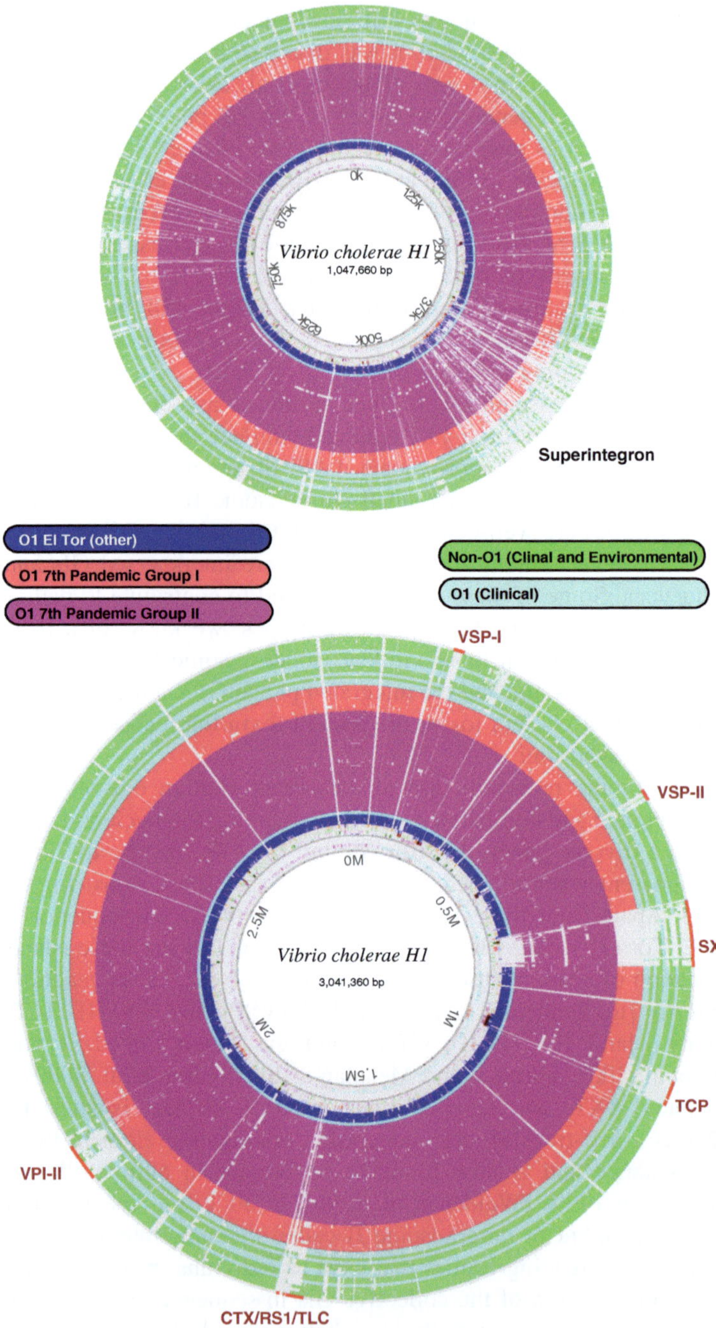

Fig. 1 Genome blast atlas created with CMG Biotools (Vesth et al. 2013) showing the aligned genomes of a panel of *V. cholerae* clinical and environmental isolates using the 2010 Haiti epidemic strain as reference. Genomes are colored by both biotype and source and also match genomes analyzed in the Fig. 2. Seventh pandemic islands and Superintegron are labeled on both chromosomes

bacterial phylogenies. The core genome is demonstrated to be one the optimum datasets for determining phylogenic relationships (Rokas et al. 2003) and is appreciably more practical in determining phylogenetic reconstruction than using 16S/23S rRNA or a handful of essential housekeeping genes, especially when applied to examine closely related taxa. An initial comparative study of 23 diverse *V. cholerae* strains found 2,432 common core genes or orthologues and 6,953 total unique genes in the pan genome (Chun et al. 2009). This core genome assemblage from both O1 and non-O1 strains integrated essential and nonessential genes and excluded the major virulence islands. This report proposed 7th pandemic strains were one of 12 lineages in this group that share a very similar backbone and hence probably all originated from a common ancestor. One major difference between the predicted lineages in this study were GIs outside the core genome and it was proposed that a driving force in diversity of *V. cholerae* can be attributed to horizontal gene transfer of GIs. In similar work, Vesth et al. examined the core and extended pan genomes of 32 *Vibrio* isolates represented by 12 species (Vesth et al. 2010). Of the 18 represented *V. cholerae* representatives, core genes comprised nearly half the genome and the pan-genome spanned a total of 6,500 genes. The divergence within *V. cholerae* species was minor when compared to that for a broad representation of the *Vibrio* genus; the core genome decreased to only 1,000 families while the pan-genome expanded to ~20,000. When these aligned core genes were used to calculate phylogeny, *V. cholerae* strains were identified again as closely related, however, environmental or clinical *V. cholerae* strains diverged. Placement within the tree was generally correlated with virulence for the O1 strains; however the presence of these GIs did not absolutely dictate phylogeny. For example, M66-2 is a clinical isolate from 1937 Indonesia that clusters with toxigenic *V. cholerae,* but it that lacks the CTXϕ prophage, and thus may represent a direct ancestor to current pandemic/epidemic *V. cholerae* (Feng et al. 2008). This work also concluded that the clinical non-O1 strain 2740-80 appeared to be an intermediate between the clinical, toxigenic isolates, and those found generally in the environment. These features in the genomes of 2740-80 and M66-2 are relevant to the field because understanding the relationship between the core-genome variation and the influence of acquired GIs on pathogenicity is an important aim of *V. cholerae* genomics. Because these bacteria can occupy multiple niches in both the estuarine biosphere and the human gut, the fitness for certain genes or GIs may vary in these environments and concomitantly be influenced by the genetic backbone. Thus, some strains may be better adapted for the only the aquatic environment and others also more fit for survival in the human gut. Surveys of environmental strains show that only a small percentage possess the phage that encodes cholera toxin and that a minority have the GI repertoire typically found in pandemic strains (Mukhopadhyay et al. 2001; Faruque et al. 2004; Rahman et al. 2008). It is also impossible to determine if these environmental strains simply represent contamination from cholera victims or free-living aquatic isolates (see below).

Distinct subgroups within the 7th pandemic El Tor clinical strains are identified. For example, during the last couple of decades, closely related O1 El Tor subgroups responsible for periodic epidemics appeared to originate in Southeast Asia and then to emanate as waves (Mutreja et al. 2011). Within the panel of clinical O1 genomes surveyed in this work nearly all genes are identical and the total number unique Single Nucleotide Polymorphisms (SNPs) between individual strains is enough to identify subtle sublineages. To illustrate phylogeny of 7th pandemic sublineages, using ~1,100,000 nucleotides that encode a set of the unique non-redundant core genome (881 genes) in a panel of 56 strains from a number of independent studies and sources (Fig. 2b), it can be shown that the relatedness of 7th pandemic strains often correlate well with both date of isolation and geographical incidence and these construed phylogenies are similar to other independent and previous analyses. The strains isolated during the Peru epidemic of the early 1990s most closely resemble other strains isolated in Latin America during the 1990s. Separate from phylogeny based entirely on core genome analysis, this relationship is also evident in the genetic islands as unique deletions in VSP-II and by the presence of a prophage (Nusrin et al. 2009; de Sa Morais et al. 2012). Likewise, both MAK757 and M66-2 (1937, Indonesia) strains appear related and together diverge from current, more contemporary isolates. The entire group of O1 strains derived from Southern Asia (Pakistan, India, Nepal, and Thailand) in the period 2000–2011 clusters with the Haitian outbreak of 2010. Accordingly, the CDC and a number of independent investigators have concluded that the importation of *V. cholerae* into Haiti from Nepal or Southeast Asia is probable. Coincidently, a number of strains in this presented phylogenetic dataset (India 2005, Pakistan 2009, India 2010) include those isolated from stool samples in the USA from infected persons traveling abroad, thus directly demonstrating the opportunity for global dissemination of pathogenic strains. There are some exceptions; an Australian strain isolated in 1986 appears closely related to a 1910 Saudi Arabian sample. It is important to also keep in mind that single strain epidemiological oddities such as this example might find more parsimonious explanations by hypothesizing laboratory cross contamination rather than a complicated theory involving global transmission of a comparably "old" strain via either environmental or human sources. Clearly, the increased resolution of these predicted phylogenies will extend our understanding of the epidemiology. However, it is important to maintain perspective and note the similarity within pandemic O1 genomes as a group in contrast to others (Fig. 2a) when the phylogeny is extended to include a broad representation of non-O1 *V. cholerae* genomes. Thus, the occasional phylogenic mapping of a putative clinical or environmental isolate of an O1 isolate in a otherwise diverged group of non-O1 strains, can be discounted as significant if the O1 isolate lacks most or all of the essential virulence genes present on typical genetic islands. Clearly, most O1 and O139 strains that cause clinical cholera and more specifically cholera epidemics are highly related from the genomic perspective and carry highly similar collection of virulence genes encoded by accessory genetic elements (Faruque and Mekalanos 2003).

TCP and CTXϕ Variation in O1 strains In contrast to whole genome analysis, the targeted surveillance of mobile virulence islands can be applied to interrogate their role in pathogenesis. TCP (also called VPI) and CTXϕ are two virulent GIs most closely connected to cholera disease. Though acquired as separate entities,

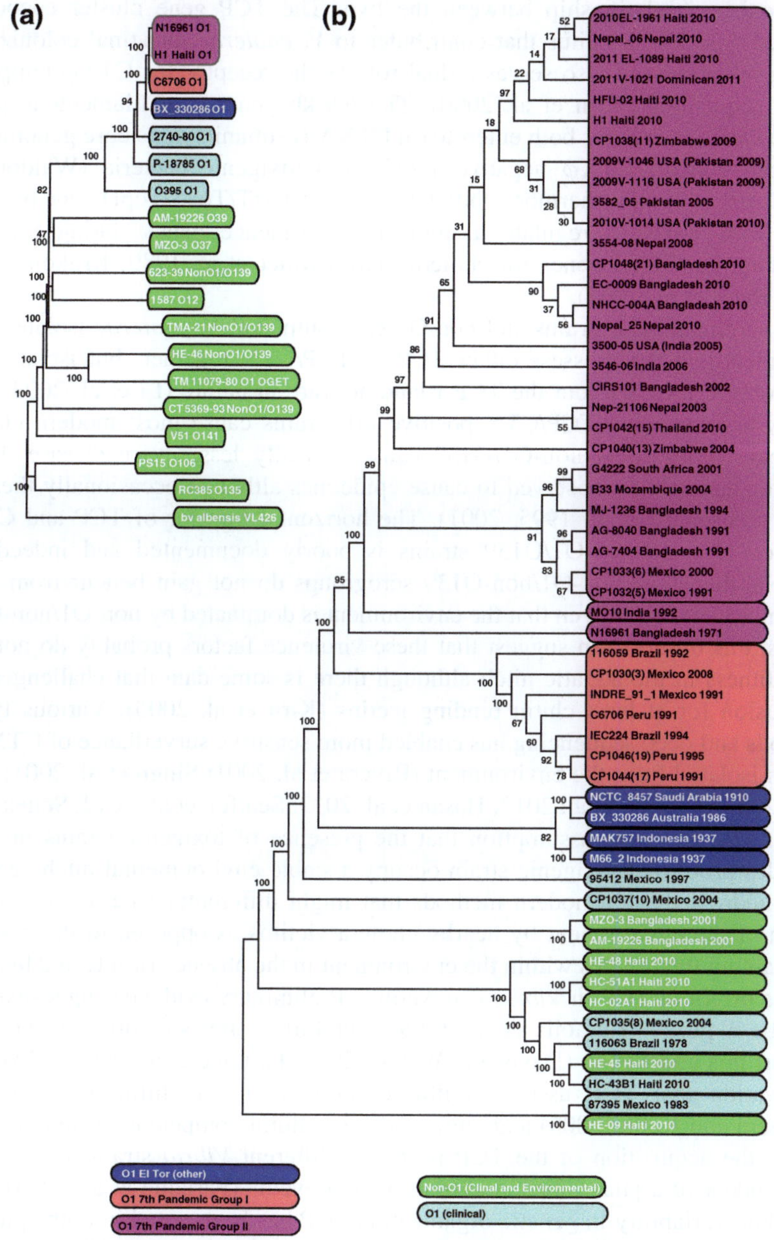

Fig. 2 The bootstrap consensus tree (Neighbor-Joining) inferred from 500 replicates for a small diverse sample of O1 and non-O1 strains (**a**) and for a collection of clinical and environmental strains (**b**). Core genomes were extrapolated using CMG-biotools 2.2, aligned using MAAFT (vs 7.127), and trees were calculated and produced using MEGA (vs 5.10). Genomes are colored by biotype and source. CMG Biotools (vs 2.2, Vesth et al. 2013), MAAFT (vs 7.127, Katoh and Standely 2013) MEGA (vs 5.10, Hall 2013)

there exists a relationship between the two. The TCP gene cluster encodes a bundled type IV-like pilus that contributes to *V. cholerae* intestinal colonization during infection and also serves a dual role as the receptor for CTXϕ temperate phage acquisition (Kirn et al. 2000). The 6.9 kb genome of filamentous phage CTXϕ carries genes for both enterotoxin CTXA/B subunits in its core genome and thus can convert CTXϕ negative *Vibrio* into toxigenic bacteria (Waldor and Mekalanos 1996). Furthermore, the TCP-encoded ToxT/ToxS/TcpH gene products work with ToxR to regulate a number of virulence genes during infection including the CTXϕ genes for cholera toxin (Miller et al. 1989; Krukonis et al. 2000; Beck et al. 2004).

Some clinical O1 strains and non-O1 environmental *V. cholerae* isolates have been identified that possess either TCP or TCP/CTX together, but isolates that carry only CTXϕ without the TCP island are rare in nature (Li et al. 2003). It is widely accepted that TCP/CTX positive O1 strains cause most modern cholera outbreaks while most non-O1/O139 cause typically less severe disease that is sporadic and seldom observed to cause epidemics although occasionally these do occur (Dalsgaard et al. 1995, 2001). The horizontal transfer of TCP and CTXϕ between O1 and non-O1/O139 strains is poorly documented and indeed this suggests that most non-O1/non-O139 serogroups do not gain benefit from these virulence elements. Given that the environment is dominated by non-O1/non-O139 strains, this observation suggest that these virulence factors probably do not promote fitness in the aquatic nitch although there is some data that challenges this conclusion for at least chitin binding lectins (Kirn et al. 2005). Various typing methods and deep sequencing has enabled more sensitive surveillance of CTXϕ in strains isolated from the environment (Rivera et al. 2001; Singh et al. 2001; Pang et al. 2007; Awasthi et al. 2012; Hasan et al. 2012; Sealfon et al. 2012; Sellek et al. 2012). The prevalent assumption that the presence of toxigenic strains in water provides proof that toxigenic strain occupy a stable environmental nitch needs to be re-addressed with modern methods that might differentiate between contamination of the environment by nearby cholera victims as opposed to these strains maintaining themselves within the environment in the absence of infected humans.

The origin of TCP in *Vibrio* is unknown. Preliminary evidence suggested TCP may be a phage (Karaolis et al. 1999), but further investigation has failed to support this conclusion (Davis and Waldor 2003; Faruque et al. 2003). Given the observation that TCP assists biofilm differentiation on chitinaceous surfaces (Reguera and Kolter 2005) and chitin induces natural competence (Meibom et al. 2005), the acquisition of the TCP island by different *Vibrio* strains could occur independent of a phage-mediated transduction events (Faruque et al. 2003).

Subtle variability in genetic organization TCP has been noted in both epidemic and nonepidemic strains (Ghosh et al. 1997; Novais et al. 1999; Mukhopadhyay et al. 2001). The ~41 kb TCP island carries a putative integrase and transposase and is integrated at the tmRNA (*ssrA)* gene in chromosome I. The region is especially A/T rich when compared to that measured in *Vibrio* species and varies among *V. cholerae* strains. Most of the highly conserved region of the TCP island encodes genes required for the biosynthesis of a type IV pilus structure and a minority of the element regulates transcription of genes both inside and outside of the TCP element. A majority of divergent sequences in TCP are either noncoding or are identified as deletions and inserted elements/transposases (Hase and Mekalanos 1998; Yu and DiRita 1999; Mukhopadhyay et al. 2001).

The TCP pilin genes share some amino acid homology and the pilin protein structure shows a novel TCP-fold with other pilin proteins found in *Nisseria, Psuedomonas,* and *Enterobacter* (Craig et al. 2003; Li et al. 2012). The major pilin (*tcpA*) gene shows more diversity in than most others in the island as there is more variance between O1 and non-O1/O139 strains (Iredell and Manning 1994; Rhine and Taylor 1994). Polymorphisms in the carboxyl terminal region of TcpA protein are predicted to be in surface-exposed TCP fibers (Boyd and Waldor 2002). Antibodies against TcpA have been found in sera of people living in cholera-endemic areas and suggesting immune response may play a role in selective pressure and may in part explain these polymorphisms (Herrington et al. 1988; Hang et al. 2003). Moreover, single mutants in TcpA are measured to affect colonization, autoagglutination, and serum-resistance suggesting TCP confers immunoprotection from complement-like activity in the intestine (Chiang et al. 1995).

The chromosomal integration structure of the CTXϕ temperate phage genome differs between classical and El Tor 7th pandemic strains and there are some identified amino acid changes at positions within key genes (Fig. 3). Integrated CTXϕ is found in the either of the chromosomes as a single copy or as a tandem array (Mekalanos 1983). In El Tor strains, CTXϕ, the adjacent RS1/RS2 regions, and TLC island are shown to be pivotal in the stable acquisition of CTXϕ and maintaining the *dif* site, a sequence important for chromosomal dimer resolution in chromosome I (Rubin et al. 1998; Hassan et al. 2010). Classical strain O395 harbors the CTXϕ on both chromosomes I and II and lacks the adjacent RS1 cassette found in El Tor strain and instead has RS2 (Waldor et al. 1997; Davis et al. 2002). RS2 and RS1 are two very similar genetic regions that encode phage replication, regulation and integration genes for the CTXϕ prophage, however RS1 possesses an additional anti-repressor gene *rstC*. Expression of *rstC* anti-repressor may be important as it is shown to relieve RtsR repression of CTX genes. Presence of *rstC* has been shown to increase CTXϕ production as much as several thousandfold and also increases the production of *rstA* transcripts, some of which certainly extend through and include *ctxAB* (Davis et al. 2002). Furthermore, the variation between the RtsR repressor in El Tor and Classical strains is sufficient to confer biotype specificity (Kimsey and Waldor 1998). The other identified class of CTXϕ variation in lies within the *ctxB* gene. These are recognized nonsynonymous variants found in either classical and El tor (and variant) strains and have been utilized as benchmarks in genomic comparisons.

First noted in Calcutta 1990 strains and Bangladesh in 2001, a growing number of 7th pandemic El Tor strains harbor atypical CTX regions (Nair et al. 2002; Raychoudhuri et al. 2009). El Tor variants have become the predominant biotype isolated in Asia, Africa, and more recently Haiti (Nair et al. 2002, 2006; Ansaruzzaman et al. 2004; Safa et al. 2006). Instead of the consensus El-Tor CTXϕ RS1 sequence, these variants carry a *ctxB* gene that possesses one or several

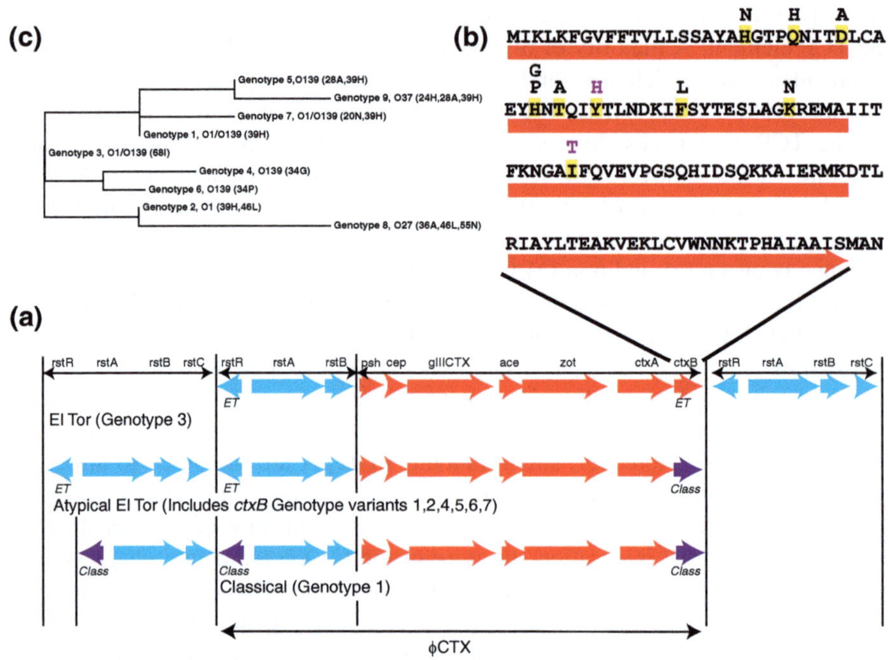

Fig. 3 Different arrangement of CTX/RS1 region in El Tor, classical and variant strains (**a**). The amino acid variation in *ctxB* gene (**b**) is used to generate phylogenic tree based on the alignment of *ctxB* variants (**c**)

nonsynonymous variants in addition to a varying number of heptad consensus repeats in the consensus upstream ToxT binding site while often maintaining the El Tor RS1 region. The variants also possess specific amino acid residues in the *ctxB* gene that are also found in classical strains. Moreover, as in classical strains, at least one of these strains possesses a second copy of CTXϕ in chromosome II. Preliminary functional and biochemical study of variants suggests they are located on exposed CtxB protein–protein interfaces within multimer CtxB pore and, therefore, could influence CtxB or CtxA binding dynamics (Shamini et al. 2011). The measured amount of cholera toxin produced by a panel of these is shown to be significantly increased when compared to classical and other El Tor strains (Ghosh-Banerjee et al. 2010; Son et al. 2011). However, the measured increase in toxin production and a concomitant hypervirulence by variants in the infant mouse model in this work were also attributed to increased levels of ToxT and TcpA.

Superintegron Integrons are natural cloning systems that consist of open reading frames that use flanking sites and site-specific recombinases/integrases to entrap and acquire gene cassettes and promoters into a larger array of genes. The super-integron is a novel integron class first discovered in *V. cholerae* and is represented in current epidemic strains as a large assemblage of these integrated genes (more than 200) that spans more than 100 kb of chromosome II (Mazel et al. 1998). Many of these ORFs code genes that have unknown function and are largely nonessential for *V. cholerae* growth or pathogenesis. They are an interesting reservoir for horizontally exchanged, yet unrelated genes and their significance is not well-understood.

The evidence for essential or important genes in the SI in *V. cholerae* is generally lacking. Microarray and RNA-seq studies measure little to almost no expression across the entire region while growing in liquid media or during infection (Larocque et al. 2005; Mandlik et al. 2011). The only measurement for upregulation of these genes is during cell growth at high density or while undergoing stress (Yildiz et al. 2004). A handful of genes do encode putative virulence factors including the mannose-fucose-resistant hemagglutinin (*mrhA*), heat-stable toxin (*sto*), and a lipoprotein gene (Ogawa and Takeda 1993; Barker and Manning 1997; MacDonald et al. 2006). However, because of its dynamic nature and variation, the SI has been most useful for genomic analysis and a fingerprint for strain comparisons. Even closely related strains are sometimes found to possess minor variability. Gene cassettes can be duplicated and present as multiple copies in separate locations, probably produced by duplication and not horizontal transfer (Rowe-Magnus et al. 2003; Feng et al. 2008).

The presence of highly conserved flanking repeat sequences in SI has proved useful for amplification-based genomic analyses. The amplification of unique genes using primers that anneal to the flanked 59 bp repeat region has been used as a molecular fingerprint to identify and profile collections of *V. cholerae* strains (Labbate et al. 2007). The examined dynamic array of MGCs for 60 strains isolated between 1961 and 2008 found more diversity in those prior to 1980s and a predominant SI structure found in most current strains since the 1990s (Gao et al. 2011).

3 Application of Genomics

Regardless of serotype or strain, the treatment of cholera disease is the same—oral and intravenous rehydration with concurrent replacement of electrolytes. Antibiotic therapy is recommended for severely ill patients but is not a first-line treatment. Though the most thorough current genomic analyses may fail to provide information relevant to the primary treatment of cholera, a case can be made for genomic surveillance in order to advance and adapt preventative measures for a number of reasons. First, the genomic content and SNPs can be compared to available sequence databases of environmental and global epidemic strains to better elucidate and determine the origin and dissemination. It is conceivable that the genome may someday be used in order to accurately predict magnitude of virulence. Second, the genomic analysis of emerging strains may be useful when evaluating the efficacy of vaccines and in their design. For example, O1 vaccine strains and strategies utilize expression and secretion of the nontoxic CtxB subunit to enhance efficacy (Thungapathra et al. 1999; Jani et al. 2002; Liang et al. 2003; Qadri et al. 2007; Yan et al. 2007). There is an emergence of the strains that encode classical-El Tor CTX islands with unique variants in the *ctxB* gene. The role of these amino acid residues during infection is unclear; incorporating this allele into vaccine strains may be useful.

New genomic tools and methods were applied to rapidly identify genomic features of the strain during the recent Haitian outbreak in 2010 (Chin et al. 2011). This represented the first cholera epidemic to be rapidly analyzed with a number of next generation sequencing platforms, even while some of these technologies were still in development. The emergence of this strain in Hispaniola, an island that had not experienced cholera in nearly 100 years posed several fundamental questions about the epidemiology and spread of *V. cholerae* that may in part be addressed with interrogation of the genomic content. It is obvious that the lack of sanitation and damaged infrastructure following the 2010 Haiti earthquake certainly exacerbated the spread of the cholera cases, but the understanding of the mode of emergence and transmission became an important aim.

One speculation was that the Haitian strain may have re-emerged from a reservoir in Latin America. Following the Peru pandemic that spread into Latin America in the 1990s, modern cholera epidemics in the Western Hemisphere have been generally sporadic but appear to be related. After the Peru pandemic, similar strains were found from Mexico to Brazil in years following and appeared to be monophyletic (Wachsmuth et al. 1993; Lam et al. 2010; Chin et al. 2011; Mutreja et al. 2011; de Sa Morais et al. 2012; Garza et al. 2012). The Latin American epidemic strains sequenced during this period possessed a unique 40 kb prophage inserted in within the alanine aminopeptidase gene (de Sa Morais et al. 2012). As a group these strains were found to be most closely resemble a strain from Angola in 1989 and other independent phylogenetic analyses also hypothesized a common African origin which is possibly linked to immigration to Lima during the corresponding period before the 1991 epidemic (Mutreja et al. 2011).

The rapid sequencing and analysis of the Haitian strain in 2010 and all subsequent work provided almost irrefutable evidence for human transmission of a clonal strain of recent Asian origin (Ali et al. 2011; Chin et al. 2011; Hendriksen et al. 2011; Reimer et al. 2011; Sjolund-Karlsson et al. 2011; Talkington et al. 2011; Frerichs et al. 2012). The Haitian strain was distinctly atypical from Latin American strains isolated during and following the Peru 1991 epidemic and possessed a hybrid Classical/El Tor CTX and ICEVchInd5 type SXT, not yet detected in the Western hemisphere and more typical of those strains isolated in Southeast Asia (Chin et al. 2011). Furthermore, an identified unique deletion in within VPS-II and an assemblage of genes found in the SI most closely matched strains previously characterized in Asia during the previous 8 years. Phylogenic clustering of a panel of El Tor isolates placed more distance between Haiti and both the Peru C6706 strain and the 1971 reference strain N16961 and highest similarity to two strains isolated in Bangladesh; a 2008 strain (M4), co-sequenced with the Haitian isolate, and CIRS101 isolated in 2002. Moreover, the first Haitian cases were noted in the isolated upper Artinobite river valley proximal to a UN camp occupied by troops from Nepal where cholera cases had been documented during the preceding months. This accidental importation and dissemination is supported by the published conclusion of several independent investigators and a UN special panel (UN 2011). Virtual definitive proof that the Haiti epidemic had an origin in Nepal came from the application of genomic analysis to isolates from obtained from Katmandu patients only weeks before the Haiti epidemic as described below.

In one of the most comprehensive and conclusive genomic analyses, the genomes of 24 Nepalese genomes were compared to ten previously sequenced genomes including three from the recent Haitian outbreak (Hendriksen et al. 2011). Using whole-genome sequence typing and phylogenetic analysis, a cluster of strains was found to be most closely related to the Haitian strains. Remarkably, two Nepal strains varied from the Hatian strains by only one or two base pair variations. Additional characterization of 77 Nepalese strains collected from ten different hospital laboratories from 2007 to 2010 clustered strains into four different groups using MLVA and *ctxB* gene typing (Shakya et al. 2012). Many of the MLVA patterns in this work matched clinical strains identified in adjacent Southeastern Asian countries and the 2008–2010 strains possessed the same CTX 3b-type toxin. A common theme in this work and other genetic studies is that regional outbreaks appear to be clonal or closely related and also resemble clinical strains isolated and identified in neighboring regions, suggesting regional dissemination. As demonstrated, it should be possible to develop phylogenies that encompass strains isolated from more regions that span multiple seasons or years to better follow evolution and dissemination of epidemic strains.

Current technology has enabled a more robust, deeper surveillance of variation in the pathogenic genome. The analytic value of these data includes understanding its rate of evolution. Recent work shows that we must be mindful in how we apply or interpret significance of measured genetic variation. Using sequence variants between an Indonesian prepandemic 1937 El Tor strain and also classical 6th and modern 7th pandemic strains Feng and colleagues attempted to calculate a "molecular clock" (Feng et al. 2008). The aim was to document changes that had occurred during the divergence of the three clones and estimate the rate of mutation. Though this dataset was limited to the Classical 6th pandemic strain O395 and two El Tor strains from 1937 to 1971, the results suggested mutation rates that were $\sim$100 times higher than had been previously assumed. In other independent work, Mutreja et al. concluded that recent epidemic strains isolated during three waves of global transmission in the last 50 years have accumulated about 2.3–3.5 SNPs/year in the core genome. The selective factors that influence this molecular or evolutionary clock include but are not limited to interactions within the host and environmental factors such as bacteriophage. Both clinical data and mathematical studies support a model where lytic phages may be important in ending outbreaks (Faruque et al. 2005a, b; Jensen et al. 2006). Recent work has evaluated genomic characterization of phages year-to-year in cholera prone areas using coupled-genomic approaches (Seed et al. 2011) and host-pathogen interactions using microarray and RNA-seq (Larocque et al. 2005; Mandlik et al. 2011).

4 Conclusions

Genomic science has greatly improved our understanding of pathogenic clones of *V. cholerae* and their relationship to relatively nonpathogenic environmental strains of this bacterial species. Clearly, gene content (largely driven by phage and GI acquisition, and superintegron and ICE element variation) defines a pathogenic O1 and O139 7th pandemic El Tor lineage of this organism that is separated distinctly from the most common ancestor of nontoxigenic non-O1/non-O139 strains present in environmental waters throughout the world (Boyd and Waldor 2002; Li et al. 2003; Pang et al. 2007; Rahman et al. 2008; Vesth et al. 2010). The suggestion that climate factors drive emergence of new pathogenic strains and genetic exchange between these distinctly different groups of *V. cholerae* (Hasan et al. 2012) is an interesting but largely speculative idea that simply has no strong support at the genome sequence level (Mekalanos et al. 2012; Katz et al. 2013) or epidemiological level (Gaudart et al. 2013a, b). Indeed, human activity (travel and poor sanitation) seems the most probable source of typical pathogenic clones globally over the last century and particularly over the three decades during which cholera has established itself as a threat to Africa, Latin America, and the Caribbean. These pathogenic clones certainly have and will undergo further evolution as they have in the case of the variant strains that now dominate cholera endemic and epidemic locales throughout the world. However, applying available genomic tools to other components in the aquatic environment (e.g. phage and microbiome) may someday define whether the key virulence genes of pathogenic *V. cholerae*, have an origin in a non-O1 *V. cholerae* (Haley et al. 2013) or even non-*Vibrio* bacterial species which may or not be pathogens of humans. Understanding the additional biological niches that *V. cholerae* virulence genes occupy will help define a better model for emergence of pathogenic clones of *V. cholerae*.

References

Ali A, Chen Y, Johnson JA, Redden E, Mayette Y, Rashid MH et al (2011) Recent clonal origin of cholera in Haiti. Emerg Infect Dis 17:699–701

Ansaruzzaman M, Bhuiyan NA, Nair BG, Sack DA, Lucas M, Deen JL et al (2004) Cholera in Mozambique, variant of *Vibrio cholerae*. Emerg Infect Dis 10:2057–2059

Awasthi SP, Asakura M, Chowdhury N, Neogi SB, Hinenoya A, Golbar HM et al (2012) Novel cholix toxin variants, an ADP-ribosylating toxin in *Vibrio cholerae* non-O1/non-O139 strains and their pathogenicity. Infect Immun 81(2):531–541

Barker A, Manning PA (1997) VlpA of *Vibrio cholerae* O1: the first bacterial member of the alpha 2-microglobulin lipocalin superfamily. Microbiology 143(Pt 6):1805–1813

Bashir A, Klammer AA, Robins WP, Chin CS, Webster D, Paxinos E et al (2012) A hybrid approach for the automated finishing of bacterial genomes. Nat Biotechnol 30(7):701–707

Beck NA, Krukonis ES, DiRita VJ (2004) TcpH influences virulence gene expression in *Vibrio cholerae* by inhibiting degradation of the transcription activator TcpP. J Bacteriol 186:8309–8316

Boyd EF, Waldor MK (2002) Evolutionary and functional analyses of variants of the toxin-coregulated pilus protein TcpA from toxigenic *Vibrio cholerae* non-O1/non-O139 serogroup isolates. Microbiology 148:1655–1666

Byun R, Elbourne LD, Lan R, Reeves PR (1999) Evolutionary relationships of pathogenic clones of *Vibrio cholerae* by sequence analysis of four housekeeping genes. Infect Immun 67:1116–1124

Chiang SL, Taylor RK, Koomey M, Mekalanos JJ (1995) Single amino acid substitutions in the N-terminus of *Vibrio cholerae* TcpA affect colonization, autoagglutination, and serum resistance. Mol Microbiol 17:1133–1142

Chin CS, Sorenson J, Harris JB, Robins WP, Charles RC, Jean-Charles RR et al (2011) The origin of the Haitian cholera outbreak strain. N Engl J Med 364:33–42

Chun J, Grim CJ, Hasan NA, Lee JH, Choi SY, Haley BJ et al (2009) Comparative genomics reveals mechanism for short-term and long-term clonal transitions in pandemic *Vibrio cholerae*. Proc Natl Acad Sci USA 106:15442–15447

Craig L, Taylor RK, Pique ME, Adair BD, Arvai AS, Singh M et al (2003) Type IV pilin structure and assembly: X-ray and EM analyses of *Vibrio cholerae* toxin-coregulated pilus and *Pseudomonas aeruginosa* PAK pilin. Mol Cell 11:1139–1150

Dalsgaard A, Albert MJ, Taylor DN, Shimada T, Meza R, Serichantalergs O, Echeverria P (1995) Characterization of *Vibrio cholerae* non-O1 serogroups obtained from an outbreak of diarrhea in Lima. Peru J Clin Microbiol 33:2715–2722

Dalsgaard A, Serichantalergs O, Forslund A, Lin W, Mekalanos J, Mintz E, Shimada T, Wells JG (2001) Clinical and environmental isolates of *Vibrio cholerae* serogroup O141 carry the CTX phage and the genes encoding the toxin-coregulated pili. J Clin Microbiol 39:4086–4092

Davis BM, Kimsey HH, Kane AV, Waldor MK (2002) A satellite phage-encoded antirepressor induces repressor aggregation and cholera toxin gene transfer. EMBO J 21:4240–4249

Davis BM, Waldor MK (2003) Filamentous phages linked to virulence of *Vibrio cholerae*. Curr Opin Microbiol 6:35–42

de Sa Morais LL, Garza DR, Loureiro EC, Nunes KN, Vellasco RS, da Silva CP et al (2012) Complete genome sequence of a sucrose-nonfermenting epidemic strain of *Vibrio cholerae* O1 from Brazil. J Bacteriol 194:2772

Dziejman M, Balon E, Boyd D, Fraser CM, Heidelberg JF, Mekalanos JJ (2002) Comparative genomic analysis of *Vibrio cholerae*: genes that correlate with cholera endemic and pandemic disease. Proc Natl Acad Sci USA 99:1556–1561

Faruque SM, Chowdhury N, Kamruzzaman M, Dziejman M, Rahman MH, Sack DA et al (2004) Genetic diversity and virulence potential of environmental *Vibrio cholerae* population in a cholera-endemic area. Proc Natl Acad Sci USA 101:2123–2128

Faruque SM, Islam MJ, Ahmad QS, Faruque AS, Sack DA, Nair GB et al (2005a) Self-limiting nature of seasonal cholera epidemics: role of host-mediated amplification of phage. Proc Natl Acad Sci USA 102:6119–6124

Faruque SM, Mekalanos JJ (2003) Pathogenicity islands and phages in *Vibrio cholerae* evolution. Trends Microbiol 11:505–510

Faruque SM, Zhu J, Asadulghani, Kamruzzaman M, Mekalanos JJ (2003) Examination of diverse toxin-coregulated pilus-positive *Vibrio cholerae* strains fails to demonstrate evidence for *Vibrio* pathogenicity island phage. Infect Immun 71:2993–2999

Faruque SM, Islam MJ, Ahmad QS, Faruque AS, Sack DA, Nair GB, Mekalanos JJ (2005b) Self-limiting nature of seasonal cholera epidemics: role of host-mediated amplification of phage. Proc Natl Acad Sci USA 102:6119–6124

Feng L, Reeves PR, Lan R, Ren Y, Gao C, Zhou Z et al (2008) A recalibrated molecular clock and independent origins for the cholera pandemic clones. PLoS ONE 3:e4053

Frerichs RR, Keim PS, Barrais R, Piarroux R (2012) Nepalese origin of cholera epidemic in Haiti. Clin Microbiol Infect 18:E158–E163

Gao Y, Pang B, Wang HY, Zhou HJ, Cui ZG, Kan B (2011) Structural variation of the superintegron in the toxigenic *Vibrio cholerae* O1 El Tor. Biomed Environ Sci 24:579–592

Garza DR, Thompson CC, Loureiro EC, Dutilh BE, Inada DT, Junior EC et al (2012) Genome-wide study of the defective sucrose fermenter strain of *Vibrio cholerae* from the Latin American cholera epidemic. PLoS ONE 7:e37283

Gaudart J, Moore S, Rebaudet S, Piarroux M, Barrais R, Boncy J et al (2013a) Environmental factors influencing epidemic cholera. Am J Trop Med Hyg 89:1228–1230

Gaudart J, Rebaudet S, Barrais R, Boncy J, Faucher B, Piarroux M et al (2013b) Spatio-temporal dynamics of cholera during the first year of the epidemic in Haiti. PLoS Negl Trop Dis 7:e2145

Ghosh-Banerjee J, Senoh M, Takahashi T, Hamabata T, Barman S, Koley H et al (2010) Cholera toxin production by the El Tor variant of *Vibrio cholerae* O1 compared to prototype El Tor and classical biotypes. J Clin Microbiol 48:4283–4286

Ghosh C, Nandy RK, Dasgupta SK, Nair GB, Hall RH, Ghose AC (1997) A search for cholera toxin (CT), toxin coregulated pilus (TCP), the regulatory element ToxR and other virulence factors in non-01/non-0139 *Vibrio cholerae*. Microb Pathog 22:199–208

Grim CJ, Hasan NA, Taviani E, Haley B, Chun J, Brettin TS et al (2010) Genome sequence of hybrid *Vibrio cholerae* O1 MJ-1236, B-33, and CIRS101 and comparative genomics with *V. cholerae*. J Bacteriol 192:3524–3533

Haley BJ, Choi SY, Hasan NA, Abdullah AS, Cebula TA, Huq A et al (2013) Genome sequences of clinical *Vibrio cholerae* isolates from an oyster-borne cholera outbreak in Florida. Genome Announc 1(6):e00966-13

Hall BG (2013) Building phylogenetic trees from molecular data with MEGA. Mol Biol Evol 30(5):1229–1235

Hang L, John M, Asaduzzaman M, Bridges EA, Vanderspurt C, Kirn TJ et al (2003) Use of in vivo-induced antigen technology (IVIAT) to identify genes uniquely expressed during human infection with *Vibrio cholerae*. Proc Natl Acad Sci USA 100:8508–8513

Hasan NA, Choi SY, Eppinger M, Clark PW, Chen A, Alam M et al (2012) Genomic diversity of 2010 Haitian cholera outbreak strains. Proc Natl Acad Sci USA 109:e2010–e2017

Hase CC, Mekalanos JJ (1998) TcpP protein is a positive regulator of virulence gene expression in *Vibrio cholerae*. Proc Natl Acad Sci USA 95:730–734

Hassan F, Kamruzzaman M, Mekalanos JJ, Faruque SM (2010) Satellite phage TLCphi enables toxigenic conversion by CTX phage through dif site alteration. Nature 467:982–985

Heidelberg JF, Eisen JA, Nelson WC, Clayton RA, Gwinn ML, Dodson RJ et al (2000) DNA sequence of both chromosomes of the cholera pathogen *Vibrio cholerae*. Nature 406:477–483

Hendriksen RS, Price LB, Schupp JM, Gillece JD, Kaas RS, Engelthaler DM et al (2011) Population genetics of *Vibrio cholerae* from Nepal in 2010: evidence on the origin of the Haitian outbreak. MBio 2:e00157-11

Herrington DA, Hall RH, Losonsky G, Mekalanos JJ, Taylor RK, Levine MM (1988) Toxin, toxin-coregulated pili, and the toxR regulon are essential for *Vibrio cholerae* pathogenesis in humans. J Exp Med 168:1487–1492

Iredell JR, Manning PA (1994) Biotype-specific tcpA genes in *Vibrio cholerae*. FEMS Microbiol Lett 121:47–54

Jani D, Meena LS, Rizwan-ul-Haq QM, Singh Y, Sharma AK, Tyagi AK (2002) Expression of cholera toxin B subunit in transgenic tomato plants. Transgenic Res 11:447–454

Jensen MA, Faruque SM, Mekalanos JJ, Levin BR (2006) Modeling the role of bacteriophage in the control of cholera outbreaks. Proc Natl Acad Sci USA 103:4652–4657

Karaolis DK, Lan R, Reeves PR (1994) Molecular evolution of the seventh-pandemic clone of *Vibrio cholerae* and its relationship to other pandemic and epidemic *V. cholerae* isolates. J Bacteriol 176:6199–6206

Karaolis DK, Somara S, Maneval DR Jr, Johnson JA, Kaper JB (1999) A bacteriophage encoding a pathogenicity island, a type-IV pilus and a phage receptor in cholera bacteria. Nature 399:375–379

Katoh K, Standley DM (2013) MAFFT multiple sequence alignment software version 7: improvements in performance and usability. Mol Biol Evol 30:772–780

Katz LS, Petkau A, Beaulaurier J, Tyler S, Antonova ES, Turnsek MA et al (2013) Evolutionary dynamics of *Vibrio cholerae* O1 following a single-source introduction to Haiti. MBio 4(4):e00398-13

Kimsey HH, Waldor MK (1998) CTXphi immunity: application in the development of cholera vaccines. Proc Natl Acad Sci USA 95:7035–7039

Kirn TJ, Jude BA, Taylor RK (2005) A colonization factor links *Vibrio cholerae* environmental survival and human infection. Nature 438:863–866

Kirn TJ, Lafferty MJ, Sandoe CM, Taylor RK (2000) Delineation of pilin domains required for bacterial association into microcolonies and intestinal colonization by *Vibrio cholerae*. Mol Microbiol 35:896–910

Krukonis ES, Yu RR, Dirita VJ (2000) The *Vibrio cholerae* ToxR/TcpP/ToxT virulence cascade: distinct roles for two membrane-localized transcriptional activators on a single promoter. Mol Microbiol 38:67–84

Labbate M, Boucher Y, Joss MJ, Michael CA, Gillings MR, Stokes HW (2007) Use of chromosomal integron arrays as a phylogenetic typing system for *Vibrio cholerae* pandemic strains. Microbiology 153:1488–1498

Lam C, Octavia S, Reeves P, Wang L, Lan R (2010) Evolution of seventh cholera pandemic and origin of 1991 epidemic, Latin America. Emerg Infect Dis 16:1130–1132

Lam C, Octavia S, Reeves PR, Lan R (2012) Multi-locus variable number tandem repeat analysis of 7th pandemic *Vibrio cholerae*. BMC Microbiol 12:82

Larocque RC, Harris JB, Dziejman M, Li X, Khan AI, Faruque AS et al (2005) Transcriptional profiling of *Vibrio cholerae* recovered directly from patient specimens during early and late stages of human infection. Infect Immun 73:4488–4493

Li J, Egelman EH, Craig L (2012) Structure of the *Vibrio cholerae* Type IVb Pilus and stability comparison with the Neisseria gonorrhoeae type IVa pilus. J Mol Biol 418:47–64

Li M, Kotetishvili M, Chen Y, Sozhamannan S (2003) Comparative genomic analyses of the vibrio pathogenicity island and cholera toxin prophage regions in nonepidemic serogroup strains of *Vibrio cholerae*. Appl Environ Microbiol 69:1728–1738

Liang W, Wang S, Yu F, Zhang L, Qi G, Liu Y et al (2003) Construction and evaluation of a safe, live, oral *Vibrio cholerae* vaccine candidate, IEM108. Infect Immun 71:5498–5504

MacDonald D, Demarre G, Bouvier M, Mazel D, Gopaul DN (2006) Structural basis for broad DNA-specificity in integron recombination. Nature 440:1157–1162

Mandlik A, Livny J, Robins WP, Ritchie JM, Mekalanos JJ, Waldor MK (2011) RNA-Seq-based monitoring of infection-linked changes in *Vibrio cholerae* gene expression. Cell Host Microbe 10:165–174

Mazel D, Dychinco B, Webb VA, Davies J (1998) A distinctive class of integron in the *Vibrio cholerae* genome. Science 280:605–608

Meibom KL, Blokesch M, Dolganov NA, Wu CY, Schoolnik GK (2005) Chitin induces natural competence in *Vibrio cholerae*. Science 310:1824–1827

Mekalanos JJ (1983) Duplication and amplification of toxin genes in Vibrio cholerae. Cell 35(1):253–263

Mekalanos JJ, Robins W, Ussery DW, Davis BM, Schadt E, Waldor MK (2012) Non-O1 *Vibrio cholerae* unlinked to cholera in Haiti. Proc Natl Acad Sci USA 109:E3206 (author reply E7)

Miller VL, DiRita VJ, Mekalanos JJ (1989) Identification of toxS, a regulatory gene whose product enhances toxR-mediated activation of the cholera toxin promoter. J Bacteriol 171:1288–1293

Mukhopadhyay AK, Chakraborty S, Takeda Y, Nair GB, Berg DE (2001) Characterization of VPI pathogenicity island and CTXphi prophage in environmental strains of *Vibrio cholerae*. J Bacteriol 183:4737–4746

Mutreja A, Kim DW, Thomson NR, Connor TR, Lee JH, Kariuki S et al (2011) Evidence for several waves of global transmission in the seventh cholera pandemic. Nature 477:462–465

Nair GB, Faruque SM, Bhuiyan NA, Kamruzzaman M, Siddique AK, Sack DA (2002) New variants of *Vibrio cholerae* O1 biotype El Tor with attributes of the classical biotype from hospitalized patients with acute diarrhea in Bangladesh. J Clin Microbiol 40:3296–3299

Nair GB, Qadri F, Holmgren J, Svennerholm AM, Safa A, Bhuiyan NA et al (2006) Cholera due to altered El Tor strains of *Vibrio cholerae* O1 in Bangladesh. J Clin Microbiol 44:4211–4213

Novais RC, Coelho A, Salles CA, Vicente AC (1999) Toxin-co-regulated pilus cluster in non-O1, non-toxigenic *Vibrio cholerae*: evidence of a third allele of pilin gene. FEMS Microbiol Lett 171:49–55

Nusrin S, Gil AI, Bhuiyan NA, Safa A, Asakura M, Lanata CF et al (2009) Peruvian *Vibrio cholerae* O1 El Tor strains possess a distinct region in the *Vibrio* seventh pandemic island-II that differentiates them from the prototype seventh pandemic El Tor strains. J Med Microbiol 58:342–354

Ogawa A, Takeda T (1993) The gene encoding the heat-stable enterotoxin of *Vibrio cholerae* is flanked by 123-base pair direct repeats. Microbiol Immunol 37:607–616

Pang B, Yan M, Cui Z, Ye X, Diao B, Ren Y et al (2007) Genetic diversity of toxigenic and nontoxigenic *Vibrio cholerae* serogroups O1 and O139 revealed by array-based comparative genomic hybridization. J Bacteriol 189:4837–4849

Pascual M, Bouma MJ, Dobson AP (2002) Cholera and climate: revisiting the quantitative evidence. Microbes Infect 4:237–245

Qadri F, Chowdhury MI, Faruque SM, Salam MA, Ahmed T, Begum YA et al (2007) Peru-15, a live attenuated oral cholera vaccine, is safe and immunogenic in Bangladeshi toddlers and infants. Vaccine 25:231–238

Rahman MH, Biswas K, Hossain MA, Sack RB, Mekalanos JJ, Faruque SM (2008) Distribution of genes for virulence and ecological fitness among diverse *Vibrio cholerae* population in a cholera endemic area: tracking the evolution of pathogenic strains. DNA Cell Biol 27:347–355

Raychoudhuri A, Patra T, Ghosh K, Ramamurthy T, Nandy RK, Takeda Y et al (2009) Classical *ctxB* in *Vibrio cholerae* O1, Kolkata, India. Emerg Infect Dis 15:131–132

Reguera G, Kolter R (2005) Virulence and the environment: a novel role for *Vibrio cholerae* toxin-coregulated pili in biofilm formation on chitin. J Bacteriol 187:3551–3555

Reimer AR, Van Domselaar G, Stroika S, Walker M, Kent H, Tarr C et al (2011) Comparative genomics of *Vibrio cholerae* from Haiti, Asia, and Africa. Emerg Infect Dis 17:2113–2121

Rhine JA, Taylor RK (1994) TcpA pilin sequences and colonization requirements for O1 and O139 *Vibrio cholerae*. Mol Microbiol 13:1013–1020

Rivera IN, Chun J, Huq A, Sack RB, Colwell RR (2001) Genotypes associated with virulence in environmental isolates of *Vibrio cholerae*. Appl Environ Microbiol 67:2421–2429

Rokas A, Williams BL, King N, Carroll SB (2003) Genome-scale approaches to resolving incongruence in molecular phylogenies. Nature 425:798–804

Rowe-Magnus DA, Guerout AM, Biskri L, Bouige P, Mazel D (2003) Comparative analysis of superintegrons: engineering extensive genetic diversity in the Vibrionaceae. Genome Res 13:428–442

Rubin EJ, Lin W, Mekalanos JJ, Waldor MK (1998) Replication and integration of a *Vibrio cholerae* cryptic plasmid linked to the CTX prophage. Mol Microbiol 28:1247–1254

Russell AJ (1925) A statistical approach to the epidemiology of cholera in Madras presidency. Proc Natl Acad Sci USA 11:653–657

Safa A, Bhuyian NA, Nusrin S, Ansaruzzaman M, Alam M, Hamabata T et al (2006) Genetic characteristics of Matlab variants of *Vibrio cholerae* O1 that are hybrids between classical and El Tor biotypes. J Med Microbiol 55:1563–1569

Sealfon R, Gire S, Ellis C, Calderwood S, Qadri F, Hensley L et al (2012) High depth, whole-genome sequencing of cholera isolates from Haiti and the dominican republic. BMC Genom 13:468

Seed KD, Bodi KL, Kropinski AM, Ackermann HW, Calderwood SB, Qadri F et al (2011) Evidence of a dominant lineage of *Vibrio cholerae*-specific lytic bacteriophages shed by cholera patients over a 10-year period in Dhaka, Bangladesh. MBio 2:e00334-10

Sellek RE, Niemcewicz M, Olsen JS, Bassy O, Lorenzo P, Marti L et al (2012) Phenotypic and genetic analyses of 111 clinical and environmental O1, O139, and non-O1/O139 *Vibrio cholerae* strains from different geographical areas. Epidemiol Infect 140:1389–1399

Shakya G, Kim DW, Clemens JD, Malla S, Upadhyaya BP, Dumre SP et al (2012) Phenotypic and genetic characterization of *Vibrio cholerae* O1 clinical isolates collected through national antimicrobial resistance surveillance network in Nepal. World J Microbiol Biotechnol 28:2671–2678

Shamini G, Ravichandran M, Sinnott JT, Somboonwit C, Sidhu HS, Shapshak P et al (2011) Structural inferences for cholera toxin mutations in *Vibrio cholerae*. Bioinformation 6:1–9

Singh DV, Matte MH, Matte GR, Jiang S, Sabeena F, Shukla BN et al (2001) Molecular analysis of *Vibrio cholerae* O1, O139, non-O1, and non-O139 strains: clonal relationships between clinical and environmental isolates. Appl Environ Microbiol 67:910–921

Sjolund-Karlsson M, Reimer A, Folster JP, Walker M, Dahourou GA, Batra DG et al (2011) Drug-resistance mechanisms in *Vibrio cholerae* O1 outbreak strain, Haiti, 2010. Emerg Infect Dis 17:2151–2154

Son MS, Megli CJ, Kovacikova G, Qadri F, Taylor RK (2011) Characterization of *Vibrio cholerae* O1 El Tor biotype variant clinical isolates from Bangladesh and Haiti, including a molecular genetic analysis of virulence genes. J Clin Microbiol 49:3739–3749

Talkington D, Bopp C, Tarr C, Parsons MB, Dahourou G, Freeman M et al (2011) Characterization of toxigenic *Vibrio cholerae* from Haiti, 2010-2011. Emerg Infect Dis 17:2122–2129

Thungapathra M, Sharma C, Gupta N, Ghosh RK, Mukhopadhyay A, Koley H et al (1999) Construction of a recombinant live oral vaccine from a non-toxigenic strain of *Vibrio cholerae* O1 serotype inaba biotype E1 Tor and assessment of its reactogenicity and immunogenicity in the rabbit model. Immunol Lett 68:219–227

Trucksis M, Michalski J, Deng YK, Kaper JB (1998) The *Vibrio cholerae* genome contains two unique circular chromosomes. Proc Natl Acad Sci USA 95:14464–14469

UN (2011) United Nation Final Report of the Independent Panel of Experts on the Cholera Outbreak in Haiti, May 4, 2011. In: (ed.), Vol. pp. United Nations. Available at http://www.un.org/News/dh/infocus/haiti/UN-cholera-report-final.pdf. Accessed March 2012

Vesth T, Lagesen K, Acar O, Ussery D (2013) CMG-biotools, a free workbench for basic comparative microbial genomics. PLoS ONE 8:e60120

Vesth T, Wassenaar TM, Hallin PF, Snipen L, Lagesen K, Ussery DW (2010) On the origins of a *Vibrio* species. Microb Ecol 59:1–13

Wachsmuth IK, Evins GM, Fields PI, Olsvik O, Popovic T, Bopp CA et al (1993) The molecular epidemiology of cholera in Latin America. J Infect Dis 167:621–626

Waldor MK, Mekalanos JJ (1996) Lysogenic conversion by a filamentous phage encoding cholera toxin. Science 272:1910–1914

Waldor MK, Rubin EJ, Pearson GD, Kimsey H, Mekalanos JJ (1997) Regulation, replication, and integration functions of the *Vibrio cholerae* CTXphi are encoded by region RS2. Mol Microbiol 24:917–926

Waldor MK, Tschape H, Mekalanos JJ (1996) A new type of conjugative transposon encodes resistance to sulfamethoxazole, trimethoprim, and streptomycin in *Vibrio cholerae* O139. J Bacteriol 178:4157–4165

Weber JT, Mintz ED, Canizares R, Semiglia A, Gomez I, Sempertegui R et al (1994) Epidemic cholera in Ecuador: multidrug-resistance and transmission by water and seafood. Epidemiol Infect 112:1–11

Yamaichi Y, Iida T, Park KS, Yamamoto K, Honda T (1999) Physical and genetic map of the genome of *Vibrio parahaemolyticus*: presence of two chromosomes in *Vibrio* species. Mol Microbiol 31:1513–1521

Yan M, Liu G, Diao B, Qiu H, Zhang L, Liang W et al (2007) A *Vibrio cholerae* serogroup O1 vaccine candidate against CTX ET Phi infection. Vaccine 25:4046–4055

Yildiz FH, Liu XS, Heydorn A, Schoolnik GK (2004) Molecular analysis of rugosity in a *Vibrio cholerae* O1 El Tor phase variant. Mol Microbiol 53:497–515

Yu RR, DiRita VJ (1999) Analysis of an autoregulatory loop controlling ToxT, cholera toxin, and toxin-coregulated pilus production in *Vibrio cholerae*. J Bacteriol 181:2584–2592

When, How, and Where can Oral Cholera Vaccines be Used to Interrupt Cholera Outbreaks?

John Clemens and Jan Holmgren

Abstract Cholera continues to be a major global health problem, at times causing major and prolonged outbreaks in both endemic and nonendemic settings in developing countries. While improved water quality, sanitation, and hygiene (WASH) will provide the ultimate solution to prevention of this disease burden, this is a far-off goal for most developing countries. Oral cholera vaccines (OCVs) have been demonstrated to be effective in the control of cholera outbreaks, and constitute useful tools to be used in conjunction with efforts to improve WASH. Two killed OCVs are prequalified by WHO for purchase by UN agencies for international use. Recently, WHO has launched a global stockpile of killed OCVs for use to control outbreaks. Rational deployment of OCV from this stockpile will require consideration of costs, feasibility, disease epidemiology, and the protective characteristics of the vaccine deployed, as well as effective and rapid coordination of processes and logistics used to make decisions on deployment and delivery of the vaccine to the population in need. Despite not having data on all the questions of relevance as to how to use OCVs to control cholera outbreaks in different settings, there is clearly more than enough evidence to initiate their use, as answers to remaining questions and refinement of policies will mainly come with experience.

J. Clemens (✉)
ICCDR,B, Dhaka, Bangladesh
e-mail: jclemens@icddrb.org

J. Clemens
UCLA School of Public Health, Los Angeles, USA

J. Holmgren
University of Gothenburg, Gothenburg, Sweden

Current Topics in Microbiology and Immunology (2014) 379: 231–258
DOI: 10.1007/82_2013_353

Published Online: 9 January 2014

Contents

1 Introduction

Cholera, an acute watery diarrheal disease caused by *Vibrio cholerae* O1, and less commonly by *V. cholerae* O139 remains a major global health problem (Sack et al. 2004). It causes epidemics, often well publicized in the wake of natural disasters and other humanitarian emergencies, as well as less well-publicized endemic disease, though the latter accounts for the major portion of the global disease burden. Cholera vaccines have been developed since the late nineteenth century, not long after the cholera vibrio was discovered. Early generation vaccines were killed whole cells (WCs) delivered parenterally. These vaccines were in widespread use for nearly 100 years without adequate evaluation of their safety and protection. When rigorous trials were finally undertaken in the 1960s, the trials found that those vaccines that were acceptably non-reactogenic failed to confer either high-grade or long-term protection. Based on this evidence, in 1973 the 26th World Health Assembly amended the International Health Regulations by removing the requirement for cholera vaccination on the certificate for international travel. WHO also recommended against the use of these vaccines for control of cholera globally (Clemens et al. 1994).

While parenteral cholera vaccines were experiencing their demise as public health tools, considerable progress was being made in the understanding of natural immunity to cholera. It had been well recognized that in cholera-endemic populations, natural cholera infections confer protection against recurrent cholera. The same was observed in North American volunteers who were challenged and re-challenged experimentally with cholera. The basis for this protection was determined to be mucosal immunity, primarily IgA secretory antibodies directed to the lipopolysaccharide (LPS) O antigen of cholera organisms, and to a lesser extent to cholera toxin. Antibacterial and antitoxin antibodies were found to protect synergistically. Importantly, it was found that the most efficient way to induce this mucosal immunity is by oral delivery of vaccine antigens (Holmgren et al. 1992; Svennerholm and Holmgren 1976; Svennerholm et al. 1984). Attention thus turned to the development of orally administered cholera vaccines (OCVs). Despite the ensuing development of safe and effective OCVs, these vaccines have until recently failed to be embraced as public health tools for developing countries. The reasons have been several. Some have cited vaccine expense, moderate levels of vaccine protection, and the logistic challenges associated with vaccine storage and administration. Also mentioned have been concerns that delivery of these vaccines might interfere with other control efforts in the context of cholera outbreaks, and the expectation that global efforts to improve water quality, hygiene, and sanitation (WASH) will soon control cholera.

Unfortunately, the past decade has not witnessed a decline in cholera incidence or mortality. To the contrary, we have observed unusually large and protracted outbreaks in Angola, Zimbabwe, Central and West Africa, Somalia, and Haiti. Further, cholera has now become endemic in Haiti, after nearly a century in which cholera was not reported in this country (Harris et al. 2010). Global statistics on cholera published by WHO, with their acknowledged limitations, have shown no decline in global cholera burden (WHO 2012a, b, c). A recent analysis of global cholera disease burden estimated that there are approximately 2.8 million cholera cases and 91,500 cholera deaths in cholera-endemic countries, and 87,000 cases and 2,500 deaths in cholera epidemics (Ali et al. 2011), and these figures may be conservative. In this context, the international public health community has recently expressed interest in using new generation OCVs in concert with non-vaccine interventions as public health tools to control cholera. This interest has been spurred in part by the development, licensure, and international qualification by WHO of the first low-cost OCV, which has been found to be safe and effective in a large trial in India (Sur et al. 2009). As well, WHO has recently committed to the creation of a global stockpile of OCVs that can be deployed for the control of cholera outbreaks (WHO 2012, b, c). It is still be debated how best to use such a vaccine stockpile, or other reserves of OCVs. In this chapter, we review the available vaccines and their characteristics and outline factors that should be considered in the targeting of the vaccines for control of cholera outbreaks, including the use of a vaccine stockpile.

2 Currently Licensed OCVs

Currently licensed OCVs consist either of genetically attenuated live organisms or of killed cholera WCs, with or without the addition of cholera toxin B subunit (CTB). Three vaccines are currently licensed: a vaccine consisting of recombinant CTB together with O1 serogroup killed WCs (Dukoral^{TM}), a vaccine containing both O1 and O139 serogroup killed WCs, but no CTB (produced as Shanchol^{TM} in

India and mORCVAX^{TM} in Vietnam), and a genetically attenuated version of an originally virulent O1 serogroup classical Inaba strain (Orochol^{TM} and Mutachol^{TM}) (Shin et al. 2011).

2.1 rCTB-WC Oral Vaccine (Dukoral^{TM})

Developed in Sweden, this killed oral vaccine contains O1 serogroup formalin- or heat-killed WCs representing both the classical and El Tor biotypes and the Ogawa and Inaba serotypes, together with recombinant cholera toxin CTB (rCTB); it is the first oral cholera vaccine to have achieved international licensure and prequalification by WHO for purchase by United Nations agencies (Holmgren et al. 1992). Its composition reflects the appreciation that antibacterial and antitoxic immunity confer synergistic protection against cholera (Svennerholm and Holmgren 1976; Svennerholm et al. 1984). The vaccine is licensed for persons 2 years of age and older; a two-dose regimen is given to persons aged 5 years and older, while a three-dose regimen is recommended for younger persons with doses being given 1–6 weeks apart. The vaccine is coadministered with a bicarbonate buffer to prevent destruction of the rCTB by gastric acid (Clemens et al. 1986). A large randomized, placebo-controlled trial in a rural Bangladeshi population with endemic cholera demonstrated that an earlier version of the vaccine (with chemically extracted rather than recombinant CTB), given in a three-dose regimen, was safe and conferred 85 % protection against cholera for 4–6 months after dosing; protection declined to 62 % at one year and 57 % during the second year, becoming negligible thereafter (Clemens et al. 1990). Additional analyses of the trial found two doses to be as protective as three doses. Short-term cross-protection against LT-ETEC was also demonstrated (Clemens et al. 1988). Reanalysis of the trial found that the vaccine conferred indirect ("herd") protection to both non-vaccinees and vaccinees (Ali et al. 2005). The high level of short-term protection against cholera was later confirmed in a randomized, placebo-controlled trial of a two-dose regimen of rCTB-WC in Peruvian military volunteers, who, in contrast to the Bangladeshi population, were presumed to have lacked previous natural exposure to cholera and thereby also natural immunity to cholera (Sanchez et al. 1994).

2.2 Bivalent Killed WC-only OCV (Shanchol^{TM} and mORCVAX^{TM})

In addition to its evaluation of CTB-WC cholera vaccine, the trial in Bangladesh of killed OCVs demonstrated the safety and long-term protection by a killed WC-only OCV, lacking CTB. Motivated by these findings, in the late 1980s the Vietnamese government, led by Professor DD Trach, initiated cooperation with

Sweden to develop and produce an inexpensive WC-only OCV in Vietnam (Clemens et al. 1990). A two-dose monovalent, O1 serogroup, killed WC-only OCV, containing killed cholera strains similar but not identical to those in Dukoral™, was developed in Vietnam and found to be safe and to confer 66 % protection against cholera at 8–10 months following vaccination in an open field trial in Hue, Vietnam (Trach et al. 1997, 2002). This vaccine, which was licensed in Vietnam as ORCVAX™ in 1997, had the additional advantage of not requiring coadministration of oral buffer. It was subsequently made bivalent (O1 and O139), and over 20 million doses have been administered in Vietnam's public health programs to date (Lopez et al. 2008).

Though used widely in Vietnam, this vaccine was not suitable for international use because of several production and standardization problems, and because the Vietnamese national regulatory authority (NRA) was not approved by WHO (2004). To enable internationalization of an improved version of this inexpensive and easily produced vaccine, in 2004 the International Vaccine Institute (IVI) in Seoul, Korea initiated a program to modify the constituent strains, production technology, quality control procedures, and standardization assays for the vaccine, and to transfer this modified bivalent WC-only OCV to Shantha Biotechnics in India, whose NRA is WHO-approved. The O1 serogroup constituents of this O1–139 bivalent vaccine were the same as those in Dukoral™, albeit in different quantities, so that the total O1 serogroup LPS content of Shanchol™ is approximately twice that of Dukoral™. Because the vaccine does not contain CTB, no concomitant oral buffer is required. A large, randomized, placebo-controlled trial of this vaccine among 66,900 nonpregnant residents aged 1 year and older in Kolkata, India found a two-dose regimen of the vaccine, given approximately 2 weeks apart, to be safe and to confer 66 % protection against O1 serogroup cholera with no decline of protection during 3 years of follow-up (Sur et al. 2009). Further analysis of this trial has revealed sustained protection at 5 years after vaccination as well as evidence of vaccine herd protection (Clemens, unpublished data; Ali et al. 2013).

All episodes of cholera in the Kolkata trial were due to a newly emergent El Tor biotype that elaborates classical biotype cholera toxin. This vaccine was licensed as Shanchol™ in India in 2009 for persons aged 1 year and older, and was subsequently prequalified by WHO for purchase by UN agencies. It is available at $1.85 per dose to the public sector in developing countries. In addition, the improved vaccine production technology has been transferred back to Vietnam, where it is licensed by VaBiotech as mORCVAX™.

2.3 Live Oral CVD-103HgR Vaccine (Orochol^{TM} or Mutachol^{TM})

To date, CVD 103-HgR is the only genetically attenuated, live OCV to have achieved licensure. Developed by Professors James Kaper and Myron Levine at the University of Maryland, this vaccine is derived from the virulent O1 serogroup, Inaba serotype, classical biotype strain 569B. The basis for its attenuation is a deletion in the gene encoding cholera toxin A subunit, while still expressing CTB. The strain was further engineered to be Hg-resistant to serve as a diagnostic marker (Kaper and Levine 1990). Given as single dose with oral buffer, this vaccine was tested in Phase 1–2 studies that enrolled over 4,000 volunteers and was found to be safe at doses of up to 5×10^9 viable organisms. Doses of $2–8 \times 10^8$ viable organisms were found to be reliably immunogenic and protective against an experimental challenge with both Inaba and Ogawa cholera vibrios in North American volunteers; protection was seen against challenges as early as 1 week and as late as 24 weeks after dosing (Tacket et al. 1992, 1999; Suharyonom et al. 1992; Su-Arehawaratana et al. 1992; Levine et al. 1988). However, when tested in developing countries, serum vibriocidal antibody responses to a 10^8 dose were substantially lower in magnitude than those seen in US volunteers. Accordingly, when CVD103-HgR entered Phase 3 testing for efficacy in a cholera-endemic setting, the dose selected for testing was 5×10^9. In this trial, performed in North Jakarta, Indonesia, 67,508 persons aged 2–41 years were randomized to a single dose of CVD103-HgR or placebo. Vaccine efficacy against treated episodes of O1 serogroup cholera was 14 % at 4 years of follow-up, and no significant protection was observed during any year of follow-up (Richie et al. 2000).

CVD103-HgR was licensed as Orochol^{TM} (also as Mutachol^{TM}) by the then Swiss Serum and Vaccine Institute (now Crucell) as a single-dose vaccine at a dose of 2×10^8 viable organisms for travelers aged 2 years and older. A dose of 2×10^9 is offered in a different presentation (Orochol E^{TM}) that is intended for use in developing countries, but to date no developing country has used this product in routine public health programs. It is given as a single dose with a booster dose recommended 6 months later. A post-licensure study of mass immunization with a single dose of 2×10^9 viable organisms, given following the onset of an epidemic in Micronesia, found that vaccination was feasible and was associated with a 79 % reduction in the risk of cholera (Calain et al. 2004). However, because this was not a double-blinded, randomized, controlled trial and because the findings of this study were at variance with those of the trial in North Jakarta, the findings will require confirmation in future studies. Another post-licensure study with a similar dose found the vaccine to be safe, albeit associated with lower immune responses, in HIV-infected adults in Mali (Perry et al. 1998). Although the vaccine is still licensed, production has been suspended by the manufacturer, and the vaccine has not yet been prequalified by WHO.

Table 1 Factors to consider when deciding on deployment of oral cholera vaccines to control a cholera outbreak

Epidemiological setting for vaccination
Burden of cholera morbidity and mortality
Protective characteristics of the vaccine
Clinical effectiveness of the vaccine
Balance between costs and effects

3 Issues to Consider in the Use of OCVs for Outbreaks

The decision to use OCVs, and how to use them, for controlling cholera outbreaks requires consideration of several factors, among which there is a complex interplay (Table 1).

3.1 Epidemiological Setting

While there is no formal definition of a cholera "outbreak", the term loosely refers to temporally defined increases in cholera incidence in specific populations. In developing countries, outbreaks of cholera occur in two distinct settings: endemic and epidemic. Endemic cholera occurs as a result of ingestion of cholera vibrios from their permanent environmental reservoirs and does not require exogenous introduction into a population. As determination of transmission routes is not practical in most settings, a pragmatic definition of endemic cholera has been proposed by WHO as cholera recurring in time and place, with occurrences in a defined population in at least three of the past 5 years (WHO 2010). Endemic cholera is well illustrated by cholera occurring in the Ganges delta of India and Bangladesh. Outbreaks of endemic cholera tend to be influenced by environmental and climatic variables, and usually occur in a recurrent seasonal pattern. In contrast, outbreaks of epidemic cholera, initiated by exogenous introduction of cholera vibrios, usually occur unpredictably, as illustrated by the recent major epidemic in Haiti as well as outbreaks that have been documented in fairs, feasts, pilgrimages, and such complex emergencies as refugee crises and natural disasters (Mintz et al. 1994; Harris et al. 2010).

The difference in predictability between outbreaks in endemic versus epidemic settings frames different approaches to use of OCVs. In predictable, endemic settings, OCVs can be delivered either preemptively, in anticipation of outbreaks, or reactively, in response to the outbreaks. In contrast, while it is known that epidemic cholera can occur following complex emergencies, such as refugee crises, earthquakes, and floods, not all such emergencies are followed by cholera outbreaks, and we lack a validated instrument to accurately differentiate those emergencies that are at very high risk for outbreaks versus those at lower risk. Thus, preemptive delivery of OCVs in such emergencies cannot be justified on the basis of evidence, leaving

Table 2 Features distinguishing epidemic from endemic cholera (from Clemens et al. 1994)

Feature	Epidemic	Endemic
Occurrence	Not predictable	Predictable
Preexisting natural immunity	Uncommon	Common
Clinical severity	Greater	Lesser
Asymptomatic infections	Less common	More common
Higher risk in children	No	Yes
Modes of transmission	Few	Many
Nonhuman reservoirs	Uncommon	Common

reactive vaccination once outbreaks are identified as the only practical option. Because a greater potential preventive impact can be anticipated with appropriately timed preemptive vaccination than with reactive vaccination once the outbreak has started, preemptive use of OCVs in endemic settings has been relatively non-controversial, as reflected in recent WHO recommendations. In contrast, reactive vaccination has been questioned as an effective strategy, although recent WHO recommendations allow for reactive vaccination "as an additional control measure, depending on local infrastructure and following a thorough investigation of the current and historical epidemiological situation, and clear identification of the geographical areas to be targeted" (WHO 2010).

Several additional features distinguish endemic from epidemic cholera (Table 2). Routes of transmission for epidemic cholera tend to be few in number, so that, when sources are identified via epidemiologic studies, simple water-sanitation-hygiene (WASH) interventions can often be designed. Conversely, in endemic cholera, routes and sources of transmission are multiple, making simple WASH interventions less likely to succeed by themselves and strengthening the argument for vaccination. In endemic settings, cholera occurs against the background of age-related acquisition of preexisting natural immunity, owing to past cholera exposures. In contrast, in epidemic settings, cholera tends to occur in populations with little preexisting immunity. These features help to explain the greater level of clinical severity in epidemic than in endemic cholera. They also provide an explanation for young age groups, with less background immunity, having highest rates of cholera in endemic settings, while the incidence of cholera tends to be age-independent in epidemic settings. Thus, in endemic settings, a case can be made to limit targeting of vaccination to younger persons, whereas general populations constitute the appropriate target in epidemic settings.

3.2 Burden of Cholera Morbidity and Mortality

It would seem obvious that use of OCVs should be reserved for settings with high cholera incidence and high cholera mortality. However, operationalization of this concept is complex. Despite the recurrent, apparently predictable pattern of

Table 3 Duration of recent cholera outbreaks in specific areas

Location	Year(s)	Duration
Pohnpei, Federated States of Micronesia (Calain et al. 2004)	2000/2001	9 months
Lusaka, Zambia (Sasaki et al. 2008)	2003/2004	27 weeks
Angola (various areas) (WHO 2007, 2008)	2006/2007	15 months
Harare, Zimbabwe (Mukandavire et al. 2011)	2008/2009	>9 months
Haiti (various areas) (Ministere de la Santa Publique et de la population 2012)	2010	18+ months

endemic cholera, several factors conspire to make targeting of OCVs in such settings challenging. Country level statistics on cholera reported to WHO are known to be underestimates, at times severe, due to limitations in laboratory capabilities in making microbiological diagnoses, weaknesses in health information systems, and economic disincentives for countries to report cholera. Moreover, endemic cholera may exhibit great geographical heterogeneity within a country, so that countrywide and regionwide statistics may not be applicable to all areas. As well, cholera in endemic settings may exhibit major year-to-year variations in disease incidence (Glass et al. 1982). Adding to the complexity is the fact that high cholera incidence does not necessarily equate to high cholera mortality, which depends on how well served a population is with cholera treatment facilities. Indeed, it is in places where treatment is lacking that cholera is often underdiagnosed and underappreciated as a public health problem. All of this means that decisions to vaccinate against endemic cholera will frequently have to be made on the basis of local knowledge about the incidence and case-fatality of cholera, however, incomplete.

As already mentioned, epidemic cholera is usually unpredictable. Most cholera epidemics occur in countries afflicted by natural or political emergencies, such as earthquakes, floods, warfare, and refugee crises. In many such situations already fragile or inadequate water, sanitation, and health care systems collapse, leading not only to a cholera outbreak but also to an overloaded or collapsed health care system, with resulting high case-fatality rates. In situations where a cholera outbreak additionally occurs in a setting that has previously been cholera-free for a long time, as was the case for the major cholera outbreak in Haiti in 2010, the situation is further worsened by the lack of the natural immunity that develops with age in cholera-endemic settings, leading to increased morbidity and mortality, which tends to occur with equal rares in young and old alike (Table 3).

3.3 Protective Characteristics of the OCVs

Several protective characteristics of the OCV to be used should be considered when deliberating on whether to deploy an OCV to control an outbreak. Table 4 summarizes several of these features for the two currently available, WHO-prequalified OCVs, Dukoral™ and Shanchol™.

Table 4 Features of the two licensed and available oral cholera vaccines (after Shin 2011)

Feature/characteristic	rCTB-WC (Dukoral™ Crucell)	WC-only (Shanchol™ Shantha Biotech; mORCVAX™ VaBiotech)
Cellular constituents	O1 serogroup El and classical biotypes	O1 serogroup El and Classical biotypes; O139 serogroup
Number of doses in primary regimen	2 doses given 1–6 weeks apart (3 doses for children 2–5 years of age)	2 doses given 14 days apart
Need for booster dose and frequency	After 2 years (every 6 months for children 2–5 years of age)	After 3 years
Minimal age of use according to license	2 years old	1 year old
Safety/tolerability	High, including in HIV+ individuals	High, presumably including HIV+ individuals (given similarity of the vaccine to Dukoral™)
Administration during pregnancy contraindicated	No	No
Time of onset of protection after full dosing	No data (presumed 1 week)	No data (presumed 1 week)
Protective efficacy	57 % at 2 years after vaccination	80 % at 5 years after vaccination
Protection against clinically severe cholera	Greater than against clinically mild cholera	No demonstrated difference in protection against clinical cholera by severity
Protection greater in 5+ year olds than in younger persons?	Yes	Yes
Protection by biotype	Greater against classical than against El Tor cholera; protection also against newly emergent hybrid El Tor cholera	Data available only for El Tor cholera; protection also against newly emergent hybrid El Tor cholera
Confers herd protection?	Yes	Yes
Confers cross-protection against LT-ETEC	Yes	No
Requires coadministration with liquid buffer?	Yes	No
Storage temperature and shelf life	2–8 °C; 3 years	2–8 °C; 2 years
WHO prequalified?	Yes	Shanchhol™: yes mORCVAX™: no
Price per dose to the public sector	\$5.25 (negotiated price for WHO)	Shanchol: \$1.85 mORCVAX: \$0.75 (projected)

The magnitude of vaccine protection is of clear importance. Vaccine protection is typically expressed by the term "protective efficacy" (PE), calculated as the relative reduction of disease incidence in individual vaccinees attributable to their receipt of the vaccine. This value is generally quoted as 60–70 % for both vaccines at 1 year after immunization. However, this cited PE is itself insufficient for making decisions for several reasons. One reason is that PE, by expressing the relative reduction of disease owing to vaccination, does not provide an index of absolute index of vaccine protection, such as the number of persons who need to be vaccinated to prevent one case of cholera. For example, in an outbreak whose incidence is three cases per 1,000 persons, a 100 % protective vaccine will require vaccination of 333 persons to prevent a single case. In contrast, in an outbreak whose incidence is 50/1,000, as may occur in a refugee camp or urban slum (WHO 2012a, b, c), use of a 50 % protective vaccine will require vaccination of only 40 persons to prevent each case.

A second reason is that enhanced levels of short-term protection may be of importance to the decision to use OCVs to control cholera outbreaks. While protection by Shanchol™ exhibits no enhancement in the short-term, protection by Dukoral™ is markedly higher (ca. 85 %) in the 4–6 months after dosing when antitoxic immunity induced by its CTB component is at hand in addition to the antibacterial immunity induced by the whole-cell vaccine components. Such enhanced short-term protection could be a major asset for a vaccine deployed in a short-lasting outbreak. Conversely, longer term protection may also be of relevance when vaccinating against an outbreak in an endemic setting, or in epidemics whose duration is long, an increasingly frequent phenomenon (Table 4) (Reyburn et al. 2011).

Third, the onset of protection should also be considered. Reactive use of an OCV in an outbreak will be more effective the sooner after initiation of vaccination that protection begins. Both Dukoral™ and Shanchol™ have two-dose regimens (three doses for young children given Dukoral™, with doses separated by 1–6 weeks for Dukoral™ and 2 weeks for Shanchol™). Although there are no efficacy data on how early protection begins for either vaccine, protection is thought to begin 4–7 days after the second dose for each vaccine (e.g., a minimum of ca. 2 weeks after initiating vaccination with Dukoral™ and ca. 3 weeks after the first dose of Shanchol™). For a short-lasting outbreak of only a few weeks' duration, the overall impact of reactive vaccination would be predicted to be minimal with either vaccine, especially considering the time required to recognize the outbreak and to acquire and deliver the OCV (Naficy et al. 1998). Recently, however, it has been appreciated for Shanchol™ that serum vibriocidal antibody responses after the first of the two dose regimen are robust, even higher than after the second dose (Kanungo et al. 2009), hinting that protection may begin even before the second dose. This prediction will be tested in a large-scale, randomized, and placebo-controlled trial to be conducted in Bangladesh.

Fourthly, because PE only reflects direct protection of vaccinees, and does not consider the indirect protective effects of a vaccine via herd protection, it may fail to capture the overall preventive impact of using OCVs at the population level.

Herd protection occurs when a vaccine not only protects vaccinated persons by eliciting immunity to cholera in *individual vaccinees*, but also protects nonvaccinated persons and enhances protection of vaccinated persons by interrupting transmission in *populations* of people, some of whom have been vaccinated. Vaccine herd protection by Dukoral™ and by an early generation killed WC-only OCV were demonstrated in the large Phase III trial of these vaccines done in rural Bangladesh, as well as in a recent demonstration project of Dukoral™ done in Zanzibar (Ali et al. 2005, 2008; Khatib et al. 2012). Data from the former were then used to parameterize a dynamic cholera transmission model for rural Bangladesh. The model showed that use of vaccine with the characteristics of Dukoral™ in rural Bangladesh could nearly extinguish the occurrence of cholera at vaccine coverage level of only 60 %, due to the combined direct and indirect effects of the vaccine (Longini et al. 2007). More recently, further analysis of the Phase III trial of Shanchol™ undertaken in urban Kolkata has also demonstrated both direct and herd protective effects of this vaccine (Ali et al. 2013).

A fifth issue is that OCVs may cross-protect against noncholera pathogens. Because it contains CTB, which is structurally similar to the B subunit of heat-labile enterotoxin (LT) of toxigenic *Escherichia coli* (ETEC), Dukoral™ protects against not only cholera but also against diarrhea due to LT-expressing ETEC. In the Phase III trial of Dukoral™ in Bangladesh, for example, recipients of the vaccine experienced a 67 % reduction of all treated episodes of LT-ETEC and an 86 % reduction of severe LT-ETEC during the initial 3 months after vaccination (Clemens et al. 1988), an observation that has been confirmed in Europeans traveling to ETEC-endemic areas (Peltola et al. 1991). Because ETEC diarrhea is common in most populations experiencing cholera, this added benefit should be taken into account. Conversely, because Shanchol™ does not contain B subunit, it is not predicted to cross-protect against ETEC.

A sixth issue is the clinical spectrum of cholera that is prevented by vaccination. Although it was argued in the past that a deficiency of parenteral cholera vaccines was that they failed to prevent asymptomatic cholera infections, the relevance of this observation to public health impact is unclear (Benenson 1976). On the other hand, it is unarguable that for an OCV to have a major public health impact, it should prevent clinically severe cholera. Both Dukoral™ and Shanchol™ prevent cholera severe enough to require treatment, and thus both are predicted to prevent cholera mortality. In the Phase III trial of Dukoral™, for example, vaccination conferred 26 % protection against all-cause mortality (Clemens et al. 1988). Moreover, there is clear evidence for Dukoral™ that vaccination has an enhanced preventive impact on treated episodes with severe dehydration. For example, in a demonstration project in Beira, Mozambique, Dukoral conferred 84 % protection against all treated cholera episodes and 95 % protection against treated episodes with severe dehydration during 6 months of follow-up (Lucas et al. 2005). In contrast, Shanchol™ exhibited no enhanced protection against those treated cholera episodes presenting with severe dehydration, as opposed to treated episodes of lesser severity, in the Phase III efficacy trial of this vaccine in Kolkata (Clemens, unpublished data).

A seventh consideration relevant to use of OCVs in outbreaks is that protection may vary substantially by host and pathogen characteristics. Protection by both Dukoral™ and Shanchol™ varies by age, being less for young children than for persons vaccinated at older ages. Although in the Phase III trial in Bangladesh Dukoral™ provided almost 100 % protection for children vaccinated at 2–5 years for the first 4–6 months after vaccination, at 2 years of follow-up PE for Dukoral™ was 40 % for this age group as compared to 70 % for older persons (Clemens et al. 1990). At 2 years of follow-up of the Phase III trial of Shanchol™ in Kolkata, India, PE was 50 % for children vaccinated at 1–4 years of age and 80 % for persons vaccinated at older ages (Sur et al. 2009). While these figures appear similar, and recognizing that there are limitations to comparing the results for PE for different vaccines tested in different trials, it is of relevance that the results for Dukoral™ reflect protection against both classical and El Tor cholera, whereas those for Shanchol™ represent protection against only El Tor cholera, the only biotype circulating in Kolkata during the trial. When parsed out by biotype, Dukoral™ protected less well against El Tor cholera at 2 years of follow-up (30 % in 2–5 year olds and 60 % in older persons) (Clemens, unpublished data). As noted earlier, however, absolute rather than relative protection is of great relevance to public health deliberations about using a vaccine, so that in circumstances in which cholera rates are much higher in under-five year olds, as is the case in endemic situations, even these lower values for PE may correspond to a major public health impact.

Another host characteristic that modifies OCV protection is ABO blood group. In the Phase III trial of killed OCVs in Bangladesh, persons who received either Dukoral™ or a killed WC-only OCV exhibited lower levels of protection against cholera if they had O blood group than if they had other ABO groups (Clemens et al. 1989). Populations with a higher prevalence of O blood type, such as those residing in the Ganges delta, would thus be expected to benefit less from vaccination than those with low blood group O prevalence rates.

Yet another host characteristic of importance is preexisting natural immunity to cholera. As noted earlier, outbreaks of epidemic cholera typically affect populations that have experienced little cholera in the past, as was the case in the 2010 outbreak of cholera in Haiti (Harris et al. 2010). It cannot be assumed that vaccine protection will be equivalent in these populations and in populations that have substantial levels of preexisting immunity due to previous natural exposure to cholera. Most evaluations of the protection of both Shanchol™ and Dukoral™ against naturally occurring cholera have been undertaken in populations with endemic cholera and presumably high levels of preexisting immunity. An exception was a trial of Dukoral™ that confirmed a high level of short-term protection against El Tor cholera in Peruvian military volunteers, who were all of blood group O and were presumed to have not at the time of the trial had previous natural exposure to cholera (Sanchez et al. 1994). Field evaluations of these vaccines in populations lacking such immunity constitute an important priority for the future.

Phenotypic characteristics of cholera also may modify vaccine protection. As mentioned earlier, Dukoral™ has been observed to protect less well against classical El Tor biotype than against El Tor classical biotype serogroup O1 cholera. Both Dukoral™ and Shanchol™, however, have shown protection against the newly emergent hybrid El Tor cholera vibrios that expresses classical biotype cholera toxin (Lucas et al. 2005; Sur et al. 2009), which now accounts for all cholera cases in many areas of Asia and Africa, as well as in Haiti.

3.4 Effectiveness of the OCVs

The effectiveness of OCVs when used to control cholera outbreaks has several dimensions (Table 4). One is clinical acceptability. Neither Dukoral™ nor Shanchol™ has been associated with side-effects when given to healthy, non-pregnant individuals. A small, controlled observational study suggested that Dukoral™ inadvertently administered to pregnant women was not associated with adverse pregnancy outcomes (Hashim et al. 2012). Since its licensure, over 15 million doses of Dukoral™ been sold. Post-licensure studies have revealed no safety concerns about use of the vaccine during pregnancy. Small studies have also demonstrated the safety of Dukoral™ when given to persons who are infected by HIV, a feature of great importance in view of the logistical impossibility of testing for HIV in order to target HIV-negative individuals during mass OCV campaigns conducted to control cholera outbreaks (Lewis et al. 1994; Ortigao-de-Sampaio et al. 1998). Although there are no data on the safety of Shanchol™ when administered to HIV-infected or pregnant individuals, the similarities of the WC constituents of Dukoral™ and Shanchol™, and the fact that they are both killed oral vaccines, make it likely that Shanchol™ will be deemed safe when administered to these two patient populations, although studies directly addressing these issues are needed.

Another aspect of clinical effectiveness is the logistic and programmatic feasibility of administering OCVs in outbreak situations. Preemptive delivery of killed OCVs has been demonstrated to be feasible in endemic settings in Beira, Mozamibique (Dukoral™), Orissa, India (Shanchol™), and Dhaka, Bangladesh (Shanchol™); in stable refugee camps in Uganda and Sudan deemed at high risk for cholera (Dukoral™); and in a complex emergency created by the 2007 tsunami in Aceh, Indonesia (Dukoral™) (Cavailler et al. 2006; Dorlencourt et al. 1999; Chaignat et al. 2008; Qadri, personal communication). As well, reactive delivery of Shanchol™ was successfully accomplished in major outbreaks in mass immunization campaigns in Guinea (Medecins sans Frontieres 2013), and Haiti (Ivers et al. 2012). Similarly, ORCVAX™, an earlier generation WC-only OCV similar to Shanchol™, has successfully been delivered reactively in multiple cholera outbreaks in Vietnam, including a large-scale recent outbreak in northern Vietnam (Anh et al. 2011). While these experiences illustrate that both Dukoral™ and Shanchol™ can be delivered to control cholera outbreaks under realistic public health conditions, it is recognized that the need to coadminister Dukoral^{TM} with relatively large volumes of buffer solution, which is not required for Shanchol^{TM}, creates greater supply demands for Dukoral^{TM} and also makes delivery of this vaccine slower and more cumbersome.

Regardless of the safety and feasibility of delivery of these vaccines, it is important that the protection conferred under the demanding and often chaotic circumstances of a cholera outbreak be established. The degree of protection of a vaccine in public health practice (effectiveness) cannot necessarily be predicted from results of prelicensure randomized trials (efficacy), which are usually conducted under idealized circumstances (Clemens et al. 1996). Several vagaries of public health practice, such as broadened criteria for targeting persons for vaccination, and problems encountered with vaccine storage and administration, can lead to a reduction of vaccine impact in relation to that predicted on the basis of prelicensure trials. Conversely, the indirect, or herd protective effects of vaccines, which are typically not measured in prelicensure trials, may substantially enhance vaccine impact beyond that expected on the basis of trials. Thus, it is important to base recommendations on use of OCVs on impacts actually observed in practice.

The protective effectiveness of Dukoral^{TM}, delivered preemptively, has been evaluated in practical public health settings in two sites with endemic cholera, one, in a population with a high prevalence of HIV in Mozambique (Lucas et al. 2005) and the other in Zanzibar (Ali et al. 2005, 2008). Each study confirmed levels of PE observed in earlier clinical trials (Clemens et al. 1990). In addition, the Zanzibar evaluation confirmed results of an earlier reanalysis of a Phase III trial that Dukoral^{TM} was capable of conferring herd protection. In aggregate, these studies suggest that the protective impact of using this vaccine in practice will be greater than that expected on the basis of estimates of PE from individually randomized, Phase III trials. To date, no study has evaluated the impact of Dukoral^{TM} when delivered reactively in outbreaks in either endemic or epidemic settings.

No studies of the protective effectiveness of Shanchol^{TM} have been completed to date. As mentioned earlier, Vietnam has used an earlier generation, locally produced, killed WC-only OCV since the early 1990s. A prolonged epidemic of cholera in Hanoi in 2007–2008 provided an opportunity to assess protection conferred by reactive vaccination, which was given as a two-dose regimen to persons aged 10 years and older in January, 2008. A case-control study of cholera occurring between April and June, 2008 revealed 76 % PE by the vaccine in this public health setting (Anh et al. 2011). As well, an effectiveness trial of a locally produced earlier generation killed WC-only OCV delivered preemptively to persons aged 1 year and older in central Vietnam revealed 50 % protection during an epidemic occurring 3–5 years after vaccine campaigns (Thiem et al. 2006).

An important aspect of the effectiveness of OCVs in control of cholera outbreaks is their potential to synergize with concomitant WASH interventions to prevent cholera. Traditionally, provision of clean water, adequate sanitation, and promotion of personal and household hygiene have been the cornerstones of WHO's approach to prevent cholera in outbreak response efforts. In addition to making intuitive sense, use of such interventions to prevent cholera has been

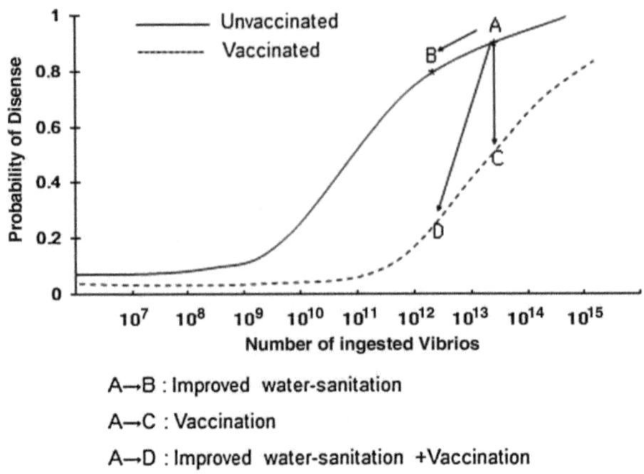

Fig. 1 Hypothetical relationship between the impact of oral cholera vaccines and improvements in water quality-hygiene-sanitation on the risk of cholera, by the size of ingested cholera inoculum. The figure presents two hypothetical curves relating the ingested inoculum of cholera organisms to the probability of diarrhea after ingestion. The *top curve* corresponds to a unvaccinated individual and the *bottom curve* to a vaccinated individual. The *top curve* roughly describes the lower risk of symptomatic cholera after WASH interventions, which act to decrease the frequency and/or dose of ingestion of cholera vibrios (movement from state *A* to state *B*). The bottom curve reflects the same for vaccinated individuals (movement from state *C* to state *D*). The effect of OCVs should be to decrease the probability of becoming ill, at any (or at least most) ingested doses (movement from state *A* to state *C*). Because of these relationships the combined effects of WASH interventions and OCVs should combine to produce a greater preventive effect than either intervention alone (movement from state *A* to state *D*)

documented in a limited number of intervention studies in the Philippines (Azurin and Alverin 1974) and India (Deb et al. 1986). While deployment of OCVs and implementation of WASH interventions have in the past been caste as competitive with one another, there is a good theoretical basis to consider them as complementary, if not synergistic (Fig. 1). A large-scale, cluster-randomized community introduction project of Shanchol™ given with or without a concomitant WASH intervention is now being conducted in urban Dhaka, Bangladesh and will test this prediction (Qadri, personal communication).

While we do not have a great deal of empiric evidence on the protective effectiveness of OCVs as reactive interventions when used in cholera outbreaks, several attempts have been made to predict the effects of hypothetical deployment of OCVs reactively, using mathematical models. One analysis considered hypothetical reactive vaccination with Dukoral™ for persons aged 2 years and above in cholera outbreaks in three settings: Zimbabwe, which was an epidemic setting in 2008/2009; Kolkata, India a setting with endemic cholera considered in respect to its outbreaks in 2003–2005; and Zanzibar, another endemic setting in which outbreaks between 1997 and 1998 were evaluated. The analysis found that prompt initiation of a two-dose regimen of this vaccine would have had a significant impact on outbreaks occurring in all three settings. Moreover, the predicted impact in the two endemic settings were likely conservative as the 2-year expected duration of vaccine protection would also act to prevent cases in subsequent outbreaks (Reyburn et al. 2011). Five modeling analyses were conducted for the recent outbreak of cholera in Haiti (Chao et al. 2011; Andrews and Basu 2011; Bertuzzo et al. 2011; Tuite et al. 2011; Date et al. 2011). All five found a protective impact, albeit at different levels. The most complete analysis incorporated direct as well as herd vaccine protection, targeted (to high-risk populations) versus nontargeted reactive vaccination, and the interaction of vaccination with varying levels of improvement of hygiene, and estimated the impact on the total epidemic, including cases occurring before vaccination was could be initiated (Chao et al. 2011; Andrews and Basu 2011). This model predicted that if the 30 % of the population deemed at high risk for cholera had been vaccinated reactively shortly after recognition of the epidemic with a vaccine having the characteristics of Shanchol™, and if this high-risk population's level of hygiene had been improved by a modest 10 %, a 55 % reduction in all cholera cases in the outbreak would have occurred.

3.5 Balance Between Costs and Effects of Using OCVs

Increasingly, decisions about deploying health interventions are being greatly influenced by analyses of the balance between costs and the impacts of the intervention, expressed monetarily or as a health metric. As pointed out elsewhere (WHO 2010), a number of cost-effectiveness analyses of the use of cholera vaccines have been published over the years, but most have been flawed by such features as unrealistic assumptions about vaccine targeting strategies, failure to account for all costs, or failure to account for vaccine herd protective effects, the last feature having been appreciated only since 2006 (Ali et al. 2005). As well, it has been persuasively argued that cost-effectiveness may not be terribly relevant to decisions about deploying OCVs in the wake of major emergencies, such as earthquakes, refugee crises, hurricanes, and tsunamis, as other relief efforts in these situations are typically very costly and are instituted without regard to cost-effectiveness (Sack 2003).

The most comprehensive, modern cost-effectiveness analyses of OCVs have been done for preemptive vaccination with OCVs against endemic cholera. One was done for specific sites in Kolkata, India; Beira, Mozambique; Matlab, Bangladesh; and Jakarta, Indonesia; the other was done from the perspective of major WHO regions affected by endemic cholera. The site-specific analyses for a vaccine with the characteristics of Shanchol™ found that, when herd effects are taken into account, mass vaccination of 1–14 year olds and of all individuals aged 1 year and over were both cost-effective, as measured by a cost per DALY gained under three times the GDP per capita of the country. Moreover, programs of childhood vaccination in Beira and Kolkata were very cost effective (cost per DALY gained less than the GDP per capita) (Jeuland et al. 2009). However, this analysis may have been a bit optimistic as it assumed a price per dose of $1, rather than the $1.85 price for Shanchol™ that has now been established by the manufacturer. A Global Investment Case for a vaccine with the characteristics of Shanchol™ estimated vaccine cost-effectiveness for 33 countries projected to be early adopters of the vaccine over the next several years. The analysis, which assumed a price per dose of $1.85 (albeit with a gradually declining price over time as more producers enter the market) and also took vaccine herd effects into account, found the vaccine to be very cost-effective for programs targeting 1–14 year olds as well as for all persons aged 1 year and over for the African, Southeast Asian, and Eastern Mediterranean regions (International Vaccine Institute 2012). Vaccinating 1–14 year olds was more cost-effective than vaccinating older persons.

4 A Cholera Vaccine Stockpile for Use in Cholera Outbreaks

In 1999, WHO recommended the pre-emptive use of OCV in emergency situations at high risk for a cholera outbreak, associated with a recommendation that an initial 2 million dose OCV stockpile should be established for use in endemic and emergency settings (WHO 1999). For various reasons, reflecting different opinions both within and outside WHO, these recommendations were not implemented. Concerns leading to inaction were raised about high vaccine costs, limitations in vaccine availability, logistic challenges associated with vaccine storage and administration, and logistic problems in administering a two-dose vaccine. Concerns were also expressed that vaccination might interfere with other WHO-recommended control efforts in cholera outbreaks. There was also an underlying optimism in some quarters that through intensified global efforts to improve WASH, the control of cholera together with many other enteric infections could soon be achieved.

Still, the past decade has not witnessed any decline in cholera incidence or mortality. To the contrary, there have been many unusually large and protracted outbreaks in Angola, Zimbabwe, Central and West Africa, Somalia, and Haiti. Indeed, cholera has now become endemic not only in many parts of Africa but also in Haiti, after nearly a century in which cholera was not reported in this country (Harris et al. 2010).

In view of this situation, the 64th World Health Assembly in 2011 called for an integrated, comprehensive strategy of cholera prevention and control, recommending the use of OCV "where appropriate, in conjunction with other recommended prevention and control methods". A follow-up consultation meeting concluded that an OCV stockpile for outbreak control should be established as soon as possible, and a Technical Working Group (TWG) was convened to develop a framework for the implementation of such a stockpile. Its report was recently published (WHO 2012a, b, c), providing criteria and guidelines on many important aspects relating to the establishment and use of such a stockpile: criteria for choice of stockpiled vaccines and their deployment; the appropriate size, storage and financing of an initial OCV stockpile and the management, partnership and evaluation processes required; and the decision-making procedure and operational issues.

The TWG established several minimum criteria for releasing OCV from a stockpile for reactive vaccination to control epidemics. These include laboratory-confirmed evidence of an outbreak, the availability of a country action plan, and availability of adequate vaccine storage capacity and administration materials to undertake vaccination campaigns (Costa 2009; WHO 2012a, b, c). Some additional recommendations regarding the OCV stockpile and its use include:

(1) *Complementation, not replacement of other control measures.* Establishment of an OCV stockpile should not detract attention from the key established responses to cholera outbreaks. These include (i) detection, diagnosis, and treatment of cases with oral rehydration and antibiotic treatment; (ii) establishment of a safe water supply; (iii) implementation of adequate waste disposal, sanitation, and hygiene; and (iv) communication and social mobilization. It is also emphasized that the creation of an initial, necessarily small, OCV stockpile and its use will not in itself constitute sufficient preparedness for a large and/or sustained cholera epidemic.
(2) *Vaccine properties criteria.* The TWG has identified a number of criteria to guide the choice of vaccine(s) to be stockpiled (see Table 5). These criteria are divided into those for vaccines that should be considered for the initial stockpile, and the partly sharpened criteria that may be requested of the next-generation stockpiled OCVs. The criteria for the first-generation stockpile essentially describe the established properties of both of the two WHO-prequalified OCVs, Dukoral™ and Shanchol™. The criteria for the 2nd-generation stockpile identifies some modified characteristics that are proposed to guide the development of the next-generation OCVs: one-dose rather than two-dose vaccine, heat-stable vaccine, <2-week onset of protection after vaccination, and no age limitations for vaccine administration.
(3) *Criteria for release of stockpiled vaccine.* A set of epidemiological criteria that should inform a decision to release stockpile vaccine in response to an outbreak are identified in the TWG report. Importantly, the report states that stockpiled vaccine will be deployed only *after* the reporting of a culture-confirmed cholera outbreak in any given area, and then *only* if the impact of the vaccination campaign is estimated to be potentially high. The OCV stockpile should be targeted at epidemics in low-income countries.
(4) *Governance, storage, and procurement of OCV stockpile.* It is recommended that the International Coordinating Group (ICG) *decision-making body* that oversees the meningococcal and yellow fever vaccine stockpile should extend its mandate to include OCV. For OCV decisions this group—which comprises MSF, IFRC, UNICEF, and WHO—should be nested within a wider group of organizations (e.g., technical, commercial, civil society, funding) that can

Table 5 Proposed criteria for candidate stockpile OCVs for immediate use, and modification requirements for subsequent medium-term stockpiled vaccine by WHO's Technical Working Group on creation of an oral cholera vaccine stockpile (WHO 2012a, b, c)

	Candidate oral cholera vaccine requirements	
	For immediate stockpile	For medium-term stockpile
Confers protection against	O1 El Tor (Inaba and Ogawa)	O1 El Tor (Inaba and Ogawa)
Number of doses required for protection	2 doses	1 dose
Indication ages	≥2 years	All age groups
Safety/tolerability profile	Only mild, short-term side-effects acceptable	Only mild, short-term side- effects acceptable
Immunocompromised persons (including HIV infection) and pregnancy contraindicated?	No known risk of whole-cell killed vaccines in pregnant women and immune-compromised individuals	Safe and immunogenic for administration
Time of onset of protection after full vaccination	2–4 weeks	<2 weeks
Efficacy 6 months after vaccination	≥50 %	≥50 %
Minimum duration of sustained protection	1 year	1 year
Ability to confer herd protection?	Desirable but not necessary	Desirable but not necessary
Formulation	Single formulation for all ages, including very young children	Single formulation for all ages, including very young children
Buffer acceptable?	Yes	Yes
Can be administered with local water (with or without chlorination)?	Yes	Yes
Presentation and packaging	Multi-vial packaging or single-dose vials	Multi-vial packaging or single-dose vials or multi-dose vials
Cold chain requirements	2–8 °C	Heat stable
Minimum shelf life	2 years	3 years
Country registration	Preferable but not necessary (authorization to use still needed)	Preferable but not necessary (authorization to use still needed)
WHO prequalification	Necessary	Necessary

inform the partnership on their specific areas of expertise. A *vaccine request* may be made by any national or international organization, and the ICG should then make a decision within 48 h. As with existing stockpiles of meningococcal and yellow fever vaccines, country receipt of OCV should then be within 7 days of approval of a request. *Storage* of stockpile vaccine should be the responsibility of the manufacturer. The OCV stockpile should initially comprise a 3-year supply of 2 million doses per year, which could later increase in size. The stockpile should be maintained on a rotating stock basis. Initial donor contributions should be sought to *finance* vaccine procurement, country preparedness, and planned operational costs for the first 2–3 years. A revolving fund should be established to assure longer term financial stability. A reserved rather than prepaid stockpile is preferred. *A Procurement Reference Group* should be established by the UNICEF Supply Division (UNICEF/SD) to advise on technical issues regarding vaccine and stockpile specifications.

(5) *Monitoring and evaluation.* The TWG report prescribes that a rigorous system of short- and long-term monitoring and evaluation should be embedded within the OCV stockpile mechanism. WHO should establish a stockpile evaluation group to define and implement the detailed monitoring required. As experience and data accrue, the results of this evaluation should enable continuous improvement in the structure and functioning of the stockpile.

While these recommendations reflect the collective views of WHO expert groups, it has to be kept in mind that they are based on expert opinion and are not formally evidence-based. Reactive cholera vaccination still largely remains "terra incognito" with regard to strategies, logistics and real-life impact. It is also clear that use of these criteria will entail a great deal in the way of subjective judgment. This is especially true for the requirement that stockpile vaccine will be deployed only "*when the impact of the vaccination campaign is estimated to be potentially high*". Factors considered by the WHO expert group as likely indicators of a high potential impact of OCV deployment after an outbreak is identified include: (1) high susceptibility of the population to cholera, as reflected by a paucity of cholera cases in the past 2–3 years (and thus a low level of preexisting population immunity to cholera) or high attack rates when past outbreaks have occurred; (2) high vulnerability of the population, as reflected in high case-fatality rates in past outbreaks, the occurrence of cholera in refugee camps, internally displaced people or slums in the affected areas, or the occurrence of cholera in areas with high levels of population movements, high population density, or poor access to clean water, sanitation, or health care; and (3) high risk of spatial extension of the outbreak, as reflected in a short (weeks, not months) time elapsed and a low attack rate since the beginning of the outbreak, a low proportion of health units in the affected districts reporting cholera since the start of the outbreak, or reporting of cases early in the anticipated epidemic season (WHO 2012a, b, c). This last consideration reflects the recognition that although cholera outbreaks have traditionally been thought to be short-lasting, often only a few weeks in duration, several recently reported cholera outbreaks have been very prolonged and widespread (Table 3) (Ministere de la Santa Publique et de la population 2012; WHO 2007, 2008; Mukandavire et al. 2011; Calain et al. 2004; Sasaki et al. 2008; Shultz et al. 2009). Predicting which outbreaks that will be prolonged would obviously have major implications for reactive vaccination strategies.

Another incompletely defined area that may need to be revisited concerns the proposed practical management and financing of the stockpile. It appears to make good sense to let the ICG, already fulfilling such a role for the meningococcal and yellow fever vaccines stockpiles, be the decision-making body also for OCV. However, the proposal that for OCV, the ICG should *"be nested within a wider group of organizations* (e.g., *technical, commercial, civil society, funding) that can inform the partnership on their specific areas of expertise"* might easily be a roadblock or at least very difficult to operationalize. If the ICG is expected to have formal consultations with this broader group, this would make it difficult for ICG to fulfill its obligation to communicate a decision within 48 h after a vaccine request. More reasonably, in practice the ICG should try to consult with other organizations and entities on a case-by-case basis to ensure that its decisions are guided by complementary know-how, especially on local conditions of relevance for the requested vaccine deployment.

It also remains uncertain to which extent the stockpile, initially comprising two million doses per year and maintained on a rotating stock basis, can be built up solely on "*a reserved rather than prepaid*" basis. The idea behind this proposal is that were vaccine reserved for the stockpile not requested, it could still be used commercially by the manufacturer and thus not entail any costs for the stockpile fund. The problem today is that there is still a very small global commercial market for OCVs, probably below 2 million doses per year. It remains to be seen whether the manufacturer(s) will accept the risk to increase their OCV production for expected use in a stockpile without any guaranteed orders. The longer term maintenance of an expanded OCV stockpile would certainly be greatly facilitated if the market for OCVs, currently largely restricted to travelers, could be expanded through the introduction of OCVs in the control of endemic cholera in high-exposure countries. If prophylactic cholera vaccination were used routinely in populations with high cholera endemicity it should also, in addition to its impact on the endemic cholera situation, reduce the risk of epidemic cholera outbreaks in these populations, since most such outbreaks do indeed occur in countries and populations where cholera is already highly endemic.

Finally, much remains to be learnt from the use of stockpiled vaccine on how best to target vaccination for outbreak response when vaccine supply is limited. Illustrative dilemmas include whether to target vaccination to the affected area or focus on surrounding areas to prevent epidemic spread and whether to focus on densely populated urban high-risk areas or more remote rural areas with higher mortality risk due to poor access to effective treatment. A mathematical cholera transmission model has been used to assess the expected impact of different vaccination strategies if they had been used in the Haiti cholera outbreak in 2010, comparing reactive overall mass vaccination with reactive high-exposure vaccination and reactive ring vaccination (Chao et al. 2011). Not surprisingly, with limited vaccine quantities, concentrating vaccination in high-risk areas would always be the most efficient strategy, and this approach would be even more effective when combined with a campaign to also improve hygiene and sanitation. It was also found important that vaccination be started in high-risk subpopulations within 5 days after the first two cases had appeared in them; waiting for several more cases or having a longer delay seriously diminished the modeled effectiveness of vaccination. The importance of a rapid response was also evident in a retrospective analysis of a number of cholera outbreaks in Zimbabwe, Kolkata (India), and Zanzibar (Tanzania): the results indicate that reactive vaccination with a two-dose cholera vaccine can substantially reduce the number of cholera cases, the more the larger and longer the epidemic is, and the impact was found to be more than doubled if vaccination can be completed within ca 10 weeks ("rapid response") as compared to 21 weeks ("delayed response") after the start of the outbreak (Reyburn et al. 2011).

Another important issue, in addition to those relating to the logistics in mobilizing and deploying vaccine from the stockpile, would be to assess whether protection by existing OCVs with two-dose regimens begins after intake of the first dose. In cholera-endemic areas where partial natural immunity is built up progressively by age, a single-dose regimen may be sufficient to elicit a protective intestinal immune response in some individuals. It would also be important, outside the direct use of the stockpile but of great relevance to it, to establish reasonable in vitro serological correlates of protection that can be used to expand or modify indications and regimens for current and future OCVs. For use of the OCV stockpile such correlates would be invaluable for studies that could extend age indications and acceptable limits of thermal storage and shelf life. Both of the WHO-prequalified OCVs, Dukoral™ and Shanchol™, are based on heat-stable vaccine components that withstand storage at temperatures up to 37 °C for months, and although the formally approved shelf life of these vaccines is limited to 3 and 2 years, respectively, studies with Dukoral™ have indicated unimpaired safety and immunogenicity of vaccine in humans after storage for almost 15 years (Holmgren, unpublished). Likewise, immunization with two full doses of Dukoral™ in infants 6 months of age in Bangladesh was well tolerated and fully immunogenic indicating that OCV can be safely administered at least down to this age (Ahmed et al. 2009).

5 Concluding Remarks

OCVs are now components of the public health tool box—alongside provision of adequate WASH and treatment—for the control of cholera outbreaks. Deployment of these vaccines preemptively in populations with high levels of cholera endemicity is relatively non-controversial, though the definition of what is "high" may be debated. As illustrated by analyses of hypothetical reactive vaccination in Zanzibar and Kolkata (Reyburn et al. 2011), reactive vaccination in endemic setting, although not an optimal strategy, can also be justified, in view of the multiyear duration of protection conferred by both Dukoral™ and Shanchol™ and the likelihood that vaccination will not only help contain the current outbreak, but the future occurrence of cholera as well. In endemic settings, a case can be made for targeting children aged 1–14 years for vaccination if resources for vaccination are constrained.

When it comes to vaccinating to control unpredictable outbreaks in epidemic settings, models predict a significant impact if reactive vaccination is initiated relatively soon after recognition of the outbreak and is targeted to high-risk populations, provided that the outbreak is relatively prolonged. At present, however, we lack validated tools for predicting the scale and duration of outbreaks after they have begun, and research to develop such tools is greatly needed. Careful evaluation of the results of using the newly created global cholera vaccine stockpile will be helpful in this respect. Preemptive vaccination in the wake of complex emergencies occurring in populations without documented endemic cholera is a much less certain strategy, as we lack validated tools for predicting in which situations cholera is likely to occur.

We currently have two OCVs that are commercially available and approved by WHO for international use: Shanchol™ and Dukoral™. Both are killed oral vaccines with excellent safety profiles, although additional studies of safety when the vaccines are given to pregnant women or persons infected by HIV are needed. Protection by Dukoral™ has been observed among adults in Peru who lacked natural immunity from past cholera exposure (Sanchez et al. 1994); we lack such data for Shanchol™, which has only been evaluated for protection in populations with preexisting natural immunity. The ability to protect immunologically naïve persons is of importance when considering whether to vaccinate in outbreaks occurring in epidemic as opposed to endemic settings, and should be a priority for evaluations of the newly created OCV stockpile. Other factors influencing the choice of Dukoral™ versus Shanchol™ include Shanchol's™ lower expense, simpler dosing regimens (two doses for all age groups), and longer duration of protection and, conversely, Dukoral's™ greater short-term efficacy against cholera and its cross-protection against LT-ETEC.

Despite not having data on all the questions of relevance to use of OCVs to control outbreaks, there is clearly enough evidence to initiate their use, as answers to the questions will come with experience. In this spirit, non-governmental organizations involved in the control of cholera outbreaks, such as MSF and Partners in Health, have used Shanchol™ recently in Africa and Haiti. Evaluations of these experiences, as well as the additional experiences that will be provided by use of the newly created global cholera vaccine stockpile, offer the opportunity to gather this needed evidence and to refine our approaches to vaccinating in the future.

References

Ahmed T, Svennerholm A-M, Al Tarique A, Sultana GNN, Qadri F (2009) Enhanced immunogenicity of an oral inactivated cholera vaccine in infants in Bangladesh obtained by zinc supplementation and by temporary withholding breast-feeding. Vaccine 27:1433–1439

Ali M, Emch M, von Seidlein L, Yunus M, Sack D, Rao M, Holmgren J, Clemens J (2005) Herd immunity conferred by killed oral cholera vaccines in Bangladesh. Lancet 366:44–49

Ali M, Emch M, Yunus M, Sack D, Lopez Al, Holmgren J, Clemens J (2008) Vaccine herd protection of Bangladeshi infants and young children against cholera: implications for vaccine deployment and person-to-person transmission. Pediatr Infect Dis J 27:33–37

Ali M, Lopez A, Yu Y, Kim Y, Sah B, Maskery B, Clemens J (2011) Global burden of cholera. Bull World Health Organ 90:209–218

Ali M, Sur D, Kanungo S, Sah B, Manna B, Puri M, Wierzba T, Donner A, Nair G, Bhattacharya S, Dhingra M, Deen J, Lopez A, Clemens J (2013) Herd protection by a bivalent-killed whole-cell oral cholera vaccine in the slums of Kolkata, India. Clin Infect Dis 56:1123–1131

Andrews J, Basu S (2011) Transmission dynamics and control of cholera in Haiti: and epidemic model. Lancet 377:1248–1255

Anh D, Lopez A, Thiem V, Grahek S, Duong T, Park J, Kwon H, Favorov M, Hien V, Clemens J (2011) Use of oral cholera vaccines in an outbreak in Vietnam: a case control study. PLoS Negl Trop Dis5:e1006

Azurin J, Alverin M (1974) Field evaluation of environmental sanitation measures against cholera. Bull WHO 51:19–26

Benenson A (1976) Review of the experience with whole-cell and somatic antigen vaccines. In: Symposium on cholera. US-Japan cooperative medical science program. Sapporo, Japan, pp 228–252

Bertuzzo E, Mari L, Righetto L et al (2011) Prediction of the spatial evolution and effect of control measures for the unfolding Haiti cholera outbreak. Geophys Res Lett 38:L06403

Calain P, Chaine J, Johnson E et al (2004) Can oral cholera vaccination play a role in controlling a cholera outbreak? Vaccine 22:2444–2451

Cavailler P, Lucas M, Perroud V et al (2006) Feasibility of a mass vaccination campaign using a two dose oral cholera vaccine in an urban cholera-endemic setting in Mozambique. Vaccine 24:4890–4895

Chaignat C-L, Monti V, Soepardi J et al (2008) Cholera in disasters: do vaccines prompt new hopes? Expert Rev Vaccines 7:431–435

Chao D, Halloran E, Longini I (2011) Vaccination strategies for epidemic cholera in Haiti with implications for the developing world. Proc Nat Acad Sci 10:7081–7085

Clemens J, Jertborn M, Sack D, Stanton B et al (1986) Effect of neutralization of gastric acid on immune responses to oral B subunit killed whole cell cholera vaccine. J Infect Dis 154:175–178

Clemens JD, Sack D, Harris JR, Chakraborty J, Khan MR, Stanton B, Ali M, Ahmed F, Yunus M, Kay B, Khan MU, Rao MR, Svennerholm A–M, Holmgren J (1988) Impact of B subunit killed whole–cell and killed whole–cell–only oral vaccines against cholera upon treated diarrhoeal illness and mortality in an area endemic for cholera. Lancet 2:1375–1378

Clemens J, Sack D, Harris J, Chakraborty J, Neogy P, Stanton B, Huda N, Khan MU, Kay BA, Khan MR, Ansaruzzaman M, Yunus M, Rao MR, Svennerholm A–M, Holmgren J (1988) Cross–protection by B subunit–whole cell cholera vaccine against diarrhoea associated with heat labile toxin–producing enterotoxigenic *Escherichia coli*: results of a large–scale field trial. J Infect Dis 158:372–377

Clemens J, Sack D, Harris J, Chakraborty J, Khan MR, Huda S, Ahmed F, Gomes J, Rao M, Svennerholm A–M, Holmgren J. ABO blood groups and cholera: new oCTBervations on specificity of risk and modification of vaccine efficacy. J Infect Dis 159:770–773

Clemens J, Sack DA, Harris J, van Loon F, Chakraborty J, Ahmed F, Rao MR, Khan MR, Yunus M, Huda N, Stanton B, Kay B, Walter S, Eeckels R, Svennerholm A-M, Holmgren J (1990) Field trial of oral cholera vaccines in Bangladesh: results from long-term follow-up. Lancet 335:270–273

Clemens J, Spriggs D, Sack D (1994) Public health considerations for the use of cholera vaccines in cholera control programs. In: Wachsmith IK, Blake P, Olsvik O. *Vibrio cholera* and cholera: molecular to global perspectives. ASM Press, Washington pp 425–442

Clemens J, Brenner R, Rao M, Lowe C (1996) Evaluating new vaccines for developing countries: efficacy or effectiveness? J Am Med Assoc 275:390–397

Clemens J, Sack DA, Harris J, van Loon F, Chakraborty J, Ahmed F, Rao MR, Khan MR, Yunus M, Huda N, Stanton B, Kay B, Walter S, Eeckels R, Svennerholm A-M, Holmgren J (1999) Field trial of oral cholera vaccines in Bangladesh: results from long-term follow-up. Lancet 335:270–273

Costa A (2009) Establishing a cholera vaccine stockpile: What do we need? Focus on neglected tropical infectious diseases: integrating vaccines into global cholera control efforts. Annecy, France

Date K, Vitari A, Hyde T, Mintz E, Donavaro-Holladay M, Henry A, Tappero J, Roels T, Abrams J, Burkholder B, Ruiz-Matus C, Andrus J, Dietz V (2011) Considerations for oral cholera vaccine use during outbreak after earthquake in Haiti, 2010–2011. Emerg Inf Dis 17:2105–2112

Deb B, Sircar B, Senoupta P, De S, Mondal S, Gupta D, Saha N, Ghosh S, Mitra U, Pal S (1986) Studies on interventions to prevent El Tor cholera transmission in urban slums. Bull WHO 64:127–1231

Dorlencourt F, Legros D, Paquet C, Neira M, Ivanoff B, Le Saout E (1999) Effectiveness of mass vaccination with WC/rCTB cholera vaccine during an epidemic in Adjumani district. Uganda Bull World Health Org 77:949–950

Glass R, Becker S, Huq I, Stoll B, Khan MU, Merson M, Lee J, Black R (1982) Endemic cholera in rural Bangladesh, 1966-80. Amer J Epidemiol 116:959–970

Harris J, LaRocque R, Charles R et al (2010) Cholera's western front. Lancet 376:1961–1965

Hashim R, Khatib A, Enwere G, Park J, Reyburn R, Ali M, Chang N, Kim D, Ley B, Thriemer K, Lopez A, Clemens J, Deen J, Shin S, Schaetti C, Hutubessy R, Aguado T, Kieny M, Sack D, Obaro S, Shaane A, Ali S, Sahah A, von Seidlein L, Jiddawi M (2012) Safety of recombinant cholera toxin B subunit, killed whole cell (rCTB-WC) oral cholera vaccine in pregnancy. PLoS Neglect Trop Dis 6:e1743

Holmgren J, Svennerholm AM, Jertborn M, Clemens J et al (1992) An oral B subunit-killed whole cell vaccine against cholera. Vaccine 10:911–914

International Vaccine Institute (2012) An investment case for the accelerated introduction of oral cholera vaccines. International vaccine institute. Seoul, Korea

Ivers I, Farmer P, Pape W (2012) Oral cholera vaccines and integrated cholera control in Haiti. Lancet 379:2026–2028

Jeuland M, Cook J, Poulos C, Clemens J, Whittington D (2009) Cost-effectiveness of new generation oral cholera vaccines: a multi-site analysis. Value Health 12:899–908

Kanungo S, Paisley A, Lopez AL, Bhattacharya M, Manna B, Kim DR, Han SH, Attridge S, Carbis R, Rao R, Holmgren J, Clemens JD, Sur D (2009) Immune responses following one and two doses of the reformulated, bivalent, killed, whole-cell, oral cholera vaccine among adults and children in Kolkata India: A randomized, placebo-controlled trial. Vaccine 27:6887–6893

Kaper JB, Levine MM (1990) Recombinant attenuated *Vibrio cholerae* strains used as live oral vaccines. Res Microbiol 141: 901–906

Khatib A, Ali M, von Seidlein L, Kim D, Hashim R, Reyburn R, Ley B, Thriemer K, Enwere G, Hutubessy R, Aguado MT, Kieny M-P, Wierzba T, Ali S, Saleh A, Clemens J, Jiddawi M, Deen J (2012) Effectiveness of an oral cholera vaccine in Zanzibar: findings from a large mass vaccination campaign and observational cohort study. Lancet Infect Dis [Epub ahead of print]

Levine M, Kaper J, Herrington D et al (1988) Safety, immunogenicity, and efficacy of recombinant live oral cholera vaccines, CVD 103 and CVD 103-HgR. Lancet 1:467–704

Lewis D, Gilks C, Ojoo S et al (1994) Immune response following oral administration of cholera toxin B subunit to HIV-1-infected UK and Kenyan subjects. AIDS 8:779–785

Longini I, Nizam A, Ali M, Yunus M, Shenvi N, Clemens J (2007) Controlling endemic cholera with oral vaccines. PLoS Med 4:e336

Lopez Al, Clemens J, Deen J, Jodar L (2008) Cholera vaccines for the developing world. Hum Vaccines 4:165–169

Lucas M, Deen JL, von Seidlein L, Wang X-Y, Ampuero J, Puri M, Ali M, Ansaruzzaman M, Amos J, Cavallier P, Guerin P, McChesney M, Mahoudeau C, Kahozi P, Chaignat C-Barreto A, Songane F, Clemens JD (2005) The effectiveness of an internationally licensed, two dose oral cholera vaccine when given in a mass vaccination campaign in Beira, Mozambique. N Engl J Med 352:757–767

Medecins sans Frontieres (2013) Cholera epidemic escalates along Sierra Leone and Guinea border. www.doctorswithoutborders.org. WeCTBite Accessed 30 Jan 2013

Ministere de la Santa Publique et de la population (2012) Rapport journalier MSPP du 01 Avril 2012. Port au Prince. http://www.mspp.gouv.ht/site/index.php. Accessed 1 Oct 2012

Mintz E, Popovic T, Blake P. Transmission of *Vibrio cholera* 01. In: Wachsmith IK, Blake P, Olsvik O. *Vibrio cholera* and cholera: molecular to global perspectives. ASM Press, Washington, pp 425–442

Mukandavire Z, Liao S, Wang J, Gaff H, Smith DL, Glenn Morris J (2011) Estimating the reproductive numbers for the 2008–2009 cholera outbreaks in Zimbabwe. Proc Nat Acad Sci USA 108:8767–8772

Naficy A, Rao M, Paquet C, Antona D, Sorkin A, Clemens J. Treatment and vaccination strategies to control cholera in Sub-Saharan refugee settings. J Amer Med Assoc. 1998; 279: 521-5.

Ortigao-de-Sampaio M, Shattock R, Hayes R et al (1998) Increase in plasma viral load oral cholera immunization of HIV-infected subjects. AIDS 12:F145–F150

Peltola H, Siitonen A, Kyronseppa H, Simula I, Hilal M, Ksonen P, Ktaaja M, Cadoz M (1991) Prevention of travellers' diarrhea by oral B subunit/whole cell cholera vaccine. Lancet 338:1285–1289

Perry C, Plowe C, Koumare B, Bougoudogo F et al (1998) A single dose of live oral cholera vaccine CVD 103Hg-R is safe and immunogenic in HIV-infected and HIV-noninfected adults in Mali. Bull World Health Organ 76:63–71

Reyburn R, Deen J, Grais R, Bhattacharya S, Sur D, Lopez A, Jiddawi M, Clemens J, von Seidlein L (2011) The case for reactive oral cholera vaccinations. PLoS Negl Trop Dis 5(1):e952

Richie EE, Punjabi NH, Sidharta YY et al (2000) Efficacy trial of single-dose live oral cholera vaccine CVD 103-HgR in North Jakarta, Indonesia, a cholera-endemic area. Vaccine 18:2399–2410

Sack D (2003) When should cholera vaccine be used in cholera endemic areas? J Health Popul Nutr 21:299–303

Sack DA, Sack RB, Nair GB, Siddique AK (2004) Cholera. Lancet 363:223–233

Sanchez J, Vasquez B, Begue R, Meza R, Castellares G, Cabezas C, Watts D, Sadoff J, Taylor D (1994) Protective efficacy of oral whole cell-recombinant B subunit cholera vaccine in Peruvian military recruits. Lancet 344:1273–1276

Sasaki S, Suzuki H, Igarashi K, Tambatamba B, Mulenga P (2008) Spatial analysis of risk factor of cholera outbreak for 2003-2004 in a peri-urban area of Lusaka, Zambia. Am J Trop Med Hyg 79:414–421

Shin S, Desai S, Sah BK, Clemens J (2011) Oral vaccines against cholera. Clin Infect Dis 52:1343–1349

Shultz A, Omollo JO, Burke H et al (2009) Cholera outbreak in Kenyan refugee camp: risk factors for illness and importance of sanitation. Am J Trop Med Hyg 80:640–645

Su-Arehawaratana P, Singharaj P, Taylor DN et al (1992) Safety and immunogenicity of different immunization regimens of CVD 103-HgR live oral cholera vaccine in soldiers and civilians in Thailand. J Infect Dis 165:1042–1048

Suharyono M, Simanjuntak C, Witham N et al (1992) Safety and immunogenicity of single-dose live oral cholera vaccine CVD 103-HgR in 5–9-year-old Indonesian children. Lancet 340:689–694

Sur D, Lopez A, Kanungo S, Paisley A, Manna B, Al M, Niyogi S, Park JK, Sarkar B, Pur M, Kim D, Deen J, Holmgren J, Carbis R, Rao R, Nguyen TV, Donner A, Ganguly NK, Nair GB, Bhattacharya SK, Clemens JD (2009) Protection and safety of a modified, killed whole cell

oral cholera vaccine in India: a cluster-randomized, double-blind, placebo-controlled trial. Lancet 374:1694–702
Svennerholm AM, Holmgren J (1976) Synergistic protective effect in rabbits of immunization with *Vibrio cholerae* lipopolysaccharide and toxin/toxoid. Infect Immun 13:735–740
Svennerholm AM, Jertborn M, Gothefors L et al (1984) Mucosal antitoxic and antibacterial immunity after cholera disease and after immunization with a combined B subunit-whole cell vaccine. J Infect Dis 149:884–893
Tacket CO, Losonsky G, Nataro JP et al (1992) Onset and duration of protective immunity in challenged volunteers after vaccination with live oral cholera vaccine CVD 103-HgR. J Infect Dis 166:837–841
Tacket CO, Cohen MB, Wasserman SS et al (1999) Randomized, double-blind, placebo-controlled, multicentered trial of the efficacy of a single dose of live oral cholera vaccine CVD 103-HgR in preventing cholera following challenge with *Vibrio cholerae* O1 El Tor Inaba three months after vaccination. Infect Immun 67:6341–6345
Thiem VD, Deen JL, von Seidlein L, Do GC, Dang DA, Park JK, Ali M, Danovaro-Holliday MC, Nguyen DS, Nguyen TH, Holmgren J, Clemens JD (2006) Long-term effectiveness against cholera of oral killed whole-cell vaccine produced in Vietnam. Vaccine 24:4297–4303
Trach DD, Clemens JD, Ke NT et al (1997) Field trial of a locally produced, killed, oral cholera vaccine in Vietnam. Lancet 349:231–235
Tuite AR, Tien J, Eisenberg M, Earn D, Ma J, Fishman D (2011) Cholera epidemic in Haiti, 2010: using a transmission model to explain spatial spread of disease and identify optimal control interventions. Ann Internal Med 154:593–601
WHO (1999) Potential use of oral cholera vaccines in emergency situations. Report of a meeting, Geneva, 12–13 May 1999, WHO 1999 (CDS/CSR/EDC/99.4)
WHO (2007) Cholera 2006. Wkly Epidemiol Rec 82:273–284
WHO (2008) Cholera 2007. Wkly Epidemiol Rec 83:261–284
WHO (2010) Cholera vaccines: WHO position paper. Wkly Epidemiol Rep 85:117–128
WHO (2012a) Cholera 2011. Wkly Epidemiol Bull 87:289–304
WHO (2012b) WHO consultation on oral cholera vaccine (OCV) stockpile strategic framework: potential objectives and possible policy options. WHO/IVB/12.05
WHO (2012c) WHO Technical working group on creation of an oral cholera vaccine stockpile. WHO/HSE/PED/2012.2
Trach DD, Cam PD, Ke NY (2002) Investigations into the safety and immunogenicity of a killed oral cholera vaccine developed in Viet Nam. Bull World Health Organ 80:2–8
World Health Organization Expert Committee on Biological Standardization (2001) Guidelines for the production and control of inactivated oral cholera vaccines. WHO Tech Rep Ser 924:129–149

Index

Current Topics in Microbiology and Immunology (2014) 379: 259–263
DOI: 10.1007/978-3-642-55404-9

MIX
Papier aus verantwortungsvollen Quellen
Paper from responsible sources
FSC® C105338

If you have any concerns about our products,
you can contact us on
ProductSafety@springernature.com

In case Publisher is established outside the EU,
the EU authorized representative is:
Springer Nature Customer Service Center GmbH
Europaplatz 3, 69115 Heidelberg, Germany

Printed by Libri Plureos GmbH
in Hamburg, Germany